Liver Cirrhosis: From Pathophysiology to Disease Management

Liver Cirrhosis: From Pathophysiology to Disease Management

Liver Cirrhosis: From Pathophysiology to Disease Management

Editor: Dallas Bowman

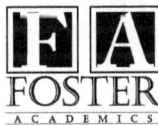

FA
FOSTER
A C A D E M I C S

www.fosteracademics.com

www.fosteracademics.com

FA
FOSTER
ACADEMICS

Cataloging-in-Publication Data

Liver cirrhosis : from pathophysiology to disease management / edited by Dallas Bowman.
    p. cm.
Includes bibliographical references and index.
ISBN 978-1-63242-679-6
1. Liver--Cirrhosis. 2. Liver--Pathophysiology. 3. Liver--Diseases.
4. Disease management. I. Bowman, Dallas.
RC848.C5 L58 2019
616.3624--dc23

Foster Academics,
118-35 Queens Blvd., Suite 400,
Forest Hills, NY 11375, USA

ISBN 978-1-63242-679-6 (Hardback)

Contents

Permissions

List of Contributors

Index

Preface

Liver cirrhosis is a condition of the liver in which normal liver parenchyma is replaced by scar tissue, thereby causing long-term damage to the liver. It is always preceded by fatty liver and hepatitis. The disease progresses gradually over months or years. In its initial stages, there are often no symptoms, but as it progresses, symptoms such as tiredness, itchiness, swelling in the lower legs, yellow skin, spider-like blood vessels on the skin and fluid build up in the abdomen start to occur. Liver cirrhosis may lead to hepatic encephalopathy, liver cancer and bleeding from dilated stomach veins or from dilated veins in the esophagus. Cirrhosis may be caused by alcohol, hepatitis B and C, and non-alcoholic fatty liver disease. Though liver damage is irreversible, treatment can slow down the progression of the disease and reduce complications. Generally, antibiotics, laxatives, medications for hepatitis, chelation therapy, etc. may be prescribed depending on the underlying cause of the disease. This book provides comprehensive insights into liver cirrhosis. It provides significant information of the clinical aspects of liver cirrhosis from pathophysiology to disease management. It is appropriate for students seeking detailed information in this area as well as for experts.

The researches compiled throughout the book are authentic and of high quality, combining several disciplines and from very diverse regions from around the world. Drawing on the contributions of many researchers from diverse countries, the book's objective is to provide the readers with the latest achievements in the area of research. This book will surely be a source of knowledge to all interested and researching the field.

In the end, I would like to express my deep sense of gratitude to all the authors for meeting the set deadlines in completing and submitting their research chapters. I would also like to thank the publisher for the support offered to us throughout the course of the book. Finally, I extend my sincere thanks to my family for being a constant source of inspiration and encouragement.

Editor

Impact of Glyoxalase-I (Glo-I) and Advanced Glycation End Products (AGEs) in Chronic Liver Disease

Marcus Hollenbach

Abstract

Inflammation caused by oxidative stress (ROS) is a main driver for development of chronic inflammatory liver disease leading to fibrosis and cirrhosis. An important source of ROS constitutes methylglyoxal (MGO). MGO is formed as a by-product in glycolysis, threonine catabolism, and ketone bodies pathway leading to formation of advanced glycation end products (AGEs). AGEs bind to their receptor for AGEs (RAGE) and activate intracellular transcription factors, such as nuclear factor-κB (NF-κB), resulting in production of pro-inflammatory cytokines and ROS. The enzymes glyoxalase-I (Glo-I) and glyoxalase-II (Glo-II) form the glyoxalase system and are essential for the detoxification of methylglyoxal (MGO). This chapter highlights Glo-I and (R)AGE in chronic liver disease with focus on fibrosis and cirrhosis. AGEs and RAGE have been shown to be upregulated in fibrosis, and silencing of RAGE reduced the latter. In contrast, recent study highlighted reduced expression of Glo-I in cirrhosis with consecutive elevation of MGO and oxidative stress. Interestingly, modulation of Glo-I activity by ethyl pyruvate resulted in reduced activation of hepatic stellate cells and reduced fibrosis in CCl_4 model of cirrhosis. In conclusion, Glo-I and R(AGE) are important components in development and progression of chronic liver disease and constitute interesting therapeutic target.

Keywords: ethyl pyruvate cirrhosis, fibrosis, methylglyoxal, AGEs

1. Introduction

Oxidate stress (reactive oxygen species, ROS) with consecutive and repetitive inflammation is responsible for development of chronic liver disease. Different etiologies of liver disease lead to damage of hepatocytes, release of pro-inflammatory cytokines, and finally activation of hepatic stellate cells (HSC). Activated HSC transform to myofibroblasts and lead to deposition of collagen, which in turn result in fibrosis and finally cirrhosis. Several molecular mechanisms are involved in this complex interplay, nevertheless the critical step is the activation of HSC by ROS. This chapter focuses on the glyoxalase-I (Glo-I) and related advanced glycation end products (AGEs) with their receptor for AGEs (RAGE) playing an important role in generation and detoxification of ROS. Current knowledge of Glo-I and (R)AGE in chronic liver disease with key aspect to fibrosis and cirrhosis will be highlighted.

2. Pathogenesis of fibrosis and cirrhosis

End-stage liver diseases are mainly caused by viral hepatitis, alcoholism, nonalcoholic fatty liver disease or steatohepatitis (NAFLD/NASH), or rare autoimmune and hereditary disorders. The followed repetitive liver injury caused inflammation, finally resulting in fibrosis and irreversible cirrhosis. Thereby, liver cirrhosis belongs to the global burden of disease responsible for more than one million deaths p.a. [1]. In cirrhosis, altered liver anatomy and reduced liver function are pathognomonic. Development of cirrhosis is characterized by the appearance of regenerative nodules, hepatocyte ballooning, accumulation of fibrotic tissue, disturbed microcirculation, angiogenesis and sinusoidal collapse with defenestration and development of a basement membrane [2]. These alterations of liver architecture lead to reduced liver function and elevation of intrahepatic resistance demonstrated by increased portal pressure with development of ascites and esophageal varices [3, 4]. Nevertheless, portal hypertension is being caused by both structural alterations of liver microarchitecture and hepatic endothelial dysfunction. The latter is characterized by an imbalance of vasoactive components. In fact, there is an hyperresponsiveness and overproduction of vasoconstrictors (mainly endothelin-1 (ET-1)) and an hyporesponsiveness and reduction of vasodilators (mainly nitric oxide (NO)) in the vascular bed of the liver [5–7]. Despite this hypoactive endothelium in hepatic microcirculation, portal hypertension leads to arterial vasodilation, formation of collateral vessels, and hyporesponsiveness to vasoconstrictors due to hyperactive endothelium in splanchnic and systemic circulation with increased NO production. Finally, these alterations result in elevated blood flow to portal vein and a vicious circle of disease [8–11].

The underlying molecular mechanism for development of fibrosis, cirrhosis, and portal hypertension has been intensively investigated over the last decades. Since the liver is formed by parenchymal cells (mainly hepatocytes (HEP)) and nonparenchymal cells (Kupffer cells (KC), hepatic stellate cells (HSC), and liver sinusoidal endothelial cells (LSEC)), both are involved in the development of fibrosis and cirrhosis. Nevertheless, HSC are the main cell type responsible for accumulation of fibrosis and increased intrahepatic vascular resistance. HSC are pericytes surrounding the sinusoids in the space of Disse. HSC are quiescent but became activated upon various stimuli and transform to myofibroblasts [12]. This activation process is a complex interplay between parenchymal and nonparenchymal cells and triggered via inflammatory processes [13]. For instance, deleterious agents (alcohol, LPS) have direct hepatotoxic effects to hepatocytes and trigger the production of reactive oxygen species (ROS). The release of ROS, DNA, and damage-associated molecular pattern (DAMP) leading to activation of KC and innate immune system followed by subsequent production of pro-inflammatory cytokines such as TNF-α and IL-6 as well as pro-fibrotic factors [14–16]. Also, alcohol consumption increases permeability of the gut resulting in increased levels of portal endotoxins (LPS) with consecutive activation of KC resulting in liver injury and inflammation [17, 18]. Furthermore, inflammation triggers the classical complement pathway activation via C1q [19], followed by production of pro-inflammatory cytokines, and inhibits components of innate immune system. As a consequence of these induced inflammatory processes, activated KC stimulate HSC subsequently leading to fibrosis [20]. This stimulation can result directly by the deleterious agent [21] or via transforming growth factor beta (TGF-β)-dependent mechanisms [22] leading to secretion of TNF-α, IL-6, TIMP-1, MCP-1, collagen-I, and α-SMA [23–25] and finally collagen deposition.

As mentioned above, pro-inflammatory factors (TNF-α, IL-1β, IL-6) are also involved in the activation of HSC. In this regard, activation of the transcription factor nuclear factor-κB (NF-κB) and subsequent overexpression of pro-inflammatory cytokines are important pathways. NF-κB, thereby, is activated by growth factors, cytokines, bacterial and viral factors, and ROS and regulates by itself pro-inflammatory cytokines (like COX-2 or IL-6) [26, 27].

Beside the production of collagen and accumulation of fibrotic tissue, HSC are involved in increased intrahepatic vascular resistance not only via structural changes. Transformation of HSC to myofibroblasts was accompanied by stimulation of rho kinase leading to activation of contractile filaments of HSC and subsequently vasoconstriction of sinusoids [28].

Another key player in the development of fibrosis comprises LSEC. They form the first line of defense protecting the liver from injury. Inflammation by LPS or ROS resulted in dysfunction of LSEC [29] indicated by disturbed sinusoidal microcirculation, defenestration, hypoxia, and pathological angiogenesis [30]. In contrast, both direct deterioration of LSEC and vasoconstriction of HSC result in impaired release of vasodilators from LSEC leading to a vicious circle of disease. In this regard, disturbed regulation of NO production in cirrhosis depends on activity of endothelial NO synthase (eNOS) and increased degradation due to phosphodiesterases, that is, PDE-5 [31]. Although eNOS expression is upregulated in sinusoidal area in cirrhosis, eNOS activity has been shown to be reduced by caveolin-eNOS binding [32] and was diminished by several post-translational modifications of the endothelial NO synthase (eNOS) [9]. In contrast, in splanchnic circulation, eNOS is upregulated [9] with increased enzyme activity in portal hypertension and regulated by phosphorylation of protein kinase B (Akt) [33]. Beside upregulation of eNOS, production of NO is also related to induction of the inducible form of the NO synthase, iNOS. iNOS is mainly stimulated by the presence of endotoxin and pro-inflammatory cytokines, all of whom occur in development of cirrhosis [34]. Indeed, recent study showed stimulation of iNOS rather than eNOS in splanchnic circulation by LPS, indicating an important role of iNOS in portal hypertension after bacterial translocation to mesenteric vessels [35]. Finally, all these alterations result in a hyperdynamic circulation with elevated blood flow to portal vein and further increase of portal pressure [8–10].

In conclusion, cirrhosis demonstrates the end stage of liver disease with disturbed liver architecture and impaired liver function. Generation of ROS and stimulation of various inflammatory pathways are critical steps in activation of HSC as the main driver for fibrosis. Despite these findings, the use of antioxidants (vitamin E, N-acetylcysteine, coenzyme Q, and others) in patients with alcoholic liver disease has failed to show an efficacy in improving disease conditions [36–38].

3. Glyoxalase system and R(AGE)

An important role in regulation and formation of ROS and oxidative stress comprises the glyoxalase system. This enzymatic system was first discovered in 1913 [39] and constitutes two cytosolic enzymes, glyoxalase-I (Glo-I, EC 4.4.1.5) and glyoxalase-II (Glo-II, EC 3.1.2.6.). Glo-I is responsible for the catalytic conversion of α-oxo aldehydes, for instance, methylglyoxal (MGO), into the hemithioacetal S-D-Lactoylglutathione using L-glutathione (GSH) as a cofactor. Further substrates of Glo-I are hydroxypyruvaldehyde, hydroxypyruvate aldehyde phosphate, glyoxal, phenylglyoxal, 4,5-dioxovalerate, alkyl and arylglyoxales [40–43]. Glo-II hydrolyzes the reaction of S-D-Lactoylglutathione to H_2O and D-lactate with regeneration of GSH (**Figure 1**). Thereby, Glo-I demonstrates the rate limiting step [42, 44], and Glo-II is of subordinate interest in inflammatory research.

MGO is the main substrate of Glo-I [45] and has been described as a reactive carbonyl compound that is formed as a by-product in glycolysis [46], ketone body metabolism, and threonine catabolism [47–49]. MGO leads to cell cytotoxicity in high concentrations through

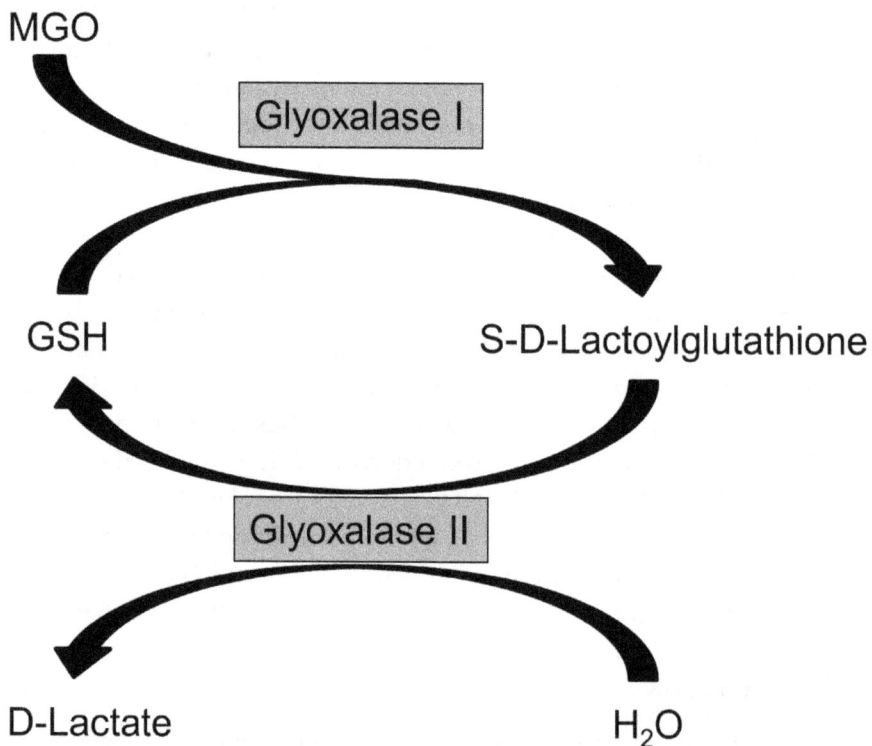

Figure 1. Glyoxalase system. Glyoxalase-I and glyoxalase-II comprise the glyoxalase system for detoxification of MGO. Glutathione is necessary as cofactor and is regenerated by Glo-II. Adapted from [43].

reaction with nucleotides, phospholipids, and proteins [50, 51], resulting in the formation of "advanced glycation end products (AGEs)" and reactive oxygen species (ROS) via AGEs or non-enzymatic reaction with hydrogen peroxide [52]. In this regard, MGO has shown to be involved in various inflammatory processes such as diabetes, aging, renal insufficiency, hypertension, or cancer [60–64].

Important MGO-derived AGEs are the non-fluorescent products 5-hydro-5-methylimidazolone (MG-H1) and tetrahydropyrimidine (THP) as well as the major fluorescent product, argpyrimidine [53, 54]. Other non-MGO-derived AGEs comprise N^{ε}-carboxymethyllysine (CML), pyrraline, or pentosidine [55]. The effects of AGEs have been allocated to their antagonistic receptor systems. The receptor for AGEs (RAGE) mediates generation of ROS, inflammation, angiogenesis, and proliferation [56, 57]. In contrast, AGE receptors (AGE-Rs), for instance, AGE-R1, are responsible for detoxification and clearance of AGEs [58]. Upon binding of AGEs to RAGE, various signal transduction pathways are activated. Recent studies showed involvement of the extracellular signal-regulated kinase 1/2 (ERK1/2), phosphoinositide 3-kinase (PI3-K)/protein kinase B (AKT), Janus kinase 2 (JAK2), and Rho GTPases, finally resulting in activation of NF-κB and production of pro-inflammatory cytokines (**Figure 3**) [59]. In addition, stimulation of RAGE resulted in activation of transforming growth factor (TGF-β) pathway and induced vascular endothelial growth factor (VEGF) overexpression [57].

In the last years, structure and genomic sequence of Glo-I was intensively analyzed. Glo-I is a dimer and consists in mammalian of two identical subunits with a molecular mass of 43–48 kDa [60]. Each subunit contains a zinc ion in its active center, whereas the apoenzyme remains catalytically inactive [45, 61]. The active center of Glo-I is localized between both monomers and comprises two structurally equivalent residues from each domain (Gln-33A, Glu-99A, His-126B, Glu-172B) and two water molecules indicating an octahedral arrangement [54, 62]. The protein sequence of Glo-I consists of 184 amino acids with post-translational modification of N-terminal Met [62].

Genomic analysis revealed three distinct phenotypes of Glo-I: GLO 1-1, GLO 1-2, and GLO 2-2 representing homo- and heterozygous expression of GLO^1 und GLO^2 [63, 64]. Gene locus of Glo-I is determined on chromosome six between centromere and human leukocyte antigen (HLA)-DR gene [65, 66]. Demographic studies showed higher distribution of GLO^1 in Alaska and lower GLO^1 allocation in southern and eastern Europe, America, Africa, and India [67].

Genetic sequencing identified association of distinct Glo-I phenotypes and Glo-I SNPs with diabetes [68], cardiovascular diseases [69], schizophrenia [70], autism [71, 72], anxiety [73], and cancer [74, 75]. These findings led to preliminary anti-tumor effects of Glo-I inhibition by siRNA or enzymatic inhibition in different cancer models [76–79]. In this regard, well-studied Glo-I inhibitors are S-ρ-bromobenzylglutathione or S-ρ-bromobenzyl-glutathione cyclopentyl diester [77, 80], methotrexate [81], indomethacin [82], troglitazone [83], and flavonoids [84, 85] showing anti-inflammatory and anti-tumor effects. Furthermore, an Glo-I inducer led to improved glycemic control and vascular function in 29 obese patients [86].

In a nutshell, Glo-I is responsible for detoxification of MGO and prevention of MGO-related formation of AGEs and ROS. Therefore, Glo-I and (R)AGE are involved in different pathophysiological inflammatory processes.

4. Glo-I and R(AGE) in fibrosis, cirrhosis, and NAFLD/NASH

4.1. Glo-I

To date, although Glo-I revealed an important role in inflammation, data about Glo-I in chronic liver disease remain preliminary. In an experimental approach of CCl_4-induced cirrhosis, Glo-I was analyzed *in vivo* and *in vitro* [87]. Wistar rats were treated with inhalative CCl_4 three times a week to induce early cirrhosis (without ascites) after 8 weeks or advanced cirrhosis (with ascites) after 12 weeks. Furthermore, primary liver cells from cirrhotic and noncirrhotic livers were isolated via portal vein perfusion and analysis of Glo-I was performed. Glo-I could be detected in HEP, HSC, and LSEC with highest expression on protein and mRNA levels in HEP. Furthermore, Glo-I expression was reduced in early and advanced cirrhosis in both whole liver and primary liver cells (**Figure 2A**). The reduction in Glo-I expression was greater with increasing severity of liver disease. Interestingly, the reduction of Glo-I was accompanied by an increase of MGO in cirrhosis (**Figure 2B**). This accumulation of MGO would lead to increased formation of AGEs and finally augment oxidative stress with ongoing inflammation in chronic liver disease [87]. So far, the reduction of Glo-I with consecutive increase of MGO would provide an explanation for perpetuating liver inflammation in advanced stages of liver disease.

Furthermore, modulation of Glo-I activity with the anti-inflammatory drug ethyl pyruvate (EP) was performed to analyze impact of Glo-I in initiation and progression of cirrhosis. EP is an α-oxo-carbonic acid and ester of pyruvate. EP came in focus due to anti-inflammatory effects of pyruvate but low stability in aqueous solution [88]. Therefore, EP constitutes a more stable compound and exerts anti-inflammatory and protective effects in a lot of ROS-mediated models [89, 90]. Therefore, a possible molecular basis for the anti-inflammatory effects of EP was assumed to be the inhibition of specific Glo-I activity [91].

Since EP showed protective effects in acute liver failure [92–95] and development of fatty liver [96], effect of EP on activation of HSC, as it might occur in initial stadium of cirrhosis, was analyzed. Stimulation of HSC with LPS for 24 hours led to increased levels of α-SMA, indicating activation of HSC and production of collagen deposit. This stimulation could be abrogated by modulation of Glo-I activity by means of EP (**Figure 2c**). Underlying mechanisms involve stimulation of Nrf2 as well as reduction of NF-κB and ERK/pERK by EP. Additional *in vivo* experiments revealed reduced collagen deposit in Wistar rats that were treated with CCl_4 for 12 weeks and i.p. EP [87]. Furthermore, EP-treated rats revealed significantly less Sirius red staining and consequently less fibrosis compared with controls receiving saline (**Figure 2D**).

Indeed, anti-inflammatory treatment of several diseases with EP might be a promising future clinical approach. However, EP was analyzed in a clinical trial (phase-II multicenter double-blind placebo-controlled study) in high-risk patients undergoing cardiac surgery with cardiopulmonary bypass. This trial was performed in 13 US hospitals including patients with

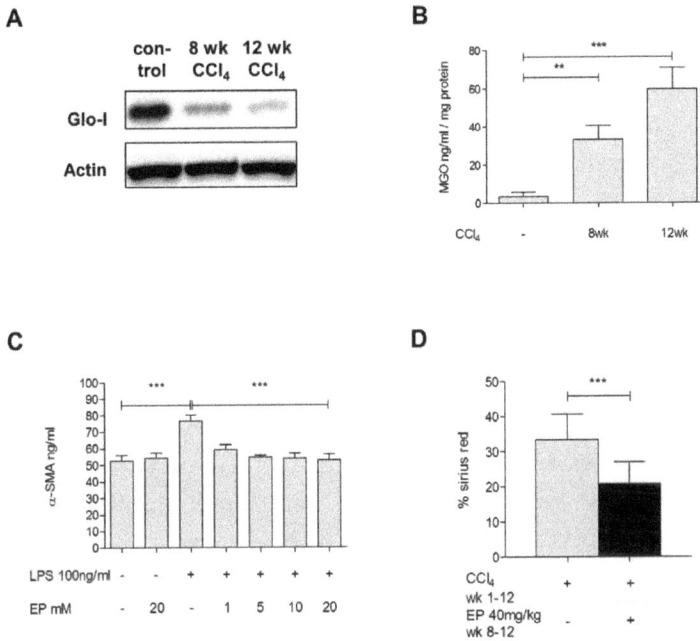

Figure 2. Glyoxalase-I in CCl$_4$-induced cirrhosis. **(A)**, Glo-I expression was reduced in early (8 week CCl$_4$-treatment) and advanced (12 week CCl$_4$-treatment) cirrhosis in Western blot. Wistar rats were treated three times per week with inhalative CCl$_4$ for induction of cirrhosis. **(B)**, MGO levels were significantly elevated in cirrhosis, indicated by ELISA-analysis. **(C)**, treatment of stellate cells (HSC) for 24 hours with LPS revealed increased production of α-SMA. Cotreatment with Glo-I modulator ethyl pyruvate (EP) abolished the LPS-induced effects. **(D)**, Wistar rats were treated with CCl$_4$ and i.p. EP or saline from week 8 to 12. Sirius red staining indicated significantly less fibrosis in EP-treated animals. * $p < 0.05$, ** $p < 0.01$, *** $p < 0.001$. Adapted from [87].

a Parsonnet risk score > 15 undergoing coronary artery bypass graft and/or cardiac valvular surgery with cardiopulmonary bypass. 102 subjects received either placebo (53) or 7.500 mg (90 mg/kg) EP (49) intravenously followed by five more doses every 6 hours. The primary endpoint was a combination of death, prolonged mechanical ventilation, renal failure, or need of vasoconstrictors. No statistically significant differences were observed between groups with regard to clinical parameters or markers of systemic inflammation [97]. Despite these disappointing results in the first clinical trial, it should be kept in mind that underlying molecular mechanisms in cardiac surgery with cardiopulmonary bypass are complex and at least partly different from ROS models showing protective effects of EP. Another clinical study design, for example, liver fibrosis, pancreatitis, septic shock, might be more promising for this interesting agent.

In summary, targeting Glo-I with EP in cirrhosis revealed an innovative therapeutic target. Nevertheless, further research needs to confirm the aforementioned results in further animal experiments and clinical trials.

4.2. AGEs

In contrast to straightforward evidence of Glo-I in chronic liver disease, several groups analyzed AGEs in liver fibrosis, cirrhosis, and NASH. In cirrhotic patients, limited amount of methylglyoxal-modified proteins were found to be elevated compared to controls [98].

Another study revealed increased levels of CML-AGEs in blood plasma of cirrhotic patients. Also, CML levels correlated with severity of disease [99]. Additional studies confirmed the observations of increased CML levels in fibrosis and cirrhosis [100, 101]. These clinical findings were supported by laboratory analysis: *in vitro* treatment of HSC with AGEs resulted in enhanced production of oxidative stress providing evidence of AGEs-involvement in fibrosis [102]. Conversely, oxidative stress was found to elevate levels of CML in rats [103] and incubation of HSC with AGEs led to elevation of α-SMA, TGF-β, and collagen-I [104]. In addition, treatment of rat hepatocyte cultures with AGEs reduced cell viability [105]. In an interesting translational study, CML-AGEs were positively correlated with liver stiffness in patients with chronic hepatitis C. *In vitro* data showed in this study enhanced cell proliferation of HSC treated with BSA-AGEs (CML) and increased production of α-SMA. In contrast, in another study, intraperitoneal administration of AGE-rat serum albumin (CML) revealed increased levels of α-SMA and fibrosis in a model of bile duct ligation [106]. Furthermore, AGEs were found to induce autophagy which subsequently contributes to the fibrosis in patients with chronic hepatitis C [107]. The finding that AGEs were elevated in fibrosis and treatment with AGEs-induced fibrosis led to an interventional approach targeting AGEs to prevent induction of chronic liver disease. Indeed, inhibition of CML resulted in attenuation of CML-induced levels of α-SMA and ROS in HSC [108].

Another model to study fibrosis belongs to metabolic liver diseases: induction of NASH by means of methionine choline deficient diet (MCD). Therefore, hepatic steatosis induced by MCD showed accumulation of CML, and CML was associated with grade of hepatic inflammation and gene expression of inflammatory markers (PAI-1, IL-8, and CRP) [109]. AGEs have also been shown to be involved in etiology of insulin resistance and diabetes [110], and rats fed with a diet rich in AGEs showed elevated oxidative stress and hepatic inflammation leading to NASH [111]. In addition, high dietary AGEs increased hepatic AGEs levels and induced liver injury, inflammation, and liver fibrosis via oxidative stress in activated HSC [112]. Another interesting study investigated the underlying mechanism of AGEs-crosstalk in NASH. AGEs induced NOX2 leading to downregulation of Sirt1/Timp3 and finally resulting in activation of TNF-α converting enzyme and inflammation. These pro-inflammatory cascades finally led to NASH and fibrosis [113]. Interventional studies on AGEs reduction in NASH also revealed promising results. The flavonoid curcumin eliminated the inflammatory effects of AGEs in HSC by interrupting leptin signaling and activating transcription factor Nrf2, which led to the elevation of cellular glutathione levels and the attenuation of oxidative stress [114]. In addition, curcumin decreased activation and proliferation of HSC by AGEs and induced gene expression of AGE-clearing receptor AGE-R1 [115]. The use of the LDL-lowering drug atorvastatin [116] or combination therapy of telmisartan and nateglinide [117] also decreased levels of AGEs in patients with NASH and dyslipidemia, leading to improvement of steatosis, nonalcoholic fatty liver disease activity score, and amelioration of insulin resistance. Another study evaluated effects of aqueous extracts from Solanum nigrum (AESN). AESN could reduce the AGE-induced expression of collagen-II, MMP-2, and α-SMA in HSC. Also, AESN improved insulin resistance and hyperinsulinemia and downregulated lipogenesis, finally preventing fibrosis [118].

Having the auspicious and conclusive effects of AGEs-lowering drugs in fibrosis in mind, it should be noted that mainly CML-AGEs were investigated. Therefore, it should be considered that CML-AGEs are rarely produced via reaction of MGO but are rather formed in lipoxidation and glycoxidation independent of MGO [119].

4.3. RAGE

The pattern recognition receptor RAGE belongs to the immunoglobulin superfamily with a molecular mass of 47–55 kDa. RAGE expression is stimulated under inflammatory conditions such as diabetes, cardiovascular diseases, or cancer [120]. RAGE has been shown to be activated by MGO- and non-MGO-derived AGEs as well as multiple ligands. Binding to RAGE results in activation of transcription factors, such as NF-κB [121], leading to the release of pro-inflammatory cytokines.

Indeed, several studies revealed participation of RAGE in fibrosis: Upon stimulation with AGE-rat serum albumin containing mainly CML, levels of RAGE, α-SMA, hydroxyproline, and Sirius red were elevated in a fibrosis model of bile duct ligation (BDL) [106, 122]. Interestingly, RAGE was found to be predominantly expressed in HSC. RAGE was stimulated in HSC during transformation to myofibroblasts, and RAGE was colocalized with α-SMA and induced by TGF-β. In addition, RAGE was expressed in filopodial membranes of myofibroblasts suggesting a role of RAGE in spreading and migration of activated HSC in fibrogenesis [123]. Further analysis provided evidence for crosstalk of RAGE and TGF-β: AGEs-induced upregulation of RAGE induced TGF-β, TNF-α, and IL-8. Interestingly, RAGE also stimulated anti-inflammatory cytokines IL-2 and IL-4 indicating a negative feedback mechanism and inhibitory crosstalk between TGF-β and RAGE [124]. In the next step, effect of RAGE inhibition on inflammation and fibrosis was discovered. First, curcumin was found to reduce, besides its AGEs-lowering effects, the gene expression of RAGE via elevation of PPAR-γ [125]. Furthermore, RAGE expression was diminished by means of RAGE siRNA in primary rat HSC resulting in downregulation of IL-6, TNF-α, and TGF-β [126]. In a following *in vivo* study, effects of repetitive RAGE siRNA in an olive oil model of fibrosis were analyzed. RAGE siRNA was injected twice weekly in the tail vein of Sprague-Dawley rats. After 6 weeks, reduced expressions of RAGE, TNF-α, IL-6, extracellular matrix, hyaluronic acid, and procollagen III were found. Also, activation of HSC and NF-κB was reduced in siRNA-treated animals attenuating the initiation and progression of fibrosis [127]. Additional studies revealed protective effects of anti-RAGE antibodies in BDL-induced acute liver injury [128, 129].

Growing evidence for implication of RAGE in fibrosis was found in NASH. Methionine choline deficient (MCD) diet caused steatosis and increased RAGE, inflammation, and fibrosis [112]. Recently, fatty acids stimulated CML accumulation and subsequently elicited RAGE induction [109]. Another group found upregulation of RAGE in the liver of aged mice with consecutive elevated oxidative stress shown by analysis of malondialdehyde. Blocking of RAGE by anti-RAGE-antibody revealed in this study prolonged survival of animals [130].

In a nutshell, various studies confirmed implication of Glo-I and (R)AGE in inflammatory liver disease and fibrosis. Especially targeting Glo-I in cirrhosis highlighted the meaning of MGO-induced liver damage and offers new therapeutic opportunities. Nevertheless, further research in this topic will uncover the exact role of Glo-I in chronic liver disease and possible translation to clinical approach (see **Figure 3**).

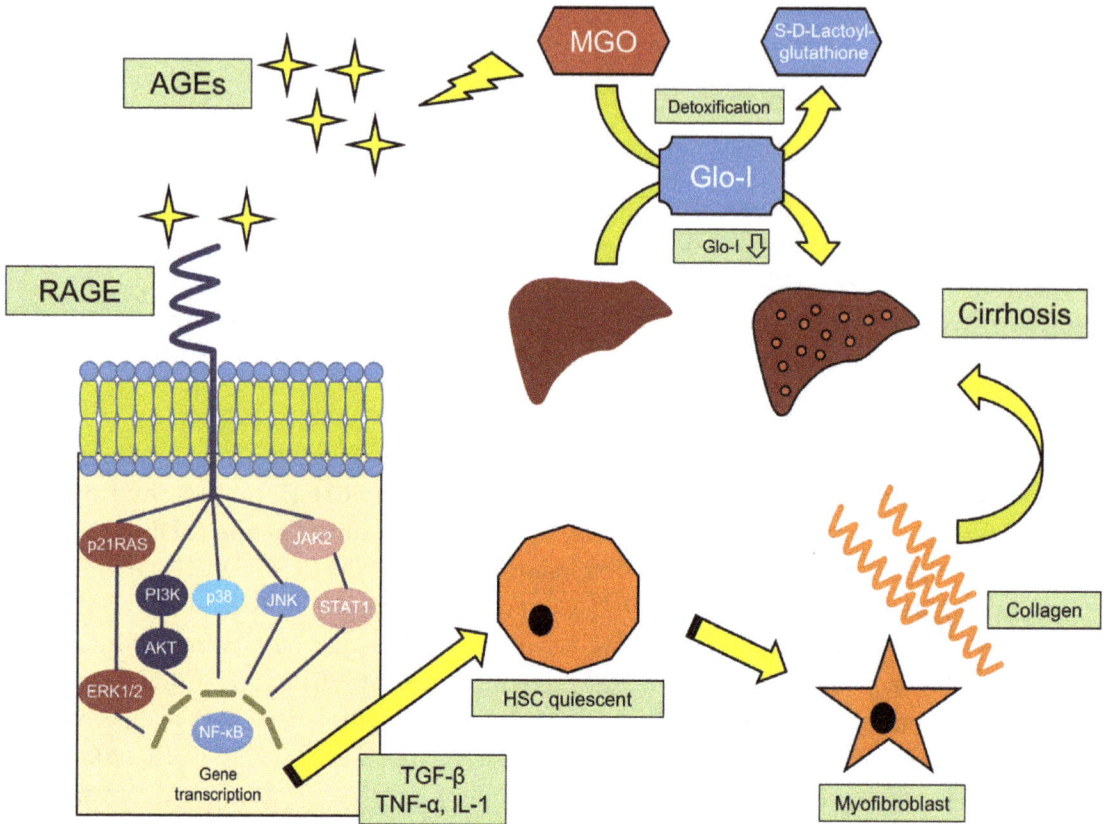

Figure 3. Impact of Glo-I and (R)AGE in cirrhosis. MGO reacts with proteins, nucleotides, and lipids leading to formation of AGEs. AGEs bind to RAGE and activate several signal pathways (including MAPK (ERK1/2, p38, JNK), PI3-K/AKT, and JAK2/STAT1), finally leading to activation of NF-κB. In a consequence, the induced production of TGF-β and pro-inflammatory cytokines activate quiescent stellate cells. HSC transform to myofibroblasts and produce pro-fibrotic factors and collagen. The collagen deposition in the liver will lead to fibrosis and finally cirrhosis. Reduction of Glo-I will perpetuate both, initiation and progression of cirrhosis due to increase of MGO and a vicious circle of disease. MGO: methylglyoxal, AGEs: advanced glycation end products, RAGE: receptor for advanced glycation end products, Glo-I: glyoxalase-I, HSC: hepatic stellate cells, MAPK: mitogen-activated protein kinase, PI3-K: phosphoinositide 3-kinase, AKT: protein kinase B, JAK2: Janus kinase 2, STAT1: signal transducer and activator of transcription-1, JNK: c-Jun N-terminal kinase, and NF-κB: nuclear factor-κB.

Abbreviations

AGEs	advanced glycation end products
AKT	protein kinase B
EP	ethyl pyruvate
ET-1	endothelin-1
Glo-I	glyoxalase-I
Glo-II	glyoxalase-II
GSH	L-glutathione
HCC	hepatocellular carcinoma

HEP	hepatocytes
HSC	hepatic stellate cells
JAK2	Janus kinase 2
JNK	c-Jun N-terminal kinase
KC	Kupffer cells
LSEC	liver sinusoidal endothelial cells
MAPK	mitogen-activated protein kinase
MCD	methionine choline deficient diet
MG-H1	5-hydro-5-methylimidazolone
MGO	methylglyoxal
NAFLD/NASH	non-alcoholic fatty liver disease/steatohepatitis
NF-κB	nuclear factor-κB
NO	nitric oxide
PI3-K	phosphoinositide 3-kinase
RAGE	receptor for advanced glycation end products
sRAGE	soluble form of RAGE
ROS	reactive oxygen species
STAT1	signal transducer and activator of transcription-1
TGF-β	transforming growth factor beta
THP	tetrahydropyrimidine

Author details

Marcus Hollenbach

Address all correspondence to: marcus.hollenbach@web.de

Department of Medicine, Neurology, and Dermatology, Division of Gastroenterology and Rheumatology, University of Leipzig, Leipzig, Germany

References

[1] Rehm J, Samokhvalov AV, Shield KD. Global burden of alcoholic liver diseases. Journal of Hepatology. 2013;**59**:160-168

[2] Novo E, Cannito S, Paternostro C, et al. Cellular and molecular mechanisms in liver fibrogenesis. Archives of Biochemistry and Biophysics. 2014;**548**:20-37

[3]   Dobbs BR, Rogers GW, Xing HY, et al. Endotoxin-induced defenestration of the hepatic sinusoidal endothelium: A factor in the pathogenesis of cirrhosis? Liver. 1994;**14**:230-233

[4]   Fernandez M, Semela D, Bruix J, et al. Angiogenesis in liver disease. Journal of Hepatology. 2009;**50**:604-620

[5]   Bosch J. Vascular deterioration in cirrhosis: The big picture. Journal of Clinical Gastroenterology. 2007;**41**(Suppl 3):S247-S253

[6]   Rockey DC. Vascular mediators in the injured liver. Hepatology. 2003;**37**:4-12

[7]   Groszmann RJ. Nitric oxide and hemodynamic impairment. Digestion. 1998;**59**(Suppl 2):6-7

[8]   Iwakiri Y. Endothelial dysfunction in the regulation of cirrhosis and portal hypertension. Liver International. 2012;**32**:199-213

[9]   Abraldes JG, Iwakiri Y, Loureiro-Silva M, et al. Mild increases in portal pressure upregulate vascular endothelial growth factor and endothelial nitric oxide synthase in the intestinal microcirculatory bed, leading to a hyperdynamic state. American Journal of Physiology-Gastrointestinal and Liver Physiology. 2006;**290**:G980-G987

[10] Groszmann RJ. Hyperdynamic circulation of liver disease 40 years later: Pathophysiology and clinical consequences. Hepatology. 1994;**20**:1359-1363

[11] Zipprich A, Loureiro-Silva MR, Jain D, et al. Nitric oxide and vascular remodeling modulate hepatic arterial vascular resistance in the isolated perfused cirrhotic rat liver. Journal of Hepatology. 2008;**49**:739-745

[12] Friedman SL. Mechanisms of disease: Mechanisms of hepatic fibrosis and therapeutic implications. Nature Clinical Practice Gastroenterology & Hepatology. 2004;**1**:98-105

[13] Friedman SL. Liver fibrosis: From bench to bedside. Journal of Hepatology. 2003;**38**(Suppl 1):S38-S53

[14] Breitkopf K, Nagy LE, Beier JI, et al. Current experimental perspectives on the clinical progression of alcoholic liver disease. Alcoholism Clinical and Experimental Research. 2009;**33**:1647-1655

[15] Hoek JB, Pastorino JG. Cellular signaling mechanisms in alcohol-induced liver damage. Seminars in Liver Disease. 2004;**24**:257-272

[16] Nagy LE. Recent insights into the role of the innate immune system in the development of alcoholic liver disease. Experimental Biology and Medicine (Maywood). 2003;**228**:882-890

[17] Hritz I, Mandrekar P, Velayudham A, et al. The critical role of toll-like receptor (TLR) 4 in alcoholic liver disease is independent of the common TLR adapter MyD88. Hepatology. 2008;**48**:1224-1231

[18] Zhao XJ, Dong Q, Bindas J, et al. TRIF and IRF-3 binding to the TNF promoter results in macrophage TNF dysregulation and steatosis induced by chronic ethanol. Journal of Immunology. 2008;**181**:3049-3056

[19] Roychowdhury S, McMullen MR, Pritchard MT, et al. An early complement-dependent and TLR-4-independent phase in the pathogenesis of ethanol-induced liver injury in mice. Hepatology. 2009;**49**:1326-1334

[20] Cubero FJ, Nieto N. Kupffer cells and alcoholic liver disease. Revista Espanola de Eenfermedades Digestivas. 2006;**98**:460-472

[21] Cubero FJ, Urtasun R, Nieto N. Alcohol and liver fibrosis. Seminars in Liver Disease. 2009;**29**:211-221

[22] Seki E, De MS, Osterreicher CH, et al. TLR4 enhances TGF-beta signaling and hepatic fibrosis. Nature Medicine. 2007;**13**:1324-1332

[23] Quiroz SC, Bucio L, Souza V, et al. Effect of endotoxin pretreatment on hepatic stellate cell response to ethanol and acetaldehyde. Journal of Gastroenterology and Hepatology. 2001;**16**:1267-1273

[24] Bai T, Lian LH, Wu YL, et al. Thymoquinone attenuates liver fibrosis via PI3K and TLR4 signaling pathways in activated hepatic stellate cells. International Immunopharmacology. 2013;**15**:275-281

[25] Novo E, Parola M. Redox mechanisms in hepatic chronic wound healing and fibrogenesis. Fibrogenesis Tissue Repair. 2008;**1**:5

[26] Jaruga B, Hong F, Kim WH, et al. Chronic alcohol consumption accelerates liver injury in T cell-mediated hepatitis: alcohol disregulation of NF-kappaB and STAT3 signaling pathways. American Journal of Physiology-Gastrointestinal and Liver Physiology. 2004;**287**:G471-G479

[27] Zima T, Kalousova M. Oxidative stress and signal transduction pathways in alcoholic liver disease. Alcoholism Clinical and Experimental Research. 2005;**29**:110S-115S

[28] Kureishi Y, Kobayashi S, Amano M, et al. Rho-associated kinase directly induces smooth muscle contraction through myosin light chain phosphorylation. Journal of Biological Chemistry. 1997;**272**:12257-12260

[29] Jagavelu K, Routray C, Shergill U, et al. Endothelial cell toll-like receptor 4 regulates fibrosis-associated angiogenesis in the liver. Hepatology. 2010;**52**:590-601

[30] Ding BS, Nolan DJ, Butler JM, et al. Inductive angiocrine signals from sinusoidal endothelium are required for liver regeneration. Nature. 2010;**468**:310-315

[31] Loureiro-Silva MR, Iwakiri Y, Abraldes JG, et al. Increased phosphodiesterase-5 expression is involved in the decreased vasodilator response to nitric oxide in cirrhotic rat livers. Journal of Hepatology. 2006;**44**:886-893

[32] Yokomori H, Oda M, Ogi M, et al. Enhanced expression of endothelial nitric oxide syn-thase and caveolin-1 in human cirrhosis. Liver. 2002;**22**:150-158

[33] Iwakiri Y, Tsai MH, McCabe TJ, et al. Phosphorylation of eNOS initiates excessive NO production in early phases of portal hypertension. American Journal of Physiology: Heart and Circulatory Physiology. 2002;**282**:H2084-H2090

[34] Vallance P, Moncada S. Hyperdynamic circulation in cirrhosis: A role for nitric oxide? Lancet. 1991;**337**:776-778

[35] Malyshev E, Tazi KA, Moreau R, et al. Discrepant effects of inducible nitric oxide syn-thase modulation on systemic and splanchnic endothelial nitric oxide synthase activity and expression in cirrhotic rats. Journal of Gastroenterology and Hepatology. 2007;**22**: 2195-2201

[36] Mezey E, Potter JJ, Rennie-Tankersley L, et al. A randomized placebo controlled trial of vitamin E for alcoholic hepatitis. Journal of Hepatology. 2004;**40**:40-46

[37] Stewart S, Prince M, Bassendine M, et al. A randomized trial of antioxidant therapy alone or with corticosteroids in acute alcoholic hepatitis. Journal of Hepatology. 2007;**47**:277-283

[38] Moreno C, Langlet P, Hittelet A, et al. Enteral nutrition with or without N-acetylcysteine in the treatment of severe acute alcoholic hepatitis: A randomized multicenter controlled trial. Journal of Hepatology. 2010;**53**:1117-1122

[39] Dakin HD, Dudley HW. An enzyme concerned with the formation of hydroxy acids from ketonic aldehydes. Journal of Biological Chemistry. 1913;**14**:155-157

[40] Weaver RH, Lardy HA. Synthesis and some biochemical properties of phosphohy-droxypyruvic aldehyde and of 3-phosphoglyceryl glutathione thiol ester. Journal of Biological Chemistry. 1961;**236**:313-317

[41] Vander Jagt DL. The glyoxalase system. In: Glutathione: Chemical, Biochemical and Medical Aspects. New York: Wiley-Interscience; 1989. pp. 597-641

[42] Mannervik B. Glyoxalase I. In: Enzymatic Basis of Detoxification. Vol. 2. New York: Academic Press; 1980. pp. 263-293

[43] Thornalley PJ. The glyoxalase system in health and disease. Molecular Aspects of Medicine. 1993;**14**:287-371

[44] Racker E. The mechanism of action of glyoxalase. Journal of Biological Chemistry. 1951;**190**:685-696

[45] Thornalley PJ. The glyoxalase system: New developments towards functional charac-terization of a metabolic pathway fundamental to biological life. Biochemical Journal. 1990;**269**:1-11

[46] Ohmori S, Mori M, Shiraha K, et al. Biosynthesis and degradation of methylglyoxal in animals. Progress in Clinical Biological Research. 1989;**290**:397-412

[47] Ray S, Ray M. Formation of methylglyoxal from aminoacetone by amine oxidase from goat plasma. Journal of Biological Chemistry. 1983;**258**:3461-3462

[48] Casazza JP, Felver ME, Veech RL. The metabolism of acetone in rat. Journal of Biological Chemistry. 1984;**259**:231-236

[49] Phillips SA, Thornalley PJ. The formation of methylglyoxal from triose phosphates. Investigation using a specific assay for methylglyoxal. European Journal of Biochemistry. 1993;**212**:101-105

[50] Vaca CE, Fang JL, Conradi M, et al. Development of a 32P-postlabelling method for the analysis of 2'-deoxyguanosine-3'-monophosphate and DNA adducts of methylglyoxal. Carcinogenesis. 1994;**15**:1887-1894

[51] Lo TW, Westwood ME, McLellan AC, et al. Binding and modification of proteins by methylglyoxal under physiological conditions. A kinetic and mechanistic study with N alpha-acetylarginine, N alpha-acetylcysteine, and N alpha-acetyllysine, and bovine serum albumin. Journal of Biological Chemistry. 1994;**269**:32299-32305

[52] Nakayama M, Saito K, Sato E, et al. Radical generation by the non-enzymatic reaction of methylglyoxal and hydrogen peroxide. Redox Report. 2007;**12**:125-133

[53] Oya T, Hattori N, Mizuno Y, et al. Methylglyoxal modification of protein. Chemical and immunochemical characterization of methylglyoxal-arginine adducts. Journal of Biological Chemistry. 1999;**274**:18492-18502

[54] Thornalley PJ. Glyoxalase I: Structure, function and a critical role in the enzymatic defence against glycation. Biochemical Society Transactions. 2003;**31**:1343-1348

[55] Singh R, Barden A, Mori T, et al. Advanced glycation end-products: A review. Diabetologia. 2001;**44**:129-146

[56] Schmidt AM, Yan SD, Yan SF, et al. The biology of the receptor for advanced glycation end products and its ligands. Biochimica et Biophysica Acta. 2000;**1498**:99-111

[57] Piperi C, Goumenos A, Adamopoulos C, et al. AGE/RAGE signalling regulation by miR-NAs: Associations with diabetic complications and therapeutic potential. International Journal of Biochemistry & Cell Biology. 2015;**60C**:197-201

[58] Lu C, He JC, Cai W, et al. Advanced glycation endproduct (AGE) receptor 1 is a negative regulator of the inflammatory response to AGE in mesangial cells. Proceedings of the National Academy of Sciences USA. 2004;**101**:11767-11772

[59] Xiang Y, Li Q, Li M, et al. Ghrelin inhibits AGEs-induced apoptosis in human endothelial cells involving ERK1/2 and PI3K/Akt pathways. Cell Biochemistry and Function. 2011;**29**:149-155

[60] Han LP, Schimandle CM, Davison LM, et al. Comparative kinetics of Mg2+-, Mn2+-, Co2+-, and Ni2+-activated glyoxalase I. Evaluation of the role of the metal ion. Biochemistry. 1977;**16**:5478-5484

[61] Sellin S, Eriksson LE, Aronsson AC, et al. Octahedral metal coordination in the active site of glyoxalase I as evidenced by the properties of Co(II)-glyoxalase I. Journal of Biological Chemistry. 1983;**258**:2091-2093

[62] Cameron AD, Olin B, Ridderstrom M, et al. Crystal structure of human glyoxalase I: Evidence for gene duplication and 3D domain swapping. EMBO Journal. 1997;**16**:3386-3395

[63] Kompf J, Bissbort S, Gussmann S, et al. Polymorphism of red cell glyoxalase I (EI: 4.4.1.5); a new genetic marker in man. Investigation of 169 mother-child combinations. Humangenetik. 1975;**27**:141-143

[64] Kompf J, Bissbort S, Ritter H. Red cell glyoxalase i (E.C.: 4.4.1.5): Formal genetics and linkage relations. Humangenetik. 1975;**28**:249-251

[65] Bender K, Grzeschik KH. Assignment of the genes for human glyoxalase I to chromosome 6 and for human esterase D to chromosome 13. Cytogenetics and Cell Genetics. 1976;**16**:93-96

[66] Kompf J, Bissbort S. Confirmation of linkage between the loci for HL-A and glyoxalase I. Human Genetics. 1976;**32**:197-198

[67] Thornalley PJ. Population genetics of human glyoxalases. Heredity. 1991;**67**(Pt 2):139-142

[68] McCann VJ, Davis RE, Welborn TA, et al. Glyoxalase phenotypes in patients with diabetes mellitus. Australian and New Zealand Journal of Medicine. 1981;**11**:380-382

[69] Gale CP, Futers TS, Summers LK. Common polymorphisms in the glyoxalase-1 gene and their association with pro-thrombotic factors. Diabetes and Vascular Disease Research 2004;**1**:34-39

[70] Bangel FN, Yamada K, Arai M, et al. Genetic analysis of the glyoxalase system in schizophrenia. Neuro-Psychopharmacology and Biological Psychiatry. 2015;**59**:105-110

[71] Barua M, Jenkins EC, Chen W, et al. Glyoxalase I polymorphism rs2736654 causing the Ala111Glu substitution modulates enzyme activity--implications for autism. Autism Research. 2011;**4**:262-270

[72] Junaid MA, Kowal D, Barua M, et al. Proteomic studies identified a single nucleotide polymorphism in glyoxalase I as autism susceptibility factor. American Journal of Medical Genetics Part A. 2004;**131**:11-17

[73] Williams R, Lim JE, Harr B, et al. A common and unstable copy number variant is associated with differences in Glo1 expression and anxiety-like behavior. PLoS One. 2009;**4**:e4649

[74] Santarius T, Bignell GR, Greenman CD, et al. GLO1-A novel amplified gene in human cancer. Genes Chromosomes Cancer. 2010;**49**:711-725

[75] Shafie A, Xue M, Thornalley PJ, et al. Copy number variation of glyoxalase I. Biochemical Society Transactions. 2014;**42**:500-503

[76] Thornalley PJ, Tisdale MJ. Inhibition of proliferation of human promyelocytic leukaemia HL60 cells by S-D-lactoylglutathione in vitro. Leukemia Research. 1988;**12**:897-904

[77] Thornalley PJ, Edwards LG, Kang Y, et al. Antitumour activity of S-p-bromobenzylgluta thione cyclopentyl diester in vitro and in vivo. Inhibition of glyoxalase I and induction of apoptosis. Biochemical Pharmacology. 1996;**51**:1365-1372

[78] Baunacke M, Horn LC, Trettner S, et al. Exploring glyoxalase 1 expression in prostate cancer tissues: Targeting the enzyme by ethyl pyruvate defangs some malignancy-associated properties. Prostate. 2014;**74**:48-60

[79] Birkenmeier G, Hemdan NY, Kurz S, et al. Ethyl pyruvate combats human leukemia cells but spares normal blood cells. PLoS One. 2016;**11**:e0161571

[80] Lo TW, Thornalley PJ. Inhibition of proliferation of human leukaemia 60 cells by diethyl esters of glyoxalase inhibitors in vitro. Biochemical Pharmacology. 1992;**44**:2357-2363

[81] Bartyik K, Turi S, Orosz F, et al. Methotrexate inhibits the glyoxalase system in vivo in children with acute lymphoid leukaemia. European Journal of Cancer. 2004;**40**:2287-2292

[82] Sato S, Kwon Y, Kamisuki S, et al. Polyproline-rod approach to isolating protein targets of bioactive small molecules: Isolation of a new target of indomethacin. Journal of the American Chemical Society. 2007;**129**:873-880

[83] Wu L, Eftekharpour E, Davies GF, et al. Troglitazone selectively inhibits glyoxalase I gene expression. Diabetologia. 2001;**44**:2004-2012

[84] Takasawa R, Takahashi S, Saeki K, et al. Structure-activity relationship of human GLO I inhibitory natural flavonoids and their growth inhibitory effects. Bioorganic & Medicinal Chemistry. 2008;**16**:3969-3975

[85] Santel T, Pflug G, Hemdan NY, et al. Curcumin inhibits glyoxalase 1: A possible link to its anti-inflammatory and anti-tumor activity. PLoS One. 2008;**3**:e3508

[86] Xue M, Weickert MO, Qureshi S, et al. Improved glycemic control and vascular function in overweight and obese subjects by glyoxalase 1 inducer formulation. Diabetes. 2016;**65**:2282-2294

[87] Hollenbach M, Thonig A, Pohl S, et al. Expression of glyoxalase-I is reduced in cirrhotic livers: A possible mechanism in development of cirrhosis. PLoS One. 2017;**12**(2):e0171260. DOI: 10.1371/journal.pone.0171260

[88] Fink MP. Ethyl pyruvate: A novel anti-inflammatory agent. Journal of Internal Medicine. 2007;**261**:349-362

[89] Fink MP. Ethyl pyruvate: A novel treatment for sepsis. Novartis Foundation Symposium. 2007;**280**:147-156

[90] Fink MP. Ethyl pyruvate. Current Opinion in Anaesthesiology. 2008;**21**:160-167

[91] Hollenbach M, Hintersdorf A, Huse K, et al. Ethyl pyruvate and ethyl lactate down-regulate the production of pro-inflammatory cytokines and modulate expression of immune receptors. Biochemical Pharmacology. 2008;76:631-644

[92] Wang LW, Wang LK, Chen H, et al. Ethyl pyruvate protects against experimental acute-on-chronic liver failure in rats. World Journal of Gastroenterology. 2012;18:5709-5718

[93] Yang R, Han X, Delude RL, et al. Ethyl pyruvate ameliorates acute alcohol-induced liver injury and inflammation in mice. Journal of Laboratory and Clinical Medicine. 2003;142:322-331

[94] Yang R, Shaufl AL, Killeen ME, et al. Ethyl pyruvate ameliorates liver injury secondary to severe acute pancreatitis. Journal of Surgical Research. 2009;153:302-309

[95] Yang R, Zou X, Koskinen ML, et al. Ethyl pyruvate reduces liver injury at early phase but impairs regeneration at late phase in acetaminophen overdose. Critical Care. 2012;16:R9

[96] Olek RA, Ziolkowski W, Flis DJ, et al. The effect of ethyl pyruvate supplementation on rat fatty liver induced by a high-fat diet. Journal of Nutritional Science and Vitaminology (Tokyo). 2013;59:232-237

[97] Bennett-Guerrero E, Swaminathan M, Grigore AM, et al. A phase II multicenter double-blind placebo-controlled study of ethyl pyruvate in high-risk patients undergoing cardiac surgery with cardiopulmonary bypass. Journal of Cardiothoracic and Vascular Anesthesia. 2009;23:324-329

[98] Ahmed N, Thornalley PJ, Luthen R, et al. Processing of protein glycation, oxidation and nitrosation adducts in the liver and the effect of cirrhosis. Journal of Hepatology. 2004;41:913-919

[99] Sebekova K, Kupcova V, Schinzel R, et al. Markedly elevated levels of plasma advanced glycation end products in patients with liver cirrhosis - amelioration by liver transplantation. Journal of Hepatology. 2002;36:66-71

[100] Yagmur E, Tacke F, Weiss C, et al. Elevation of Nepsilon-(carboxymethyl)lysine-modified advanced glycation end products in chronic liver disease is an indicator of liver cirrhosis. Clinical Biochemistry. 2006;39:39-45

[101] Zuwala-Jagiello J, Pazgan-Simon M, Simon K, et al. Elevated advanced oxidation protein products levels in patients with liver cirrhosis. Acta biochimica Polonica. 2009;56:679-685

[102] Guimaraes EL, Empsen C, Geerts A, et al. Advanced glycation end products induce production of reactive oxygen species via the activation of NADPH oxidase in murine hepatic stellate cells. Journal of Hepatology. 2010;52:389-397

[103] Lorenzi R, Andrades ME, Bortolin RC, et al. Oxidative damage in the liver of rats treated with glycolaldehyde. International Journal of Toxicology. 2011;30:253-258

[104] Iwamoto K, Kanno K, Hyogo H, et al. Advanced glycation end products enhance the proliferation and activation of hepatic stellate cells. Journal of Gastroenterology. 2008;43:298-304

[105] Hayashi N, George J, Takeuchi M, et al. Acetaldehyde-derived advanced glycation end-products promote alcoholic liver disease. PLoS One. 2013;8:e70034

[106] Goodwin M, Herath C, Jia Z, et al. Advanced glycation end products augment experimental hepatic fibrosis. Journal of Gastroenterology and Hepatology. 2013;28:369-376

[107] He Y, Zhu J, Huang Y, et al. Advanced glycation end product (AGE)-induced hepatic stellate cell activation via autophagy contributes to hepatitis C-related fibrosis. Acta Diabetologica. 2015;52:959-969

[108] Hsu WH, Lee BH, Hsu YW, et al. Peroxisome proliferator-activated receptor-gamma activators monascin and rosiglitazone attenuate carboxymethyllysine-induced fibrosis in hepatic stellate cells through regulating the oxidative stress pathway but independent of the receptor for advanced glycation end products signaling. Journal of Agricultural and Food Chemistry. 2013;61:6873-6879

[109] Gaens KH, Niessen PM, Rensen SS, et al. Endogenous formation of Nepsilon-(carboxymethyl)lysine is increased in fatty livers and induces inflammatory markers in an in vitro model of hepatic steatosis. Journal of Hepatology. 2012;56:647-655

[110] Vlassara H. Recent progress in advanced glycation end products and diabetic complications. Diabetes. 1997;46(Suppl 2):S19-S25

[111] Patel R, Baker SS, Liu W, et al. Effect of dietary advanced glycation end products on mouse liver. PLoS One. 2012;7:e35143

[112] Leung C, Herath CB, Jia Z, et al. Dietary glycotoxins exacerbate progression of experimental fatty liver disease. Journal of Hepatology. 2014;60:832-838

[113] Jiang JX, Chen X, Fukada H, et al. Advanced glycation endproducts induce fibrogenic activity in nonalcoholic steatohepatitis by modulating TNF-alpha-converting enzyme activity in mice. Hepatology. 2013;58:1339-1348

[114] Tang Y, Chen A. Curcumin eliminates the effect of advanced glycation end-products (AGEs) on the divergent regulation of gene expression of receptors of AGEs by interrupting leptin signaling. Laboratory Investigation. 2014;94:503-516

[115] Lin J, Tang Y, Kang Q, et al. Curcumin eliminates the inhibitory effect of advanced glycation end-products (AGEs) on gene expression of AGE receptor-1 in hepatic stellate cells in vitro. Laboratory Investigation. 2012;92:827-841

[116] Kimura Y, Hyogo H, Yamagishi S, et al. Atorvastatin decreases serum levels of advanced glycation endproducts (AGEs) in nonalcoholic steatohepatitis (NASH) patients with dyslipidemia: clinical usefulness of AGEs as a biomarker for the attenuation of NASH. Journal of Gastroenterology. 2010;45:750-757

[117] Miura K, Kitahara Y, Yamagishi S. Combination therapy with nateglinide and vilda-
       gliptin improves postprandial metabolic derangements in Zucker fatty rats. Hormone
       and Metabolic Research. 2010;**42**:731-735

[118] Tai CJ, Choong CY, Shi YC, et al. Solanum nigrum protects against hepatic fibrosis
       via suppression of hyperglycemia in high-fat/ethanol diet-induced rats. Molecules.
       2016;**21**:269

[119] Fu MX, Requena JR, Jenkins AJ, et al. The advanced glycation end product, Nepsilon-
       (carboxymethyl)lysine, is a product of both lipid peroxidation and glycoxidation reac-
       tions. Journal of Biological Chemistry. 1996;**271**:9982-9986

[120] Yamagishi S, Matsui T. Role of receptor for advanced glycation end products (RAGE)
       in liver disease. European Journal of Medical Research. 2015;**20**:15

[121] Barbezier N, Tessier FJ, Chango A. Receptor of advanced glycation endproducts RAGE/
       AGER: An integrative view for clinical applications. Annales de Biologie Clinique
       (Paris). 2014;**72**:669-680

[122] Lohwasser C, Neureiter D, Popov Y, et al. Role of the receptor for advanced glycation
       end products in hepatic fibrosis. World Journal of Gastroenterology. 2009;**15**:5789-5798

[123] Fehrenbach H, Weiskirchen R, Kasper M, et al. Up-regulated expression of the receptor
       for advanced glycation end products in cultured rat hepatic stellate cells during trans-
       differentiation to myofibroblasts. Hepatology. 2001;**34**:943-952

[124] Serban AI, Stanca L, Geicu OI, et al. RAGE and TGF-beta1 cross-talk regulate extracel-
       lular matrix turnover and cytokine synthesis in AGEs exposed fibroblast cells. PLoS
       One. 2016;**11**:e0152376

[125] Lin J, Tang Y, Kang Q, et al. Curcumin inhibits gene expression of receptor for
       advanced glycation end-products (RAGE) in hepatic stellate cells in vitro by elevating
       PPARgamma activity and attenuating oxidative stress. British Journal of Pharmacology.
       2012;**166**:2212-2227

[126] Xia JR, Chen TT, Li WD, et al. Inhibitory effect of receptor for advanced glycation end
       product specific small interfering RNAs on the development of hepatic fibrosis in pri-
       mary rat hepatic stellate cells. Molecular Medicine Reports. 2015;**12**:569-574

[127] Cai XG, Xia JR, Li WD, et al. Anti-fibrotic effects of specific-siRNA targeting of the
       receptor for advanced glycation end products in a rat model of experimental hepatic
       fibrosis. Molecular Medicine Reports. 2014;**10**:306-314

[128] Xia P, Deng Q, Gao J, et al. Therapeutic effects of antigen affinity-purified polyclonal
       anti-receptor of advanced glycation end-product (RAGE) antibodies on cholestasis-
       induced liver injury in rats. European Journal of Pharmacology. 2016;**779**:102-110

[129] Kao YH, Lin YC, Tsai MS, et al. Involvement of the nuclear high mobility group B1 peptides released from injured hepatocytes in murine hepatic fibrogenesis. Biochimica et Biophysica Acta. 2014;**1842**:1720-1732

[130] Kuhla A, Trieglaff C, Vollmar B. Role of age and uncoupling protein-2 in oxidative stress, RAGE/AGE interaction and inflammatory liver injury. Experimental Gerontology. 2011;**46**:868-876

2

Predictors of the Response to Tolvaptan Therapy and Its Effect on Prognosis in Cirrhotic Patients with Ascites

Tomomi Kogiso, Kuniko Yamamoto,
Mutsuki Kobayashi, Yuichi Ikarashi,
Kazuhisa Kodama, Makiko Taniai, Nobuyuki Torii,
Etsuko Hashimoto and Katsutoshi Tokushige

Abstract

Aims: The vasopressin V2 receptor antagonist, tolvaptan, has been reported to be effective in cirrhotic patients with ascites. Here, we evaluated predictors of the response to tolvaptan. *Methods*: A total of 97 patients with cirrhosis (60 males; median age, 63 years) who had been treated for ascites with oral tolvaptan were enrolled. Tolvaptan efficacy was defined as urine volume increase of $\geq$500 mL or a urine volume $\geq$2000 mL/day on the day following treatment. Normalization of the serum sodium (Na) level after 1 week of treatment and the posttreatment survival rate was analyzed. *Results*: Tolvaptan therapy resulted in effective urination in 67% of patients. A multivariate analysis revealed that the blood urea nitrogen/creatinine (BUN/Cr) ratio and urinary Na/potassium (Na/K) ratio were predictive of the tolvaptan response ($p < 0.05$). The serum Na level was 135 (121–145) mEq/L, and normal levels were recovered in 50.0% of the patients with an initial Na level of <135 mEq/L. The posttreatment survival rate was significantly higher in patients who responded to tolvaptan therapy ($p < 0.05$). *Conclusions*: The combination of the initial BUN/Cr and urine Na/K ratios and a normalized serum Na level after 1 week was predictive of a favorable outcome to tolvaptan therapy.

Keywords: vasopressin V2 receptor antagonist, tolvaptan, blood urea nitrogen/creatinine ratio, urine sodium/potassium ratio, serum sodium

1. Introduction

Ascites accumulation is commonly observed in decompensated liver cirrhosis [1]. The symptoms of ascites lead to a poor quality of life and prognosis [2]. Recently, the vasopressin V2 receptor antagonist tolvaptan has been used for ascites treatment of cirrhosis in addition to spironolac-tone ± furosemide [3, 4]. The Japanese Society of Gastroenterology published evidence-based clinical practice guidelines in 2015 [5]. Tolvaptan is recommended for use before ascites drainage or administration of albumin because of its high efficacy irrespective of the serum albumin level [6]. While the serum sodium (Na) level is low in cirrhosis, it is increased in tolvaptan-treated patients because of free water clearance without accompanying Na elimination. In contrast, con-ventional diuretics promote hyponatremia and impair renal function. Thus, tolvaptan has ben-efits for the treatment of cirrhosis.

The mechanism underlying refractory ascites caused by liver cirrhosis has been hypoth-esized as one or more of the following [7, 8]: (1) hypo-osmotic pressure due to hypoalbumin-emia; (2) a response to mesenteric and systemic vasodilation, accompanied by development of portal hypertension, which decreases the effective circulatory volume and depletes renal flow, leading to increased arginine vasopressin (AVP) release; increased AVP results in an increase in renin-angiotensin-aldosterone system activity; and (3) postsinusoidal obstruc-tion and lymphatic edema. These multiple causative factors are associated with ascites accumulation.

Approximately 70% of tolvaptan-treated patients exhibit increased urination and achieve a reduction in body weight within 7–14 days [9, 10]. In addition to this short-term efficacy, tolvaptan also exerts long-term effects [11]. However, factors that predict the response to tolvaptan and its effect on prognosis are unclear. In this study, we focused on predictors of the tolvaptan response and the outcome of tolvaptan therapy.

2. Patients and methods

2.1. Patients

This was a single-center, retrospective observational study performed between September 2013 and March 2016. We enrolled a total of 97 Japanese cirrhotic patients (60 males, 62%) who received tolvaptan 3.75–7.5 mg/day (Samsca™; Otsuka Pharmaceutical Co. Ltd., Tokyo, Japan) after hospitalization for ascites treatment. They were treated with conven-tional diuretics.

2.2. Method

The patients were classified as responders or nonresponders to tolvaptan therapy. Tolvaptan efficacy was defined as a urine volume increase of ≥500 mL or a urine volume ≥2000 mL/day on the day following tolvaptan treatment, as described by Ohki et al. with slight modi-fications [12]. The baseline characteristics of patients, including age, sex, medications, and laboratory parameters, were evaluated. We investigated the changes in body weight and the serum Na level after 1 week of treatment and evaluated laboratory parameters. Tolvaptan was not used in patients with severe renal dysfunction (estimated glomerular filtration rate <15 mL/min/1.73 m^2 or a serum creatinine [Cr] level >3.5 mg/dL) or a hepatic coma scale score >II.

This study was conducted according to the principles of the Declaration of Helsinki, and the Institutional Review Board of Tokyo Women's Medical University Hospital (Tokyo, Japan) approved the study protocol (no. 3258-R). The results of this study, including figures and tables, were published in Hepatology Research [13] and were transferred with permission.

2.3. Statistical analysis

Data are presented as medians with minimum and maximum values. Significant differences between the two groups were assessed using the Mann–Whitney U-test and χ^2 test. The Statistical Package for the Social Sciences software (SPSS Institute, 11.01.J, Chicago, IL, USA) was used for the statistical analyses. Statistical significance was considered at $p < 0.05$.

3. Results

3.1. Response to tolvaptan according to urination and body weight parameters

The median age of the 97 patients (62% male) receiving tolvaptan treatment was 63 years (range, 22–90 years; **Table 1**). The underlying liver diseases and frequency of other ascites treatments did not differ significantly. The median increase in urine volume on the day after treatment was 690 mL (range: –530 to +3490 mL), while the median urine volume was 1675 mL/day (range: 195–6630 mL/day). The distributions of urination and body weight changes and their correlations with the tolvaptan response are shown in **Figure 1(a)**. The change in body weight after 1 week of treatment was –1.5 kg (–17.2 to +6.2 kg). A total urine volume ≥2000 mL was achieved in 40% of cases and an increase in the urine volume in ~50% of cases (**Figure 1b**). Approximately 40% of cases achieved a ≥2.0 kg body weight reduction after 1 week of treatment. Overall, 67% of the cases achieved the desired level of urination. In cases who responded to tolvaptan, the platelet count, urine Na level, and urine Na/potassium (K) ratio were higher, and the blood urea nitrogen (BUN)/Cr ratio was lower (**Table 2**). The serum Na level was 135 (121–145) mEq/L, and 39.2% of cases had an Na level of <135 mEq/L.

3.2. Urination-based predictors of the response to tolvaptan

Multivariate analysis revealed that the BUN/Cr ratio (odds ratio [OR], 1.08; 95% confidence interval [CI], 1.006–1.174; $p < 0.05$) and urine Na/K ratio (OR, 0.59; 95% CI, 0.366–0.855; $p < 0.01$) were predictors of the tolvaptan response (**Table 3**). In particular, patients who satisfied both

	Total ($n = 97$)	Responder ($n = 65$)	Nonresponder ($n = 32$)	p-value
Age (years)	63 (22–90)	62 (22–90)	63 (37–84)	0.21
Sex (% of males)	62	66	53	0.21
Underlying hepatitis (%) (viral/metabolic/PBC)	37/39/9	32/43/11	47/31/6	0.29
Complication (%) (varices/HCC/hepatic encephalopathy)	67/35/23	71/35/18	59/34/31	0.37
Diuretics				
Furosemide dose (mg/day)	20 (0–160)	20 (0–160)	20 (0–80)	0.96
Spironolactone dose (mg/day)	50 (0–400)	50 (0–400)	50 (0–400)	0.97
BCAA (%)	90	89	91	0.11
Administration of albumin (%)	62	63	59	0.65
CART or drainage (%)	41	38	47	0.43
Prognosis; death or transplantation (%)	45	37	63	0.03

Notes: PBC, primary biliary cholangitis; HCC, hepatocellular carcinoma; BCAA, branched-chain amino acid; CART, cell-free and concentrated ascites reinfusion therapy.

Table 1. Baseline characteristics of the patients.

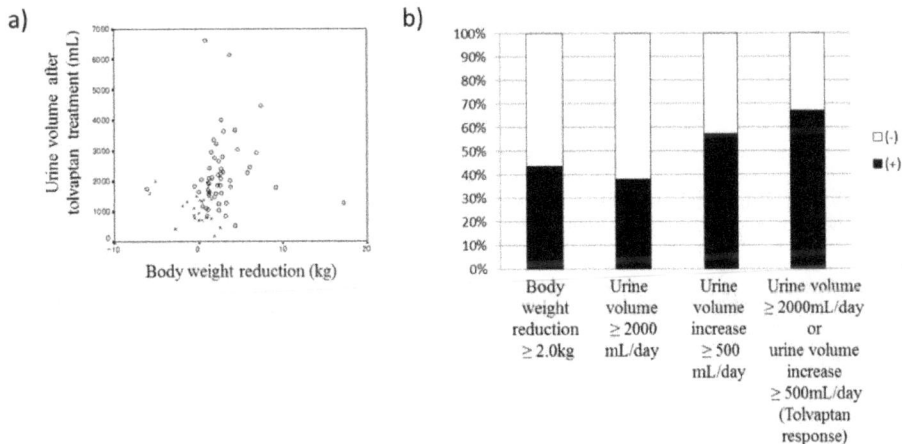

Figure 1. Urine volume and body weight response after tolvaptan treatment. (a) Distributions of urine volume after 1 day, and change in body weight after 1 week, of tolvaptan treatment. Circle, responder; cross, nonresponder. (b) The percentage of urination and body weight reduction responded to a tolvaptan therapy. Urine volume 1 day after, and change in body weight 1 week after, tolvaptan treatment was correlated with the tolvaptan response (a). A body weight reduction of ≥2.0 kg was found in 40% of cases, and a urine volume ≥2000 mL and a urine volume increase ≥500 mL were found in 67% of patients in response to tolvaptan therapy (b).

	Total (n = 97)	Responder (n = 65)	Nonresponder (n = 32)	p value
Albumin (g/dL)	2.5 (1.5–4.2)	2.5 (1.5–4.2)	2.4 (1.9–3.5)	0.88
Total bilirubin (mg/dL)	1.8 (0.3–52.4)	1.5 (0.5–33.0)	2.2 (0.3–52.4)	0.73
Platelet count (×10^4 μL^{-1})	8.6 (1.5–42.4)	9.0 (1.5–42.4)	6.4 (2.1–23.9)	0.05
Prothrombin time (%)	54.5 (16.3–90.3)	54.5 (16.3–90.3)	52.6 (22.6–89.0)	0.70
Ammonia (mg/dL)	69 (25–269)	70 (25–269)	63 (29–212)	0.97
α-Fetoprotein (ng/mL)	4 (1–29,292)	4 (1–4510)	6.5 (1–29,292)	0.36
DCP (mAU/mL)	75 (3–4994)	42 (3–4994)	324 (10–1788)	0.61
BUN (mg/dL)	23.4 (5.5–125.3)	21 (5.5–63.3)	27 (12.0–125.3)	0.02
Creatinine (mg/dL)	1.07 (0.20–3.30)	1.00 (0.42–2.12)	1.17 (0.50–3.30)	0.13
eGFR (mL/min/1.73 m²)	50.0 (15.0–250.6)	50.3 (18–250.6)	46.2 (15.0–108.6)	0.15
Serum Na (mEq/L)	135 (121–145)	136 (122–145)	133 (121–144)	0.06
Serum K (mEq/L)	4.2 (2.8–6.1)	3.9 (2.8–5.3)	4.3 (3.1–6.1)	0.06
Serum osmolarity (mOsm/L)	281 (100–317)	283 (100–317)	279 (256–299)	0.68
Urine osmolarity (mOsm/L)	404 (116–938)	405 (116–938)	388 (233–715)	0.63
Urinary Na (mEq/L)	61 (7–256)	69.5 (10–256)	39 (7–108)	<0.01
Urinary K (mEq/L)	21 (6–72)	20 (6–72)	22 (13–48)	0.72
24 h creatinine clearance (mL/min)	51.2 (7.6–124.0)	52.8 (12.4–124.0)	44.1 (7.6–92.9)	0.12
BUN/creatinine ratio	22.5 (6.83–138.5)	21 (5.5–138.5)	23.7 (14.4–48.3)	0.01
Urine Na/K ratio	2.53 (0.22–25.6)	3.31 (0.35–25.6)	2.01 (0.22–5.13)	<0.01
Child-pugh score	10 (7–14)	10 (7–13)	10 (8–14)	0.23
Model for end-stage liver disease score	14 (7–31)	14 (7–31)	16 (8–31)	0.37

Notes. DCP; des-γ-carboxy prothrombin, BUN; blood urea nitrogen; eGFR, estimated glomerular filtration rate; Na/K; sodium/potassium.

Table 2. Laboratory data at initiation of tolvaptan treatment.

Parameter	Odds ratio	95% confidence interval	p-value
BUN/Cr ratio	1.08	1.006–1.174	<0.05
Urine Na/K ratio	0.59	0.366–0.855	<0.01
Serum K	1.41	0.537–3.893	n.s
Serum Na	0.96	0.854–1.080	n.s
Platelet count	0.95	0.839–1.051	n.s

Notes. Na/K, sodium/potassium; n.s, not significant.

Table 3. Multivariate analysis of parameters predicting a urination response to tolvaptan therapy.

		Urine Na/K ratio	
		<3.09 (*n*= 47)	≥3.09 (*n* = 30)
BUN/Cr ratio	<17.5 (*n* = 23)	10/12 (83.3%)	8/8 (100.0%)
	≥17.5 (*n* = 64)	13/33 (39.4%)	19/22 (86.3%)

Notes. BUN/Cr, blood urea nitrogen/creatinine; Na/K, sodium/potassium.

Table 4. Response to tolvaptan according to BUN/Cr and urine Na/K ratios.

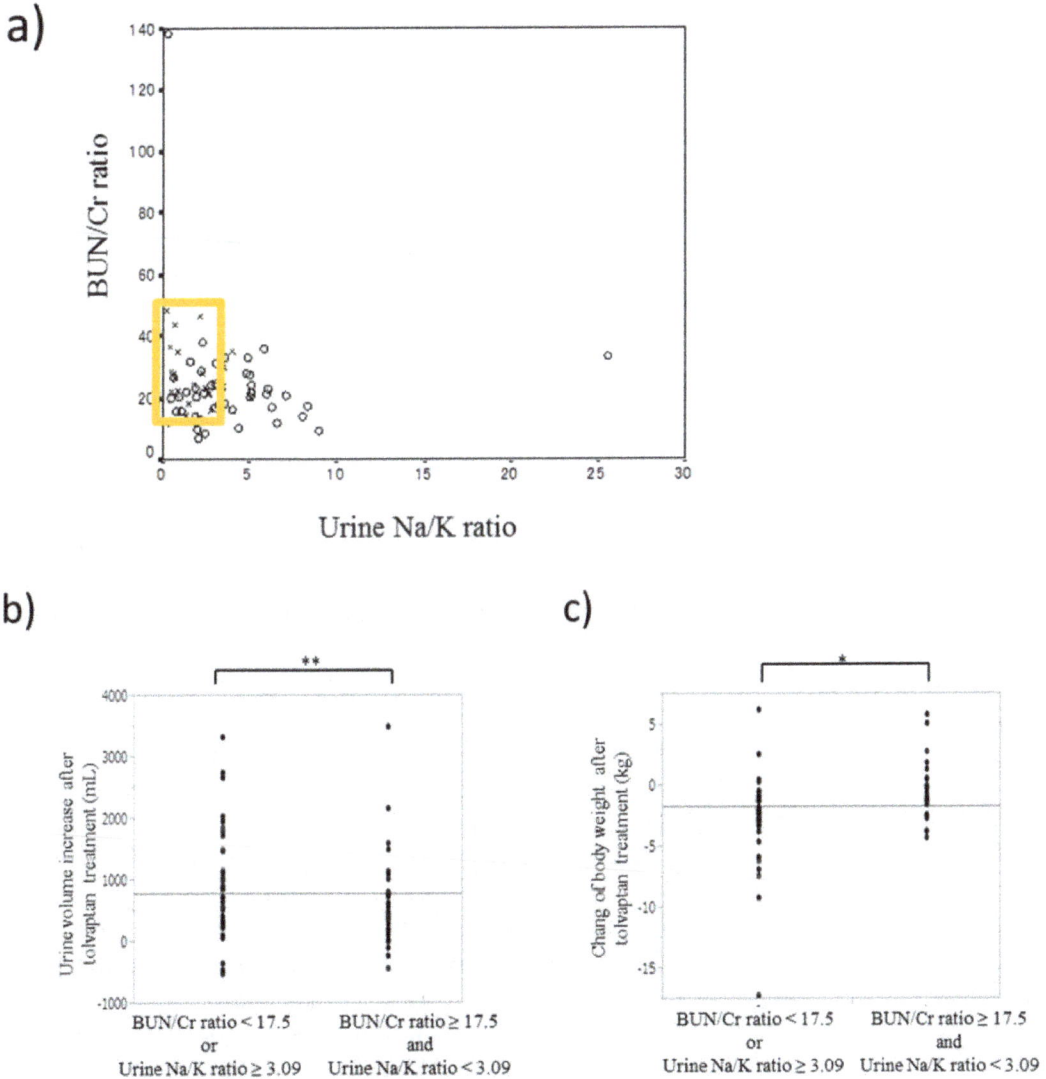

Figure 2. Distributions of the BUN/Cr ratio and urinary Na/K ratio and changes in urine volume and body weight. (a) Distributions of the BUN/Cr ratio and urinary Na/K ratio according to the tolvaptan response. Circle, responder, cross, nonresponder; framed square, BUN/Cr ratio ≥17.5, and urine Na/K ratio <3.09. Changes in (b) urine volume and (c) body weight in patients with and those without a BUN/Cr ratio ≥17.5 and urine Na/K ratio <3.09. Patients without a BUN/Cr ratio ≥17.5 and urine Na/K ratio <3.09 showed greater reductions in urine volume after 1 day (b) and in body weight after 1 week of treatment (c). BUN/Cr, blood urea nitrogen/creatinine; Na/K, sodium/potassium, *$p < 0.01$, **$p < 0.05$.

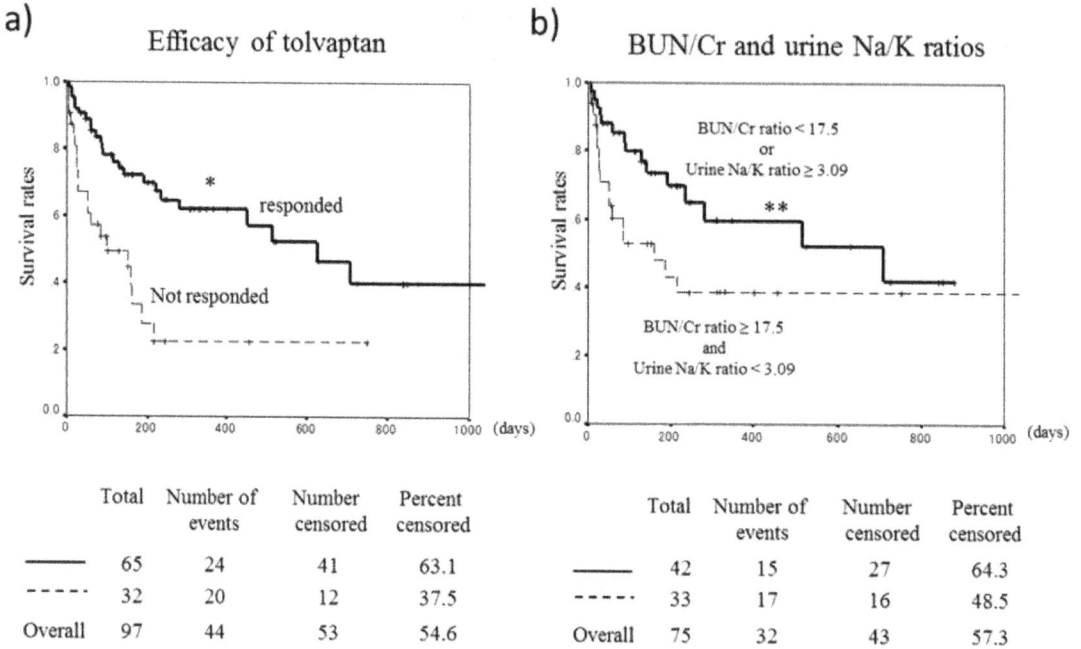

Figure 3. Survival rate of patients with and without a response to tolvaptan and the BUN/Cr and urine Na/K ratios. Patients who responded to tolvaptan therapy (a) and who did not have a BUN/Cr ratio ≥17.5 or urine Na/K ratio <3.09 (b) showed a significantly higher survival rate compared with nonresponders. BUN/Cr, blood urea nitrogen/creatinine; Na/K, sodium/potassium, *$p < 0.01$, **$p < 0.05$.

criteria of a BUN/Cr ratio <17.5 and urine Na/K ratio ≥3.09 achieved high tolvaptan response rates ($n = 8$, 100%; **Table 4**). In contrast, patients with a BUN/Cr ratio ≥17.5 and urine Na/K ratio <3.09 exhibited an extremely poor response (**Figure 2a**, framed area). In those patients who did not meet these criteria, urination and body weight reductions were observed (**Figure 2b** and **c**).

3.3. Prognosis after tolvaptan treatment

Regarding the mortality rate, 44 subjects died (45.4%). The survival rate was higher in patients who responded to tolvaptan therapy, as estimated by the Kaplan–Meier analysis (**Figure 3a**, $p < 0.01$). Patients with a BUN/Cr ratio <17.5 or urine Na/K ratio ≥3.09 showed a significantly higher survival rate than that of those who did not meet these criteria (**Figure 3b**, $p < 0.05$).

After 1 week of treatment, 70.1% of the patients achieved a normal serum Na level. These patients showed a significantly higher survival rate ($p < 0.05$). Among the patients with an initial Na level of <135 mEq/L ($n = 38$), 50.0% achieved a normal Na level after tolvaptan therapy and showed a significantly higher survival rate than that of patients without normalized Na levels ($p < 0.05$).

4. Discussion

The results suggest that the initial BUN/Cr and urine Na/K ratios and a normalized serum Na level after 1 week of treatment is predictive of a tolvaptan response in cirrhosis patients. The patients showing a response to tolvaptan in terms of increased urination or serum Na level had prolonged survival and a better prognosis.

Representative factors predicting a response to tolvaptan are shown in **Table 5**. Free water clearance [14], aquaporin-2/AVP [15], and urinary Na excretion [16] were reported to be predictors of a tolvaptan response in patients with cirrhosis. The combination of BUN/Cr and urine Na/K ratios was the first reported predictor of a tolvaptan response.

Regarding prognosis, tolvaptan reduced the rate of inhospital mortality [17] and evidenced longer mortality same as other diuretics in heart failure patients [18], although no study has assessed these parameters in cirrhotic patients. In our study, patients with a BUN/Cr <17.5 or urine Na/K ≥3.09 showed high response rates. Approximately 50.0% of tolvaptan-treated patients reached a normal serum Na level after 1 week of tolvaptan therapy. Patients who responded to tolvaptan exhibited prolonged survival compared with those who did not. Tolvaptan may improve the prognosis.

Tolvaptan has been reported to delay the onset of end-stage renal disease and to be associated with a low rate of renal function deterioration [19, 20]. Therefore, early initiation of tolvaptan is recommended to protect renal function and improve prognosis.

However, our study had limitations because hepatocellular carcinoma (HCC) affects the mortality rate of patients with cirrhosis. Therefore, HCC cases must be excluded from prognostic analyses.

Author	Journal	Year	Predictor	Disease
Imamura et al. [21]	Circ J.	2013	Urine osmolality and percentage decrease in urine osmolarity	Heart failure
Imamura et al. [22]	Circ J.	2014	Urine aquaporin-2 (AQP2)/plasma arginine vasopressin	Heart failure
Okayama et al. [23]	Am J Cardiovasc Drugs	2015	Blood urea nitrogen/creatinine (BUN/Cr) ratio	Heart failure
Shimizu et al. [24]	Nephrology (Carlton)	2015	Urine urea nitrogen/BUN ratio	Heart failure
Iwatani et al. [25]	Nephron	2015	Urine osmolarity	Chronic kidney disease
Miyaaki et al. [14]	Biomed Rep.	2015	Free water clearance	Liver cirrhosis
Nakanishi et al. [15]	J Gastroenterol.	2016	Urinary AQP2/Cr ratio	Liver cirrhosis
Chishina et al. [26]	Dig Dis.	2016	Serum BUN and serum Cr	Liver cirrhosis
Imamura et al. [27]	Int J Mol Sci.	2016	Urine AQP2	Heart failure
Kogiso et al. [13]	Hepatol Res.	2016	Serum BUN/Cr and urine sodium/potassium ratios	Liver cirrhosis

Table 5. Representative predictors of the response to tolvaptan therapy.

5. Conclusion

In addition to the combination of an initial BUN/Cr ratio <17.5 and urine Na/K ratio ≥3.09, a normalized serum Na level after 1 week of tolvaptan therapy was predictive of a favorable outcome in cirrhotic patients with hyponatremia and ascites treated with tolvaptan.

Author details

Tomomi Kogiso*, Kuniko Yamamoto, Mutsuki Kobayashi, Yuichi Ikarashi, Kazuhisa Kodama, Makiko Taniai, Nobuyuki Torii, Etsuko Hashimoto and Katsutoshi Tokushige

*Address all correspondence to: kogiso.ige@twmu.ac.jp

Department of Internal Medicine, Institute of Gastroenterology, Tokyo Women's, Medical University, Shinjuku-ku, Tokyo, Japan

References

[1] Ginés P, Quintero E, Arroyo V, Terés J, Bruguera M, Rimola A, Caballería J, Rodés J, Rozman C. Compensated cirrhosis: Natural history and prognostic factors. Hepatology. 1987;7:122-128

[2] Planas R, Montoliu S, Ballesté B, Rivera M, Miquel M, Masnou H, Galeras JA, Giménez MD, Santos J, Cirera I, Morillas RM, Coll S, Solà R. Natural history of patients hospitalized for management of cirrhotic ascites. Clinical Gastroenterology and Hepatology. 2006;4:1385-1394. DOI: 10.1016/j.cgh.2006.08.007

[3] Pérez-Ayuso RM, Arroyo V, Planas R, Gaya J, Bory F, Rimola A, Rivera F, Rodés J. Randomized comparative study of efficacy of furosemide versus spironolactone in nonazotemic cirrhosis with ascites. Relationship between the diuretic response and the activity of the renin-aldosterone system. Gastroenterology. 1983;84:961-968

[4] Sherlock S, Senewiratne B, Scott A, Walker JG. Complications of diuretic therapy in hepatic cirrhosis. Lancet. 1966;1:1049-1052

[5] Fukui H, Saito H, Ueno Y, Uto H, Obara K, Sakaida I, Shibuya A, Seike M, Nagoshi S, Segawa M, Tsubouchi H, Moriwaki H, Kato A, Hashimoto E, Michitaka K, Murawaki T, Sugano K, Watanabe M, Shimosegawa T. Evidence-based clinical practice guidelines for liver cirrhosis 2015. Journal of Gastroenterology. 2016;51:629-650. DOI: 10.1007/s00535-016-1216-y.

[6] Sakaida I, Nakajima K, Okita K, Hori M, Izumi T, Sakurai M, Shibasaki Y, Tachikawa S, Tsubouchi H, Oka H, Kobayashi H. Can serum albumin level affect the pharmacological action of tolvaptan in patients with liver cirrhosis? A post hoc analysis of previous clinical trials in Japan. Journal of Gastroenterology. 2015;50:1047-1053. DOI: 10.1007/s00535-015-1052-5.

[7] Schrier RW, Arroyo V, Bernardi M, Epstein M, Henriksen JH, Rodés J. Peripheral arterial vasodilation hypothesis: A proposal for the initiation of renal sodium and water retention in cirrhosis. Hepatology. 1988;8:1151-1157

[8] Grace JA, Herath CB, Mak KY, Burrell LM, Angus PW. Update on new aspects of the renin-angiotensin system in liver disease: Clinical implications and new therapeutic options. Clinical Science (London). 2012;123:225-239. DOI: 10.1042/CS20120030

[9] Okita K, Sakaida I, Okada M, Kaneko A, Chayama K, Kato M, Sata M, Yoshihara H, Ono N, Murawaki Y. A multicenter, open-label, dose-ranging study to exploratively evaluate the efficacy, safety, and dose-response of tolvaptan in patients with decompensated liver cirrhosis. Journal of Gastroenterology. 2010;45:979-987. DOI: 10.1007/s00535-010-0240-6

[10] Sakaida I, Yamashita S, Kobayashi T, Komatsu M, Sakai T, Komorizono Y, Okada M, Okita K; ASCITES 14-Day Administration Study Group. Efficacy and safety of a 14-day administration of tolvaptan in the treatment of patients with ascites in hepatic oedema. The Journal of International Medical Research. 2013;4:835-847. DOI: 10.1177/0300060513480089

[11] Kogiso T, Tokushige K, Hashimoto E, Ikarashi Y, Kodama K, Taniai M, Torii N, Shiratori K. Safety and efficacy of long-term tolvaptan therapy for decompensated liver cirrhosis. Hepatology Research. 2016,46.E194-E200. DOI: 10.1111/hepr.12547

[12] Ohki T, Sato K, Yamada T, Yamagami M, Ito D, Kawanishi K, Kojima K, Seki M, Toda N, Tagawa K. Efficacy of tolvaptan in patients with refractory ascites in a clinical setting. World Journal of Hepatology. 2015;7:1685-1693. DOI: 10.4254/wjh.v7.i12.1685

[13] Kogiso T, Yamamoto K, Kobayashi M, Ikarashi Y, Kodama K, Taniai M, Torii N, Hashimoto E, Tokushige K. Response to tolvaptan and its effect on prognosis in cirrhotic patients with ascites. Hepatology Research. 2016. In press. DOI: 10.1111/hepr.12822.

[14] Miyaaki H, Nakamura Y, Ichikawa T, Taura N, Miuma S, Shibata H, Honda T, Nakao K. Predictive value of the efficacy of tolvaptan in liver cirrhosis patients using free water clearance. Biomedical Reports. 2015;3:884-886. DOI: 10.3892/br.2015.521

[15] Nakanishi H, Kurosaki M, Hosokawa T, Takahashi Y, Itakura J, Suzuki S, Yasui Y, Tamaki N, Nakakuki N, Takada H, Higuchi M, Komiyama Y, Yoshida T, Takaura K, Hayashi T, Kuwabara K, Sasaki S, Izumi N. Urinary excretion of the water channel aquaporin 2 correlated with the pharmacological effect of tolvaptan in cirrhotic patients with ascites. Journal of Gastroenterology. 2016;51:620-627. DOI: 10.1007/s00535-015-1143-3

[16] Uojima H, Kinbara T, Hidaka H, Sung JH, Ichida M, Tokoro S, Masuda S, Takizawa S, Sasaki A, Koizumi K, Egashira H, Kako M. Close correlation between urinary sodium excretion and response to tolvaptan in liver cirrhosis patients with ascites. Hepatology Research. 2017;47:E14-E21. DOI: 10.1111/hepr.12716

[17] Yoshioka K, Matsue Y, Kagiyama N, Yoshida K, Kume T, Okura H, Suzuki M, Matsumura A, Yoshida K, Hashimoto Y. Recovery from hyponatremia in acute phase is associated with better in-hospital mortality rate in acute heart failure syndrome. Journal of Cardiology. 2016;67:406-411. DOI: 10.1016/j.jjcc.2015.12.004

[18] Suzuki S, Yoshihisa A, Yamaki T, Sugimoto K, Kunii H, Nakazato K, Abe Y, Saito T, Ohwada T, Suzuki H, Saitoh S, Kubota I, Takeishi Y. Long-term effects and prognosis in acute heart failure treated with tolvaptan: The AVCMA trial. BioMed Research International. 2014;**2014**:704289. DOI: 10.1155/2014/704289

[19] Kimura K, Momose T, Hasegawa T, Morita T, Misawa T, Motoki H, Izawa A, Ikeda U. Early administration of tolvaptan preserves renal function in elderly patients with acute decompensated heart failure. Journal of Cardiology. 2016;**67**:399-405. DOI: 10.1016/j.jjcc.2015.09.020

[20] Mori T, Ohsaki Y, Oba-Yabana I, Ito S. Diuretic usage for protection against end-organ damage in liver cirrhosis and heart failure. Hepatology Research. 2017;**47**:11-22. DOI: 10.1111/hepr.12700

[21] Imamura T, Kinugawa K, Minatsuki S, Muraoka H, Kato N, Inaba T, Maki H, Shiga T, Hatano M, Yao A, Kyo S, Komuro I. Urine osmolality estimated using urine urea nitrogen, sodium and creatinine can effectively predict response to tolvaptan in decompensated heart failure patients. Circulation Journal. 2013;**77**:1208-1213

[22] Imamura T, Kinugawa K, Fujino T, Inaba T, Maki H, Hatano M, Yao A, Komuro I. Increased urine aquaporin-2 relative to plasma arginine vasopressin is a novel marker of response to tolvaptan in patients with decompensated heart failure. Circulation Journal. 2014;**78**:2240-2249

[23] Okayama D, Suzuki T, Shiga T, Minami Y, Tsuruoka S, Hagiwara N. Blood urea nitrogen/creatinine ratio and response to tolvaptan in patients with decompensated heart failure: A retrospective analysis. American Journal of Cardiovascular Drugs. 2015;**15**:289-293. DOI: 10.1007/s40256-015-0121-8

[24] Shimizu K, Doi K, Imamura T, Noiri E, Yahagi N, Nangaku M, Kinugawa K. Ratio of urine and blood urea nitrogen concentration predicts the response of tolvaptan in congestive heart failure. Nephrology (Carlton). 2015;**20**:405-412

[25] Iwatani H, Kawabata H, Sakaguchi Y, Yamamoto R, Hamano T, Rakugi H, Isaka Y. Urine osmolarity predicts the body weight-reduction response to tolvaptan in chronic kidney disease patients: A retrospective, observational study. Nephron. 2015;**130**:8-12. DOI: 10.1159/000381859

[26] Chishina H, Hagiwara S, Nishida N, Ueshima K, Sakurai T, Ida H, Minami Y, Takita M, Kono M, Minami T, Iwanishi M, Umehara Y, Watanabe T, Komeda Y, Arizumi T, Kudo M. Clinical factors predicting the effect of tolvaptan for refractory ascites in patients with decompensated liver cirrhosis. Digestive Diseases and Sciences. 2016;**34**:659-664. DOI: 10.1159/000448828

[27] Imamura T, Kinugawa K. Urine aquaporin-2: A promising marker of response to the arginine vasopressin type-2 antagonist, tolvaptan in patients with congestive heart failure. International Journal of Molecular Sciences. 2016;**17**(105):1-7. DOI: 10.3390/ijms17010105

3

Correlation Between Transthoracic Contrast-Enhanced Ultrasound and Pulse Oximetry in Hepatopulmonary Syndrome Diagnosis

Andra-Iulia Suceveanu, Adrian-Paul Suceveanu,
Irinel-Raluca Parepa, Felix Voinea and Laura Mazilu

Abstract

The prevalence of hepatopulmonary syndrome (HPS) in the setting of cirrhosis ranges between 4 and 47% and its presence increases the mortality rate, especially when hypoxemia is present. Our study aim was to fix whether there is a correlation of results between two simple and non-invasive procedures such as transthoracic contrast-enhanced ultrasound (CEUS) and pulse oximetry, used for early detection of HPS in patients with liver cirrhosis, having as endpoint the improvement in their outcome. The rapid lung enhancement and delayed left ventricle enhancement of the saline solution, after at least three systolic beats during CEUS and pulse oximetry showing a $SaO_2 < 95\%$, were correlated and considered positive for the diagnosis of HPS. One hundred and sixty-five (44%) of the total of 375 patients diagnosed with liver cirrhosis enrolled in the current study, with or without respiratory symptoms (dyspnea, clubbing, distal cyanosis, cough and/or spider angioma), showed positive criteria for HPS diagnosis during CEUS. $SaO_2 < 95\%$ and $PaO_2 < 70$ mmHg were found in 123 patients (33%) during pulse oximetry investigation. Pearson correlation index showed a good correlation between lung and heart CEUS findings and pulse oximetry ($r = 0.97$) for HPS diagnosis. CEUS and pulse oximetry results correlate and rapidly diagnose HPS, a highly fatal complication of liver cirrhosis (LC), guiding the future treatment by speeding up orthotopic liver transplant OLT recommendations to improve the survival rates.

Keywords: transthoracic contrast-enhanced ultrasonography, pulse oximetry, liver cirrhosis, hepatopulmonary syndrome, hypoxemia

1. Introduction

The hepatopulmonary syndrome (HPS) represents a complication of liver cirrhosis character-ized by a gross dilatation of the pulmonary precapillary and capillary vessels, an increase in the number of dilated vessels, portopulmonary anastomoses, pleural and pulmonary arterio-venous shunts. It can be diagnosed when the triad represented by liver disease, impaired oxy-genation and intrapulmonary vascular abnormalities, referred to as intrapulmonary vascular dilatations (IPVDs) coexist [1]. The prevalence of pulmonary complications associated with liver cirrhosis ranges between 4 and 47%, worsening the evolution and prognosis, especially when hypoxemia is present [2, 3]. According to the medical literature focused on the current topic, 23% of patients with HPS have an average survival rate around 24 months, compared to 63% of patients without HPS. Survival can be further worsened in case of comorbidities or advanced age [4]. Respiratory signs and symptoms are common in patients with liver cir-rhosis, no matter the stage of the disease. Intrapulmonary vascular complications of liver cir-rhosis consist of hepatopulmonary syndrome (HPS) and portopulmonary hypertension. HPS appears when intrapulmonary blood shunting impairs arterial gas exchange [5], and por-topulmonary hypertension occurs when pulmonary arterial constriction leads to increased pulmonary arterial pressure [6]. The latter, although rare, can cause pulmonary complication, which worsens the morbidity and mortality in patients with liver dysfunction. The outcome of patients with advanced liver disease, complicated with pulmonary involvement, can be influ-enced even in the setting of orthotopic liver transplant, due to chronic hypoxemia installed during the evolution of cirrhosis influencing the prognosis. A key factor in the diagnosis of HPS is the exclusion of causes other than HPS that may be involved in cirrhosis and charac-terized by hypoxemia (cardiopulmonary abnormalities, pulmonary atelectasis, pneumonia, ascites, pulmonary edema or hepatic hydrothorax) [7]. The challenge for physicians working in the field of hepatology is to raise the idea of establishing new methods for a conventional, rapid and simple diagnosis of pulmonary involvement during the evolution of liver cirrhosis, in order to improve as much as possible the outcome of possible curative treatment.

HPS is defined by a widened alveolar-arterial oxygen gradient (age corrected) in room air, with or without hypoxemia. It results from intrapulmonary vascular dilatations in the pres-ence of hepatic dysfunction and/or portal hypertension [8, 9].

The development of pulmonary vascular dilatation has as pathogenic mechanism a pulmo-nary overproduction of endogenous nitric oxide (NO) [10]. According to studies focused on the topic in the last two decades, a theory can be formulated according to which endothelin-1 and tumor necrosis factor-α may play a role in pulmonary microvascular tone modulation [11, 12]. The contributing factors to the process of pulmonary microvascular dilatation in HPS include angiogenesis, vascular remodeling, pulmonary arteriovenous shunts and portopul-monary venous anastomoses [13, 14].

Trough this pathogenic mechanism, the rapid or direct passage of mixed venous blood into the pulmonary veins is responsible for the pulmonary vascular dilatation. The mismatch of ventilation-perfusion sequence produces a deficit in the blood oxygenation. The inhibition of hypoxic vasoconstriction produces an increased blood flow and preserved alveolar ventilation.

The alveolar-arterial oxygen tension difference—≥15, or ≥20 mmHg for patients aged >64 is considered as a very sensitive index of early arterial deoxygenation in HPS, and this difference being overload before arterial oxygen tension becomes abnormally low [8]. On the other hand, the alveolar-capillary interface is too wide to allow for complete equilibration of carbon monoxide with hemoglobin, thus being translated in reducing the diffusing capacity of the lungs for carbon monoxide.

Patients complain of symptoms correlated not only with the subsequent liver disease, but also with the respiratory signs and symptoms, usually revealing dyspnea and cyanosis. The management of these patients requires the exclusion of other causes for such respiratory symptoms, because chronic obstructive pulmonary disease and pulmonary fibrosis can coexist in approximately 30% of patients with HPS [15]. Dyspnea ("platypnea") and hypoxemia ("orthodeoxia") are characteristically worsened in the upright position and improved by lying supine, resulting from a gravitational increase in blood flow through dilated vessels in the lung bases [16].

According to the pathogenic definition, the diagnosis of HPS requires evidence of pulmonary vascular dilatation and hypoxemia, with no cardiopulmonary disease history. To stage the severity of the disease, it is required to investigate the arterial blood gas tension at rest, while breathing room air and in the sitting position. A sensitive and non-invasive tool for the detection of pulmonary vascular dilatation is the contrast-enhanced transthoracic echocardiography after injection of hand-agitated normal saline. During the first pass, microbubbles are physiologically trapped and absorbed by alveoli, and they should not be seen in the left atrium. The passage of saline microbubbles through abnormally dilated lung vessels requires more than three cardiac cycles to reach left heart chambers [17]. In contrast, the immediate enhancement of saline microbubbles in the left atrium raises the suspicion of an intracardiac right-to-left shunt [18]. The alternative to CEUS investigation is scintigraphic perfusion scanning, which uses the technetium-99-labeled albumin macroaggregates >20 μm in diameter. The uptake of tc-99-labeled albumin macroaggregated in other organs occurs in case of right-to-left shunt, while the trapping of albumin macroaggregates in pulmonary circulation is characteristic for HPS [19].

The present management of HPS lacks of efficient therapy solutions, until the OLT is available. Starting from the pathogenic mechanism, physicians investigated several classes of drugs such as β-blockers, cyclo-oxygenase inhibitors, systemic corticosteroids, cyclophosphamide, inhaled NO, and NO inhibitors, but without a real benefit in oxygenation improvement or pulmonary vascular dilatation. The only efficient treatment in case of severe and refractory hypoxemia is the oxygen supplementation, with complete resolution in more than 80%, according to study results [8, 20]. The presence of HPS offers exception points in MELD scoring and an advantage for patients to occupy better places on waiting lists for OLT [21]. Without OLT, the prognosis for HPS is poor, with mortality around 41% of patients over a mean period of 2.5 years [22]. The literature data do not provide reliable clinical predictors or diagnosis guidelines for the outcome of HPS [23].

A retrospective cohort analysis of data submitted to the United Network for Organ Sharing studied the effects of room-air oxygenation of patients with HPS and the pre- and post-transplantation outcomes. Patients with HPS were given MELD exception points and prioritized for liver transplantation due to their high pre- and post-transplantation mortality. Comparing the overall survival rates of patients with and without HPS, transplant recipients with more severe hypoxemia had increased risk of death after liver transplantation. The overall mortality was significantly lower among waitlist candidates with HPS (hazard ratio = 0.82; 95% CI: 0.70–0.96), having the OLT before the deterioration of tissue oxygenation and liver dysfunction, due to exception MELD points given, which provided an advantage for a rapid transplant [24].

The aim of our study was a possible correlation between contrast-enhanced ultrasound (CEUS) findings on heart and pulse oximetry, in order to early detect HPS, as a prognostic factor for orthotopic liver transplant (OLT) success [25].

2. Methods

Demographic data, etiology and severity scores were recorded. For the diagnosis of HPS, we used the classical triad: presence of chronic liver disease, an increased alveolar-arterial oxygen gradient, and evidence of right-to-left intrapulmonary shunt (IPS) [26]. In order to determine the HPS diagnosis, we used the classical charts provided by the guidelines for transplant candidates (**Table 1**). The diagnosis of liver cirrhosis was based on clinical, biochemical, ultrasound, and upper endoscopy criteria. The patients with liver cirrhosis were classified according to MELD scores, considering exception points according to international recommendations. The contrast-enhanced echocardiography (CEUS) [27], technetium-99m-labeled macroaggregated albumin (Tc-99m MAA) scanning [28], and pulmonary arteriography are the current imagistic tools to diagnose the IPS. We correlated transthoracic CEUS findings with pulse oxymetry as a screening test for detecting IPS in 375 patients diagnosed with liver cirrhosis between December 2009 and June 2016 in Gastroenterology Department of Clinical Emergency Hospital "St Apostle Andrew" of Constanta County.

Criteria	Data requirements
Strict HPS criteria	Alveolar-arterial gradient ≥15 mmHg, or ≥20 mmHg if age older than 60 years
	Intrapulmonary shunting on transthoracic echocardiogram or >6% shunt fraction on macroaggregated albumin scan
	No evidence of severe restrictive or obstructive pulmonary disease
Hypoxia/hypoxemia+ IP shunts	Hypoxemia defined as: • PaO_2 <70 mmHg on room air or • Pulse oximetry ≤96% (room air or supplemental O_2)
	Intrapulmonary shunting (right → left bubbles on echocardiogram after three cardiac cycles and/or free text stating "intrapulmonary shunting")
	No evidence of concurrent cardiopulmonary disease

Table 1. Inclusion criteria defining OLT waitlist candidates with HPS based on exception narrative data [28].

All patients were examined by chest X-ray and pulmonary function tests (to rule out common intrinsic pulmonary disorders such as chronic obstructive pulmonary disease). We used as a contrast agent of hand-agitated saline solution, in order to produce microbubbles with a mean diameter of up to 10 μm injected through a peripheral vein. Unlike blood, microbubbles resonate at a frequency similar to clinical transducer frequencies, which make ultrasounds to be reflected. Under normal circumstances, only the right heart chambers are opacified, and the microbubbles are trapped in the pulmonary capillaries (mean diameter, 8 μm). The presence of contrast in the left chamber suggests an arteriovenous connection. In patients with intracardiac shunts, a small amount of contrast is usually recorded in the left chambers within 1 or 2 cardiac cycles after its appearance in the right-side chambers (early shunt). On the contrary, late arrival of contrast in the left atrium after a time delay of 4–8 cardiac cycles is diagnostic for HPS (delayed shunt) and is done by the time required for passage through the pulmonary circulation [27]. Measurement of SaO_2 was performed with a portable pulse oximeter. In all patients, the measurements were performed at ambient O_2 partial pressure in supine position. We have chosen a SaO_2 value of <95% in order to detect all HPS patients with a $PaO_2 < 70$. The correlation of rapid lung enhancement and delayed left ventricle enhancement of the saline solution, after at least three systolic beats in the left ventricle during CEUS and pulse oximetry showing a $SaO_2 < 95\%$ was considered positive for the diagnosis of HPS [29].

3. Results

A total of 375 patients diagnosed with liver cirrhosis were enrolled in our study. The majority of patients were male (251/375). The average age was 66.04 years (SD 8.81). The etiology of liver cirrhosis was alcohol abuse in 39% (146/375) of patients, viral hepatitis B (VHB) in 28% (105/375) of patients, viral hepatitis C (VHC) in 21% (79/375) of patients, and the rest of 12% (45/375) having uncommon etiologies. Severity in MELD score divided our patients in three groups according to which we could fix the prognosis and the need of transplantation (**Table 2**).

According to present international recommendations, we decided upon exception points for those patients meeting the criteria for MELD exception: patients with $PaO_2 < 60$ mmHg on room air at rest in the sitting position, arterial blood gas result provided, patients with pulmonary vascular dilatation documented by a positive transthoracic contrast echocardiography, patients with absence of significant alternative pulmonary disease to explain severe hypoxemia (chest X-ray, pulmonary function tests, and chest computed tomography reports), patients with moderate or severe pulmonary function tests changes or significant chest X-ray abnormalities or MAA scan positive for intrapulmonary shunting) (**Table 3**). From the total of 375 patients studied, 165 (44%) presented respiratory symptoms. Pulse oximetry showed alterations, such as $SaO_2 < 95\%$ and $PaO_2 < 70$ mmHg in 123 patients (33%). From 375 patients diagnosed with LC, with or without present respiratory signs and/or symptoms (dyspnea, clubbing, distal cyanosis, cough and/or spider angioma) referred to CEUS examination, 105 (28%) had rapid lung enhancement and delayed left ventricle enhancement of the contrast agent (**Figures 1–3**). PaO_2 was less than 70 mmHg in all 105 HPS patients (100%) versus 12 (14.76%) of non-HPS patients ($P < 0.0001$). Pearson correlation index showed a good correlation between lung and heart CEUS findings and pulse oximetry ($r = 0.97$) in HPS diagnosis.

Variable	HPS (no, %)	Non-HPS (no, %)
Mean age (IQR)	66.04 ± 8.81 (95% CI, 58.44–74.85)	63.10 ± 10.71 (95% CI, 61.55–64.65)
Gender		
Males	128 (50.99)	123 (49.00)
Females	59 (47.58)	65 (52.41)
Race		
Caucasians	92 (87.61)	243 (90)
Blacks	2 (1.90)	1 (0.37)
Asians	11 (10.47)	26 (09.62)
Ethnicity		
Romanian	51 (48.57)	173 (64.07)
Turcs/tatars	8 (7.61)	19 (7.03)
Moldavians	4 (3.80)	9 (3.33)
Macedonians	31 (29.52)	42 (15.55)
Other	11 (10.47)	27 (10)
Primary diagnosis		
HCV	27 (25.71)	52 (19.25)
HBV	31 (29.52)	74 (27.40)
Alcohol	39 (37.14)	106 (39.25)
HVD	5 (4.76)	18 (6.66)
Autoimmune	2 (1.90)	4 (1.48)
NASH/criptogenetic	1 (0.95)	9 (3.33)
Other rare causes	–	5 (1.85)
MELD score, median (IQR)	14 (11–22)	16 (11–24)
MELD score categories		
<15	47 (44.76)	156 (57.77)
15–20	34 (32.38)	76 (28.14)
>20	14 (13.33)	38 (14.07)
MELD exceptions		
PaO_2 < 60 mmHG (22 pts)	5 (4.76)	–
PaO_2 = 51–55 mmHG (24 pts)	4 (3.80)	–
PaO_2 < 50 mmHG (26 pts)	1 (00.95	–
History of ascites	84 (80.00)	229 (84.81)
History of liver decompensations	74 (70.47)	172 (63.70)

Table 2. Baseline clinical and demographic characteristics of HPS and non-HPS patients.

PaO$_2$	Exception points for MELD scoring for HPS
56–59 mmHg	22 MELD points
51–55 mmHg	24 MELD points
<50 mmHg	26 MELD points

Table 3. Allocation of exception points for HPS in MELD scoring system [28].

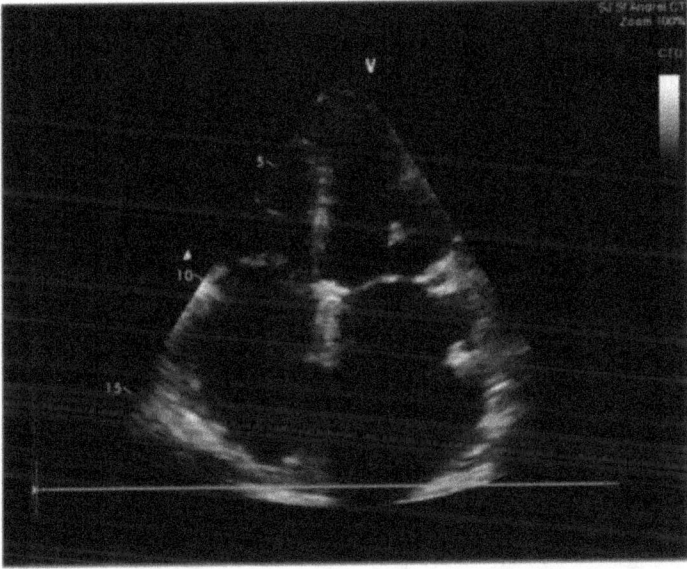

Figure 1. Contrast-enhanced echocardiogram. Apical four-chamber view before contrast injection.

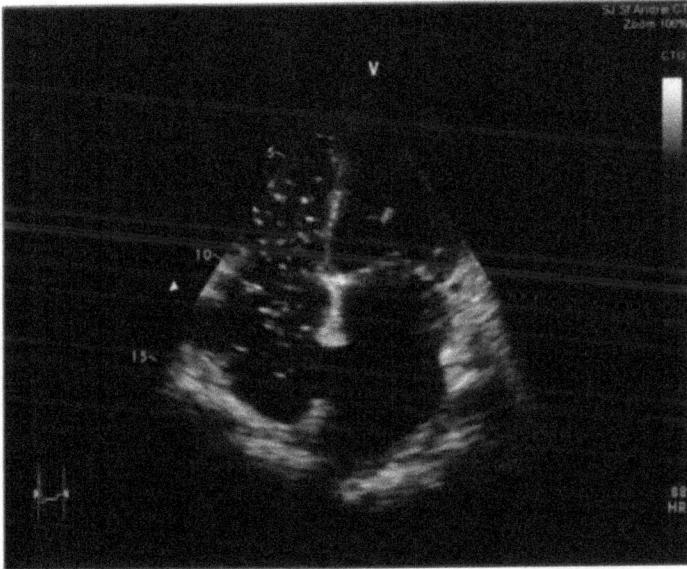

Figure 2. Contrast-enhanced echocardiogram. Apical four-chamber view after contrast injection (agitated saline) showing the presence of bubbles in the right chambers and no bubbles in the left chambers after the first sistola.

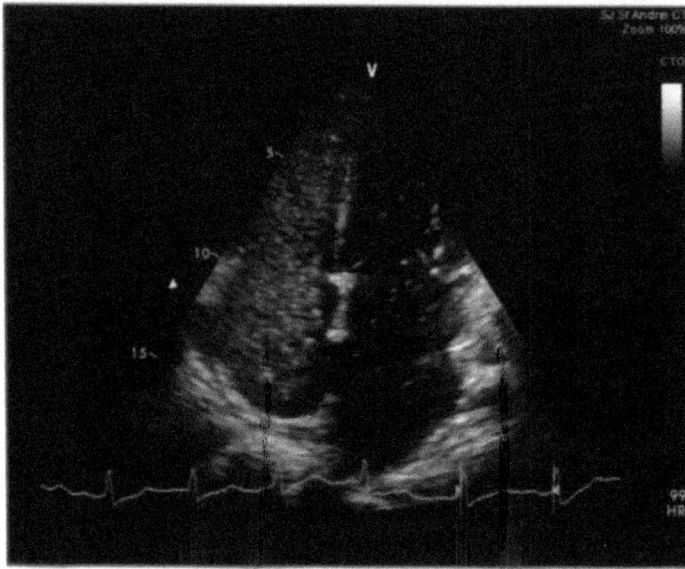

Figure 3. Contrast-enhanced echocardiogram. Apical four-chamber view after contrast injection (agitated saline) showing the presence of bubbles in the right heart chambers and the appearance of bubbles in the left heart chambers, late, after the forth sistola.

4. Discussion

HPS was defined as a triad of portal hypertension with or without hepatic dysfunction, intra-pulmonary vascular dilatation or shunting, and hypoxemia [30]. Hypoxemia was defined by PaO_2 cutoff level of less than 70 mmHg in an arterial blood sample to pick up these patients for further evaluation by CEUS. This arterial PO_2 cutoff level was suggested by previous researchers [31], who found that patients with PaO_2 of more than 70 mmHg were unlikely to have HPS.

In the current study, among 375 patients diagnosed with liver cirrhosis, 105 patients (28%) met the clinical, laboratory and imagistic criteria of HPS. HPS shows a wide variability in prevalence in different studies, ranging from 4 to 47% among cirrhotic patients [1, 4, 32], depending on the diagnostic criteria and the cutoff levels used for hypoxia. In our study, PaO_2 was less than 70 mmHg in 100% of HPS patients versus 12% of non-HPS patients, in which pulmonary function tests were used to diagnose chronic intrinsic pulmonary disease. All patients with positive CEUS findings had arterial PaO_2<70 mmHg and were qualified for the diagnosis of HPS. CEUS was proved by previous investigators to be a useful sensitive and specific screening test for HPS even in early stages of liver dysfunction and even in whom the lung scintigraphy was still negative [33]. Some authors suggested transesophageal CEUS as a gold standard [34, 35]. However, others argued that transthoracic CEUS has the same accuracy as transesophageal CEUS in determining the presence of right to left shunt. Proper timing of left atrial opacification by microbubbles during the cardiac cycle was considered a distinguishing step in the transthoracic CEUS between intracardiac and intrapulmonary shunting [36]. Transesophageal CEUS might have higher sensitivity than transthoracic CEUS because it allows the contrast to be seen when entering from the pulmonary veins [37, 38]. However, transthoracic CEUS is diagnostic in the majority of cases. In addition, esophageal varices are relatively common in these patients, and this can be considered as a relative contraindication in transesophageal CEUS performing [29, 39].

According to their correlated results, the transthoracic CEUS and pulse oximetry could be inserted in the algorithm of liver cirrhosis staging, in order to select those patients in need for a more rapid indication of OLT. Both methods provide data regarding the pulmonary dysfunction during liver cirrhosis evolution, improving the outcome after OLT, especially in HPS patients with moderate or severe hypoxemia. The presymptomatic stage of HPS can be correctly diagnosed using the combination of these two methods, making the algorithm of liver cirrhosis staging more accurate.

5. Conclusion

Our study showed a good correlation between lung and heart CEUS findings and pulse oximetry in HPS diagnosis. When correlated, these two simple, non-invasive, low-cost and rapid methods can easily diagnose HPS, a highly fatal complication of liver cirrhosis, which can worsen the outcome of patients even after OLT.

Acknowledgements

This work was accomplished with the support of Dr. Razvan Maxim, for transthoracic enhanced ultrasonography images caption, and Dr. Phillipos Manousos Goniotakis, for the English linguistic assistance.

Author details

Andra-Iulia Suceveanu[1]*, Adrian-Paul Suceveanu[1], Irinel-Raluca Parepa[3], Felix Voinea[4] and Laura Mazilu[2]

*Address all correspondence to: andrasuceveanu@yahoo.com

1 Faculty of Medicine, Department of Gastroenterology, Emergency Hospital of Constanta, Ovidius University, Constanta, Romania

2 Faculty of Medicine, Department of Internal Medicine, Emergency Hospital of Constanta, Ovidius University, Constanta, Romania

3 Faculty of Medicine, Department of Cardiology, Emergency Hospital of Constanta, Ovidius University, Constanta, Romania

4 Faculty of Medicine, Department of Surgery, Emergency Hospital of Constanta, Ovidius University, Constanta, Romania

References

[1]   Hoeper MM, Krowka MJ, Strassburg CP. Portopulmonary hypertension and hepatopul-
      monary syndrome. Lancet. 2004;**363**:1461

[2]   Martinez G, et al. Hepatopulmonary Syndrome in candidates for liver transplantation.
      Journal of Hepatology. 2001;**34**:756-758

[3]   Schenk P, et al. Hepatopulmonary syndrome: Prevalence and predictive value of various
      cut Fallon M, Abrams G. Pulmonary dysfunction in chronic liver disease. Hepatology.
      2000;**32**:859-865

[4]   Rodríguez-Roisin R, Krowka MJ. Hepatopulmonary syndrome—a liver-induced lung
      vascular disorder. The New England Journal of Medicine. 2008;**358**:2378

[5]   Fallon M, Abrams G. Pulmonary dysfunction in chronic liver disease. Hepatology.
      2000;**32**:859-865

[6]   Budhiraja R, Hassoun PM. Portopulmonary hypertension: A tale of two circulations.
      Chest. 2003;**123**:562-576

[7]   Varghese J, Ilian H, Dhanasekaran R, Singh S, Venkataraman J. Hepatopulmonary syn-
      drome—Past to present. Annals of Hepatology. 2007;**6**(3):135-142

[8]   Rodríguez-Roisin R, Krowka MJ, Hervé P, Fallon MB; ERS Task Force Pulmonary-
      Hepatic Vascular Disorders (PHD) Scientific Committee. Pulmonary-hepatic vascular
      disorders (PHD). European Respiratory Society. 2004;**24**:861-880

[9]   Zhang J, et al. Pulmonary angiogenesis in a rat model of hepatopulmonary syndrome.
      Gastroenterology. 2009;**136**:1070-1080

[10] Cremona G, Higenbottam TW, Mayoral V, et al. Elevated exhaled nitric oxide in patients
      with hepatopulmonary syndrome. European Respiratory Society. 1995;**8**:1883-1885

[11] Rabiller A, Nunes H, Lebrec D, et al. Prevention of gramnegative translocation reduces
      the severity of hepatopulmonary syndrome. American Journal of Respiratory and
      Critical Care Medicine. 2002;**166**:514-517

[12] Zhang M, Luo B, Chen SJ, Abrams GA, Fallon MB. Endothelin-1 stimulation of endothe-
      lial nitric oxide synthase in the pathogenesis of hepatopulmonary syndrome. American
      Journal of Physiology. 1999;**277**:944-952

[13] Berthelot P, Walker JG, Sherlock S, Reid L. Arterial changes in the lungs in cirrhosis of
      the liver-lung spider nevi. The New England Journal of Medicine. 1966;**274**:291-298

[14] Gómez FP, Barberà JA, Roca J, Burgos F, Gistau C, Rodríguez-Roisin R. Effects of neb-
      ulized N^G-nitro-L-arginine methyl ester in patients with hepatopulmonary syndrome.
      Hepatology. 2006;**43**:1084-1091

[15] Martínez GP, Barberà JA, Visa J, Rodriguez-Roisin R. Hepatopulmonary syndrome asso-
      ciated with cardiorespiratory disease. Journal of Hepatology. 1999;**30**:882-889

[16] Gómez FP, Martínez-Pallí G, Barberà JA, Roca J, Navasa M, Rodríguez-Roisin R. Gas exchange mechanism of orthodeoxia in hepatopulmonary syndrome. Hepatology. 2004;**40**:660-666

[17] Krowka MJ, Tajik AJ, Dickson ER, Wiesner RH, Cortese DA. Intrapulmonary vascular dilatations (IPVD) in liver transplant candidates: Screening by two-dimensional contrastenhanced echocardiography. Chest. 1990;**97**:1165-1170

[18] Raffy O, Sleiman C, Vachiery F, et al. Refractory hypoxemia during liver cirrhosis. Hepatopulmonary syndrome or "primary" pulmonary hypertension? American Journal of Respiratory and Critical Care Medicine. 1996;**153**:1169-1171

[19] Krowka MJ, Wiseman GA, Burnett OL, et al. Hepatopulmonary syndrome: A prospective study of relationships between severity of liver disease, PaO(2) response to 100% oxygen, and brain uptake after (99m)Tc MAA lung scanning. Chest. 2000;**118**:615-624

[20] Collisson EA, Nourmand H, Fraiman MH, et al. Retrospective analysis of the results of liver transplantation for adults with severe hepatopulmonary syndrome. Liver Transplantation. 2002;**8**:925-931

[21] Fallon MB, Mulligan DC, Gish RG, et al. Model for end-stage liver disease (MELD) exception for hepatopulmonary syndrome. Liver Transplantation. 2006;**12**(Suppl.):S105-S107

[22] Krowka MJ, Dickson ER, Cortese DA. Hepatopulmonary syndrome: Clinical observations and lack of therapeutic response to somatostatin analogue. Chest. 1993;**104**:515 521

[23] Sanyal AJ, Kowdley K, Vargas HE. Hepatopulmonary Syndrome, in: Keeping the Patient with End-stage Cirrhosis Alive. AASLD Postgraduate Course. 2009;134-141

[24] Goldberg DS, Krok K, Batra S, Trotter JF, Kawut SM, Fallon MB. Impact of the hepatopulmonary syndrome MELD exception policy on outcomes of patients after liver transplantation: An analysis of the UNOS database. Gastroenterology. 2014;**146**(5):1256-1265.e1

[25] Arguedas M, Abrams GA, Krowka MJ, Fallon MB. Prospective evaluation of outcomes and predictors of mortality in patients with HPS undergoing liver transplantation. Hepatology. 2003;**37**:192-197

[26] Rollán MJ, Muñoz AC, Pérez T, Bratos JL. Value of contrast echocardiography for the diagnosis of hepatopulmonary syndrome. European Journal of Echocardiography. 2007;**8**(5):408-410

[27] Gudavalli A, Kalaria VG, Chen X, Schwarz KQ. Intrapulmonary arteriovenous shunt: Diagnosis by saline contrast bubbles in the pulmonary veins. Journal of the American Society of Echocardiography. 2002;**15**:1012-1014

[28] Abrams GA, Nanda NC, Dubovsky EV, Krowka MJ, Fallon MB. Use of macroaggregated albumin lung perfusion scan to diagnose hepatopulmonary syndrome: A new approach. Gastroenterology. 1998;**114**:305-310

[29] Suceveanu AI, Mazilu L, Tomescu D, Ciufu N, Parepa IR, Suceveanu AP. Screening of hepatopulmonary syndrome (HPS) with CEUS and pulseoximetry in liver cirrhosis patients eligible for liver transplant. Chirurgia. 2013;**108**:684-688

[30] Krowka MJ. Hepatopulmonary syndrome and portopulmonary hypertension: Implications for liver transplantation. Clinics in Chest Medicine. 2005;**26**(4):587-597

[31] Hira HS, Kumar J, Tyagi SK, Jain SK. A study of hepatopulmonary syndrome among patients of cirrhosis of liver and portal hypertension. Indian Journal of Chest Diseases and Allied Sciences. 2003;**45**(3):165-171

[32] Colle I, Van Steenkiste C, Geerts A, Van Vlierberghe H. Hepatopulmonary syndrome and portopulmonary hypertension: What's new? Acta Gastro-Enterologica Belgica. 2007;**70**(2):203-209

[33] Wang YW, Lin HC. Recent advances in HPS. Journal of the Chinese Medical Association. 2005;**68**(11):500-505

[34] Clarke NR, Timperley J, Kelion AD, Banning AP. Transthoracic echocardiography using second harmonic imaging with Valsalva manoeuvre for the detection of right to left shunts. European Journal of Echocardiography. 2004;**5**(3):176-181

[35] Frazin LJ. Patent foramen ovale or pulmonary arteriovenous malformation: An appeal for diagnostic accuracy. Chest. 2007;**132**(1):5-6

[36] Viles-Gonzalez JF, Rodriguez-Roisin R. The hepatopulmonary syndrome, correspondence. The New England Journal of Medicine. 2008;**359**:866-867

[37] Vedrinne JM, Duperret S, Bizollon T, Magnin C, Motin J, Trepo C, et al. Comparison of transesophageal and transthoracic contrast echocardiography for detection of an intrapulmonary shunt in liver disease. Chest. 1997;**111**:1236-1240

[38] Nemec JJ, Davison MB, Marwick TH, et al. Detection and evaluation of intrapulmonary vascular shunt with "contrast Doppler" transesophageal echocardiography. Journal of the American Society of Echocardiography. 1991;**4**:79-83

[39] Khandheria BK, Seward JB, Tajik AJ. Transesophageal echocardiography. Mayo Clinic Proceedings. 1994;**69**:856-863

4

Ascites: Treatment, Complications, and Prognosis

Patricia Huelin, Jose Ignacio Fortea,
Javier Crespo and Emilio Fábrega

Abstract

Ascites is the most common complication in patients with cirrhosis. It can lead to several life-threatening complications resulting in a poor long-term survival outcome. Ascites is due to the loss of compensatory mechanism to maintain effective arterial blood volume secondary to splanchnic arterial vasodilatation in the progression of liver disease and portal hypertension. Refractory ascites, spontaneous bacterial peritonitis (SBP), hyponatremia, and hepatorenal syndrome (HRS) are complications that can occur with ascites, all of them leading to a worse quality of life and short-term mortality. When complication appears, liver transplantation as a definitive and curative treatment should be considered. Other common therapeutical approaches to control ascites such as diet, sodium restriction, or the use of diuretics are needed to avoid these complications, although some patients will require further treatments when ascites becomes refractory to standard treatment. This chapter will review the complex treatment of ascites, and its related complications.

Keywords: ascites, hepatorenal syndrome, hyponatremia, portal hypertension, spontaneous bacterial peritonitis

1. Introduction

Decompensated cirrhosis is the end stage of chronic liver disease of any etiology. It has a wide range of different clinical manifestations that are secondary to portal hypertension and/or liver insufficiency. Ascites is the most frequent decompensation, and it is usually the first manifestation of the disease in the majority of the patients [1]. Ascites is the accumulation of liquid inside of the peritoneal cavity, and it is developed in 60% of patients with compensated cirrhosis within 10 years during the natural course of their liver disease [1]. Hippocrates of Kos described ascites a long time ago (ca. 460–ca. 310 BC), and its treatment with large paracentesis was already performed since the ancient Greek physicians. It is still a very common problem in patients with liver cirrhosis, malignancy, or cardiovascular disease today. As in Western Europe and the United States of America, liver cirrhosis is the main cause of ascites (75–85%), and we will focus on this disease [2, 3].

The development of ascites is the consequence of the action of several complex mechanisms secondary to severe portal hypertension (i.e., hepatic venous pressure gradient (HVPG) >12 mm Hg) giving place to an impairment of hepatic, circulatory, and renal function. Portal hypertension induces the activation of the endogenous vasoactive systems, which prevent the renal excretion of an adequate amount of sodium, leading to a positive sodium balance [4]. Large evidence suggests that renal sodium retention in patients with cirrhosis is secondary to arterial splanchnic vasodilation. This causes a decrease in effective arterial blood volume with activation of arterial and cardiopulmonary volume receptors, and homeostatic activation of vasoconstrictor and sodium retaining systems (i.e., renin-angiotensin-aldosterone, vasopressin, and the sympathetic nervous systems). Renal sodium retention leads to expansion of the extracellular fluid volume and increases intestinal capillary pressure. The latter is further increased due to both portal hypertension and splanchnic arterial vasodilatation, which also disrupts the intestinal capillary permeability, and thereby contributes to the accumulation of fluid in the abdominal cavity [5]. In addition, certain polymorphisms of the aquaporin-1 gene could predispose to water retention [6].

The development of ascites is associated with a poor prognosis and impaired quality of life in patients with cirrhosis [7]. The probability of survival at 1 and 5 years after decompensation by ascites is about 50 and 20%, respectively [8]. Because of the poor survival, and other complications that will be explained later, patients with ascites should generally be considered for referral for liver transplantation [3].

2. Evaluation and initial investigations

2.1. History and physical examination

The first step in the management of every patient with a new-onset ascites is to reveal its underlying cause. A thorough history and physical examination will help narrow the differential diagnosis and reveal factors that might have been implicated in the development of ascites (e.g., nonsteroidal anti-inflammatory drugs (NSAIDs)). Risk factors for liver disease such as alcohol abuse, metabolic syndrome, or family history of hemochromatosis should be sought. Patients should also be questioned about past history of cancer, heart failure, renal disease, or tuberculosis as they may all be responsible for the development of ascites [3].

The main complaint of patients with ascites is an increase in abdominal girth, often accompanied by lower-extremity edema. Other common manifestations include dyspnea due to increasing abdominal distension and/or accompanying pleural effusions, abdominal pain, anorexia, nausea, and fatigue [9]. The accuracy of the physical examination to detect ascites is highly dependent on the amount of ascites and on the physical constitution of the patient. Accordingly, patients must have approximately 1500 mL of fluid for ascites to be detected reliably by physical examination and the presence of obesity greatly reduces its diagnostic accuracy [3]. Several signs support the presence of ascites such as the shifting dullness, fluid wave, and puddle signs. The former has 83% sensitivity and 56% specificity in detecting ascites. It is also less cumbersome and performs better than the latter two [3, 10]. The clinician should also look for other physical signs that suggest the presence of a liver disease (e.g., spider angiomas, Dupuytren contracture, palmar erythema, gynecomastia, parotid gland enlargement, or testicular atrophy) or an extra-hepatic disease (e.g. jugular venous distension related to heart failure) as the cause of ascites.

2.2. Initial investigations

The essential investigations that should follow the anamnesis and physical examination to confirm the cause of ascites include an abdominal ultrasound (to screen for morphologic evidence of cirrhosis and portal hypertension, tumors, portal vein thrombosis, and hepatic vein thrombosis), laboratory assessment of liver function, renal function, serum and urine electrolytes, and abdominal paracentesis. The latter is compulsory in order to confirm the cause of the ascites and to rule out complications such as spontaneous bacterial peritonitis (SBP). Thus, it should always be performed in a new episode of ascites grades 2 or 3, in patients hospitalized for any complication of the disease or because of worsening of ascites [2, 11]. It is a safe procedure, even in patients with prolonged prothrombin time and low platelets. Indeed, the policy of some physicians to give blood products (fresh frozen plasma and/or platelets) routinely in these patients is not data-supported [3]. Growing evidence from the last two decades has demonstrated that most patients with liver cirrhosis remain in a tenous but balanced state of hemostasis [12]. Accordingly, in a study of 1100 large volume paracentesis, there were no hemorrhagic complications despite no prophylactic correction of platelet counts as low as 19,000 cells/mm^3 (54% < 50,000) and of prolonged international normalized ratios for prothrombin time as high as 8.7 (75% > 1.5 and 26.5% > 2.0) [13]. The most common site for paracentesis is the left lower quadrant of the abdominal wall (3 cm cephalad and 3 cm medial to the anterior superior iliac spine), as in this location the wall is thinner and with a larger pool of fluid than the midline. Visible collateral must be avoided, and in patients with obesity or loculated ascites, an ecoguided paracentesis is commonly needed [3].

The analysis of the ascitic fluid includes cell count and differential, culture, biochemical analysis, and cytology. Current guidelines recommend to routinely perform only cell count and differential, ascitic fluid protein and albumin, and note the gross appearance of the fluid (i.e., water-clear, bilious, purulent, bloody, or chylous) [2, 3]. The former enables to discard SBP or suspect the presence of other type of infection (e.g., high lymphocyte count in patients with tuberculosis). Albumin measurement on the same day in serum and ascitic fluid allows the calculation of the serum-ascites albumin gradient (SAAG), which properly differentiates ascites due to portal hypertension from ascites due to other causes. If the SAAG is greater than or equal to 1.1 g/dL, ascites is ascribed to portal hypertension with an approximate 97% accuracy [14]. Importantly, SAAG accuracy is not influenced by fluid infusion and diuretic use and also remains greater or equal to 1.1 g/dL in patients with both portal hypertension and a second cause for ascites formation [3]. Measurement of SAAG is, therefore, of utmost importance in patients with new-onset ascites, but its repeated measurement is usually not needed in other scenarios (e.g., worsening or refractory ascites) [3]. **Table 1** shows the etiological classification of ascites according to the SAAG value. Further ascitic testing should be done depending on clinical judgment [3]. In patients in whom a peritoneal carcinomatosis is suspected, an ascitic fluid cytology must be performed, as it has a sensitivity as high as 96.7% if three samples from different paracentesis procedures are analyzed [15]. Bacterial culture is mandatory if infection is suspected. Cultures should be done in aerobic and anaerobic blood cultures inoculated (10 mL) at the bedside to increase their profitability (80% by this method). The utility of lactate

SAAG	Diseases	Diagnosis
≥1.1	Liver cirrhosis	Compatible image test and biopsy, known etiology of liver disease, HVPG > 10 mm Hg, liver stiffness >15 Kpa, proteins in ascites <2.5 g/L
	Budd-Chiari syndrome	Imaging test, proteins in ascites >2.5 g/L
	Sinusoidal obstruction syndrome	Appropriate clinical context (e.g. hemotopoietic stem cell transplantation), proteins in ascites >2.5 g/L
	Portal thrombosis	Imaging test, usually associated with a clinical trigger such as variceal bleeding
	Right heart failure	Right heart failure confirmed by echocardiogram, serum BNP >364 pg/mL, dilated suprahepatic veins, proteins in ascites >2.5 g/L
	Acute liver failure	Appropriate clinical context
	Massive liver metastases	Imaging test, proteins in ascites <2.5 g/L
	Myxedema	Clinical and laboratory findings of severe hypothyroidism
	"Mixed" ascites*	Imaging or other test according to clinical suspicion
<1.1	Peritoneal carcinomatosis	Positive citology, proteins in ascites >2.5 g/L, WBC >500 with PMNs<250, image test to find primary tumor (most frequent ovarian, gastric, and pancreatic origin)
	Peritoneal tuberculosis	WBC > 500 with PMNs<250 and predominance of lymphocytes, proteins in ascites >2.5 g/L, ADA >40 UI/L, positive culture or PCR, peritoneal biopsy
	Pancreatic ascitis	Ascitic amylase level usually >2000 UI/L, protein concentration in ascites variable, but normally >2.5 g/L, PMN > 250, imaging test to diagnose the underlying disease
	Bilious ascites	Elevated ascitic bilirubin levels and higher than serum, imaging test to diagnose the underlying disease
	Chylous ascites	Ascitic triglyceride level >110–200 mg/dL or higher than serum, imaging test to diagnose the underlying disease
	Nephrotic syndrome	Appropriate clinical context, proteins in ascites <2.5 g/L
	Protein-losing enteropathy	Diarrhea and other clinical symptoms due to the underlying disease, proteins in ascites <2.5 g/L
	Serositis related to connective tissue diseases	Rare manifestación of systemic lupus erythematosus, polyarteritis nodosa and Schölein-Henoch purpura. Appropriate clinical context
	Intestinal ischemia or obstruction	Imaging test

*Patients with cirrhosis and other cause (one or more) of ascites formation. Abbreviations: SAAG: serum-ascites albumin gradient; HVPG: hepatic venous pressure gradient; WCC: white blood cell; PMN: polymorphonuclear leukocyte; ADA: adenosine deaminase; PCR: polymerase chain reaction.

Table 1. Etiological classification of ascites according to the serum-ascites albumin gradient value.

dehydrogenase and glucose determination in ascitic fluid to assist in differentiating sponta-neous from secondary bacterial peritonitis is supported by limited data and the European Association for the Study of the Liver (EASL) does not recommend its performance [2]. On the contrary, an ascitic fluid carcinoembryonic antigen >5 ng/mL or ascitic fluid alkaline phos-phatase >240 units/L has been shown to be accurate in detecting gut perforation into ascitic fluid [16]. Other tests, such as amylase, triglycerides, and polymerase chain reaction (PCR) and culture for mycobacteria should be done only when there is a clinical suspicion of pancre-atic disease, chylous ascites, and tuberculosis, respectively. Finally, it is worth mentioning that serum cancer antigen 125 levels are increased in patients with ascites of any cause. Therefore, its measurement is not recommended to guide the differential diagnosis [3].

3. Treatment of ascites

Current guidelines follow the classification of ascites from the International Ascites Club, which divides patients into three groups on the basis of a quantitative criterion. Each group is also linked to a specific treatment strategy (see **Table 2**) [3, 17]. Accordingly, only patients with ascites grade 2 or more should be treated, and they can be treated as outpatients unless they have other complications [2]. The aim of the treatment of ascites is to induce negative sodium balance by reducing sodium intake and increasing sodium excretion by the adminis-tration of diuretics.

3.1. Sodium restriction

In approximately 10–20% of patients with cirrhosis and ascites, we can obtain a negative sodium balance only by reducing dietary sodium intake, particularly in those presenting with their first episode of ascites [18]. No predictive factors of response to low sodium diet have been detected. Although the level of dietary restriction should be applied according to the baseline urinary sodium excretion, a moderate restriction of salt intake is generally recom-mended (intake of sodium of 80–120 mmol/day, which corresponds to 4.6–6.9 g of salt/day). This is generally equivalent to a no-added salt diet with avoidance of preprepared meals. A more severe reduction in dietary sodium content is considered unnecessary and even

Severity and definition	Treatment and strategy
Grade 1 or mild Diagnosed exclusively by ultrasonography.	No treatment is necessary.
Grade 2 or moderate Clinically evident.	Dietary sodium restriction and diuretics. (first spironolactone 50–100 mg/day to reach weight loss: 300–500 mg/day, if needed, add furosemide 20–40 mg/day and increase both every 7 days up to 400 and 160 mg/day, respectively)
Grade 3 or large Clinically evident or tense.	Large-volume paracentesis plus albumin 8 g/L of ascites removed in first place and later dietary sodium restriction (90 mmol/day) and diuretics.

Table 2. Ascites classification and treatment [17].

potentially deleterious since it may impair nutritional status [2, 3]. Fluid restriction is not necessary unless patients have hypovolemic hyponatremia (serum sodium <130 mEq/L together with ascites and/or edema). Fluid loss and weight change are directly related to sodium balance in these patients. It is sodium restriction, not fluid restriction, which results in weight loss, as fluid follows sodium passively [2].

3.2. Diuretics

Evidence demonstrates that renal sodium retention is mainly due to increased proximal as well as distal tubular sodium reabsorption rather than due to a decrease of filtered sodium load [2, 19]. The increased reabsorption of sodium along the distal tubule is mostly related to hyperaldosteronism. As previously mentioned, patients with ascites grade 2 require diuretic treatment if there is no contraindication. The goal of treatment is to achieve an average weight loss of no more than 500 g/day in patients without peripheral edema and no more than 800–1000 g/day in those with peripheral edema.

The efficacy of diuretic therapy in the control of ascites is approximately 90% in patients without renal dysfunction [2, 19]. The diuretics most frequently used are aldosterone antagonists, mainly spironolactone, which selectively antagonizes the sodium-retaining effects of aldosterone in the renal collecting tubules, and loop diuretics, especially furosemide, that inhibit the Na + −K + −2Cl − cotransporter in the loop of Henle. It has been extensively debated whether both types of diuretics should be combined from the beginning or use aldosterone antagonists in a stepwise increase every 7 days with furosemide added only in patients not responding to high doses of aldosterone antagonists. It can be concluded that a diuretic regime based on the combination of aldosterone antagonists and furosemide is the most adequate approach for patients with recurrent ascites but not for patients with a first episode of ascites. These latter patients respond well to spironolactone 50–100 mg/day [2]. Those with recurrent episodes of ascites or peripheral edema should receive a combination of spironolactone 100 mg/day with furosemide 40 mg/day [2, 19]. If there is no response, adherence to a low sodium-diet and diuretic treatment should be confirmed through a good anamnesis and a 24-hour urine sodium excretion measurement. An ascites that is not controlled despite a natriuresis greater than 80–110 mmol/day suggests a non-adherence to a low-sodium diet [3]. Given that full-day collections are cumbersome, the measurement of urine creatinine helps determine if the collection of the 24-hour specimen has been complete. Men with cirrhosis should excrete more than 15 mg of creatinine/kg of body weight per day, and women should excrete more than 10 mg/kg/day. Less creatinine is indicative of an incomplete collection [3]. A random "spot" urine sample is also useful to assess natriuresis and is the preferable test to adjust diuretic treatment in certain scenarios such as the emergency unit. A sodium concentration that is greater than the potassium concentration correlates well with a 24-hour sodium excretion. When the urine sodium/potassium ratio is >1, the patient should be responding to the treatment. The higher the ratio, the greater the urine sodium excretion [20]. In compliant patients with poorly controlled ascites, diuretics may then be increased every 7 days by doubling doses (1:1 ratio) to a maximal dose of spironolactone (400 mg/day) and a maximal dose of furosemide (160 mg/day). Unfortunately, diuretics can also have side effects and cause fluid and electrolytes balance disturbances such as hyponatremia, dehydration, renal impairment, hyperkalemia, or hypokalemia and subsequently, hepatic encephalopathy. For all these reasons, patients should be closely followed after the onset of diuretic treatment. Thus, a clinical evaluation and measurements of serum and urine electrolytes must be performed within the first 2 weeks after starting or modifying their dose. When any of the abovementioned side effects appear, diuretics should be stopped or their dose reduced. A particular side effect of spironolactone is tender gynecomastia and muscle cramps in some patients. Amiloride, a diuretic acting in the collecting duct, is less effective than aldosterone antagonists and should be used only in those patients who develop severe side effects with aldosterone antagonists [2].

3.3. Other general measures

Treatment of the underlying disease whenever possible is of great importance as dramatic responses have been described after alcohol abstinence, antiviral, and immunosuppressive therapies in patients with alcoholic, viral and autoimmune liver diseases, respectively [3]. Nutritional therapy can ameliorate nutritional status in cirrhotic patients, reduce infection rates, and decrease perioperative morbidity [11]. Some drugs must be avoided or use with caution in patients with ascites such as NSAID due to the high risk of developing further sodium retention, hyponatremia, and renal failure. In a recent case control study, 37% of the NSAIDs-associated acute kidney injury (AKI) cases were severe and persistent with a very poor short-term outcome [21]. Interestingly, Metamizol use was more common in patients with persistent AKI than in those with transient AKI, and therefore, this drug should also be used with caution. Likewise, angiotensin converting enzyme inhibitors, angiotensin II antagonists, or a1-adrenergic receptor blockers should generally not be used in patients with ascites because of increased risk of renal impairment [2]. Bed rest was previously recommended on the basis that the upright posture could aggravate the already elevated plasma renin levels of patients with liver cirrhosis and ascites. However, it is no longer advocated as there is insufficient evidence to support its use as part of ascites treatment [2]. There is an ongoing debate about the use of nonselective betablockers in patients with refractory ascites. The current guidelines from the American Association for the Study of Liver Diseases recommend to avoid high doses of these drugs (over 160 mg/day of propranolol or over 80 mg/day of nadolol), and in patients with concomitant severe circulatory dysfunction [i.e., systolic blood pressure <90 mm Hg, serum sodium <130 mEq/L, or hepatorenal syndrome (HRS)], their dose should be decreased or the drug temporarily held [22]. Finally, in unblinded randomized clinical trials (RCTs), the long-term albumin infusion (25 g weekly for one year and 25 g every two weeks thereafter) improved survival in patients with new onset ascites [23]. However, further studies are needed before this treatment can be advocated [3].

4. Complications, prognosis, and treatment

Despite the fact that patients with ascites constitute a heterogeneous population with different prognosis depending on the degree of liver insufficiency and circulatory dysfunction, the development of ascites is an ominous sign. The probability of survival at one and five years after the diagnosis of ascites is approximately 50 and 20%, respectively, and long-term survival of more than 10 years is very rare [8]. In addition, mortality rises up to 80% within 6–12 months in patients who also develop kidney failure [1]. Patients with cirrhosis and ascites are also at high risk for other life-threatening complications of liver disease, including refractory ascites, SBP, respiratory distress, worsening of nutritional status, hyponatremia, or HRS. Accordingly, current guidelines recommend that every patient with ascites should be generally considered for referral for liver transplantation, especially when quality of life is impaired due to refractory ascites, or in the presence of SBE and HRS [2, 3]. Since 2002, the model of end-stage liver disease (MELD) score is used for patient priority in liver transplantation. However, MELD does not reflect the impact of some complications (the so-called Exceptions to MELD score) such as refractory ascites. Indeed, in some patients with this complication the latter score does not accurately reflect their poor prognosis (median survival is approximately 6 months) and their prioritization in the list should be assessed [24].

4.1. Refractory ascites

A nonnegligible number of patients with ascites (10%) develop refractory ascites due to severe sodium retention that cannot be mobilized pharmacologically either because there is no response to high diuretic dose (resistant ascites) or because side effects appear with the use of diuretics (intractable ascites). The term "recurrent ascites" defines an ascites that requires more than three admissions per year because of reaccumulation of ascites [25]. In these patients other therapeutical approaches must be used.

4.1.1. Large volume paracentesis (LVP)

Current guidelines recommend LVP as the first-line treatment in patients with refractory ascites, unless it is loculated [2, 3]. In order to minimize the number of paracentesis (LVP is usually performed every 2–4 weeks), total paracentesis is preferred and diuretic therapy can be maintained if the urine sodium is >30 mmol/day. It is a safe procedure with a complicate rate similar to diagnostic paracentesis, and it can be performed in the outpatient setting [2, 3]. LVP is defined as a volume above 5 L. Although Kao et al. arbitrarily selected this threshold in 1985 based upon the volume required to "adequately decompress the distended abdomen," the intra-individual neurohormonal changes induced by the removal of different ascitic volumes have not been examined [26, 27]. These neurohormonal changes reflect the physiopathological background of the main complication of LP, i.e., postparacentesis circulatory dysfunction (PPCD). Indeed, the removal of large volumes of ascites fluid can further decline the effective circulating volume by causing a significant drop in peripheral vascular resistance by mechanisms not fully elucidated. This hemodynamic derangement is demonstrated by a pronounced reactivation of renin-angiotensin-aldosterone and sympathetic nervous systems that can persist for months. An increase in plasma renin activity of 50% or greater is usually used to define PPCD [27, 28]. Although frequently asymptomatic, PPCD has been associated with significant detrimental effects such as re-accumulation of ascites, development of HRS and dilutional hyponatremia, and shortened survival [2]. It was first demonstrated in the 1980s that adjunctive albumin infusion can prevent PPCD occurrence and since the early 1990s, less costly alternatives to albumin have been sought, such as artificial colloid volume expanders and vasoconstrictors [28]. Despite initial uncertain results, a meta-analysis of

17 trials with a total 1225 patients demonstrated that albumin infusion after LVP is more effective than other plasma expanders (i.e., hypertonic saline, hydroxyethyl starch, and dextran-70, poly-geline) for the prevention of PPCD and showed a trend to increased survival. The rate of PPCD was 73% after paracentesis without any re-expansion, 38% when combined with an infusion of dextran or gelatin solutions and only 15–17% when taps were combined with albumin administration. Doses of albumin infusion ranged between 5 and 10 g of albumin per liter of fluid removed [28]. Current guidelines recommend 8 g/L as this has been the dose most commonly used [2, 3]. It is usually administered during or after the paracentesis. Whether lower doses could be used is currently debated as one study comparing doses of 4 vs. 8 g/L showed similar efficacy in preventing PPCD and renal impairment [29]. When less than 5 L of ascites are removed, artificial plasma expanders, saline, and albumin are equally effective [2]. The latter meta-analysis also compared albumin with vasoconstrictors (i.e., midodrine, norepinephrine, and terlipressin). The results were more variable in this subgroup (OR from 0.30 to 5.54) due to the small size of the five included trials and therefore, no definitive conclusions can be made [28]. Further studies that target survival as the primary end-point in patients with truly refractory ascites are needed to fully demonstrate whether albumin or vasoconstrictors can improve survival.

4.1.2. Transjugular intrahepatic portosystemic shunt (TIPS)

Another treatment option for patients with refractory ascites is transjugular intrahepatic portosystemic shunt (TIPS). It is a procedure in which an intrahepatic stent is inserted between the hepatic and portal veins with intent for portal decompression to avoid the recurrence of ascites [30]. The optimal portal pressure gradient (PPG) that needs to be obtained to adequately control ascites is not clear, but might be lower than the well-validated 12 mm Hg threshold for the prevention of rebleeding from esophageal varices [30]. Most of randomized clinical trials (RCTs) aimed to reduce PPG below 12 mm Hg by dilating 10-mm diameter stents to 6–8 mm with subsequent calibration up to 10 mm, depending on post-PPG and clinical response [31–34]. By this approach, marked reductions in PPG are avoided, which may be associated with an increased risk of hepatic encephalopathy and liver failure. Until today, seven RCT [31–37] and six meta-analysis [38–43] have assessed the efficacy and safety of TIPS in patients with refractory and recurrent ascites. They have consistently demonstrated that TIPS is effective in the management of this complication, but is associated with higher risk of hepatic encephalopathy compared to LVP. Thus, about 64% (range of 38–84%) had their ascites controlled (although its resolution was slow and most patients required continued administration of diuretics and salt restriction), and hepatic encephalopathy occurred in approximately 51% of patients (39% severe) treated with TIPS. This latter complication is known to increase the rate of mortality and hospitalization and to significantly affect the quality of life [30]. TIPS dysfunction due to pseudointimal hyperplasia within the parenchymal tract or within the outflow hepatic vein was another major drawback in these studies. Indeed, a significant proportion of patients (from 30 to 87%) needed TIPS revision due to malfunction. It must be emphasized that all, but one clinical trial [34], used bare stents instead of the politetrafluoroethylene-covered stents that are used today. These covered-stents have greatly improved shunt patency rates and have also reduced the incidence of hepatic encephalopathy after TIPS placement [30]. There is great controversy over the survival benefit of TIPS in refractory ascites. At the time current guidelines were published, studies had not convincingly proved that TIPS improved survival compared to repeated LVP, and consequently, it was left as a second-line therapy that had to be considered in patients with very frequent requirement of LVP or with loculated ascites [2, 3]. Among the five trials that had been published at that time, transplant-free survival was significantly improved in two (in one of them only in the multivariate analysis) [33, 36], decreased in one (probably due to technical disability) [35], and not affected in the other two [31, 37]. These discrepancies among studies were likely due to patient selection and data analysis biases. These RCTs excluded patients with advanced liver disease (as defined by serum bilirubin > 5–6 mg/dL, INR > 2, current or chronic HE > 2 by West-Heaven scale), and renal failure (as defined by serum creatinine >3 mg/dL) and thus, only 48% (median, 21–77%) of the screened patients could be included in the RCTs. Meta-analysis also contributed to this controversy. Four conventional meta-analysis did not show any benefit in survival [38–41], whereas a meta-analysis of individual patient data from four RCT showed a significant improvement in transplant-free survival at 1 and 2 years between TIPS and LVP (63 and 49% vs. 53 and 35%, $p = 0.035$) [42]. After the publication of the current guidelines, two RCT [32, 34] and another meta-analysis [43] have been published and concluded that TIPS is more effective in controlling ascites than repeated LVP and improved transplant-free survival in these patients. The RCT of Narahara et al. included 60 patients with refractory ascites treated with bare metal TIPS or LVP. The selection criteria were stricter than the previous RCT and included patients with better preserved renal and hepatic function [32]. The last RCT was recently published and included patients with recurrent ascites treated with covered-stents or LVP with inclusion criteria similar to the former RCT [34]. It can be concluded that pending further RCT with covered stents, TIPS can be recommended in patients with refractory ascites and preserved liver function (Child–Pugh score <13, MELD score <18, bilirubin <5 mg/dL, platelet count >75,000, serum sodium >130 mEq/L), aged <70, no previous episodes of hepatic encephalopathy, and neither central or large hepatocellular carcinoma nor cardiopulmonary disease [19]. In fact, some authors and scientific associations recommend TIPS as the primary therapy for refractory ascites [44–46].

4.1.3. Automated low flow pump system (Alfapump System)

The alfapump is a subcutaneous battery-operated pump to move ascites from the peritoneum to the urinary bladder. One catheter connects the pump to the peritoneal cavity, and another connects it to the urinary bladder. Every 5–10 min small volumes of ascites (generally 5–10 mL) are pumped into the urinary bladder, ranging the daily volume that can be removed between 500 mL and 2.5 L. In order to improve patient's comfort it is deactivated at night. The pump battery is charged via a charging device (Smart Charger, Sequana Medical AG, Zürich, Switzerland) that is placed over the area of the pump twice daily during no more than 20 min. It is at this time when pump function parameters (e.g., volumen transported, pressures in the bladder and abdominal cavity) are automatically transmitted to the charger. This information is forwarded to a central databank and communicated, if needed, to the treating physician, who can remotely program the system to the patient's needs or contact the patient because of possible technical issues. The current price of the device is 22,500 Euros [47].

The alfapump was conceived as an alternative treatment for refractory ascites, especially in those patients who are not candidates for TIPS [47, 48]. This system also requires a good selection process, in which issues such as compliance of the patient, nutritional status, previous abdominal surgery, urinary outlet obstruction, or local skin infections should be carefully evaluated before its implantation [47]. An initial multicenter, prospective, uncontrolled study (PIONEER) evaluated its safety and efficacy in 40 patients over a period of 6 months. It showed that the pump removed 90% of the ascites and reduced the median number of LVP, but with a significant rate of complications mainly due to infections and catheter dislodgement [49]. However, the number of complications was reduced along the study after including some changes recommended by the data safety monitoring board (i.e., antibiotic prophylaxis with norfloxacin, strict avoidance of NSAID, and the intravenous administration of albumin if ascites was aspired during the surgical intervention) [47]. A recent RCT compared the safety and efficacy of the alfapump system in comparison with LVP in 58 cirrhotic patients with refractory ascites over a 6-month period [48]. The alfapump was more effective reducing and, in many cases, eliminating (more than 50%) the need for paracentesis. It also improved the quality of life and nutritional status of the patients. Survival was similar in both groups, despite the occurrence of more adverse events (96.3 vs. 77.4%, $p = 0.057$), which were also more frequently severe (85.2% vs. 45.2%, $p = 0.002$) in the group treated with alfapump. Adverse events consisted predominantly of AKI in the immediate post-operative period, and re-intervention for pump-related issues. Device deficiencies accounted for seven re-interventions, which are an improvement compared to the results of the PIONEER study and may reflect the continual technological improvements to the alfapump system since commercialization in 2011. After the postoperative period (>7 days), the incidence of AKI and hyponatremia was similar in both groups, but more of these events required hospitalization in the alfapump group. The underlying mechanism for this renal dysfunction and hyponatremia remains unclear. In a recent prospective study that included ten patients with refractory ascites treated with the alfapump system, a marked activation of endogenous vasoconstrictor systems and impairment of kidney function after the device insertion was observed. This finding led the authors to hypothesize that treatment with alfapump might impair effective arterial blood volume mimicking a postparacentesis circulatory dysfunction syndrome and suggested a potential role of albumin in counteracting these effects [50]. Supporting this hypothesis, the authors of the RCT observed an increase in plasma renin activity at 3 months. Finally, total median cost (including implantation procedure and device, scheduled visits, lab test, medications and treatment of adverse events) was significantly higher in the alfapump group (£36970 vs. £12660, p < 0.0001). The difference was primarily due to the statistically higher cost of implantation procedure and adverse effects [48]. It can be concluded that further refinements in patient selection, patient care algorithms (including regular albumin administration), and modifications in device design are needed before the alfapump can become a truly alternative treatment for patients with refractory ascites.

4.1.4. Vaptans

Vaptans are V2 vasopressin receptor antagonists acting on the kidney and promoting solute-free water diuresis. In patients with cirrhosis, they have been studied in the setting of dilutional hyponatremia (see below section 6) and ascites. In patients with both uncomplicated and refractory ascites, satavaptan did not have a clinical benefit in controlling ascites and even increased mortality, which was related with known complications of liver cirrhosis [51, 52]. Consequently, the drug was withdrawn from development. Tolvaptan has also been used in patients with liver cirrhosis and refractory ascites. Most of the data come from observational studies in which tolvaptan seemed to improve control of ascites [53–57]. Two RCT also showed that tolvaptan was more effective than placebo for the treatment of ascites-related clinical symptoms. However, in both trials, the drug was given for only 7 days and the follow-up period was no longer than 3 weeks [58, 59]. Both issues are of great concern, given that its efficacy is lost after the discontinuation of the drug [60] and that a black-box warning by the Food and Drug Administration determined that tolvaptan should not be used for longer than 30 days, and limited its use in patients with underlying liver disease. The latter warning came from an increased risk of liver injury in a recent large clinical trial evaluating tolvaptan for a new use in patients with autosomal dominant polycystic kidney disease [61]. Therefore, the use of vaptans in cirrhotic patients with uncomplicated or refractory ascites cannot be recommended at present and required further RCT with a longer follow-up [3, 11].

4.1.5. Vasoconstrictors

Since arterial splanchnic vasodilation plays a major role in the pathogenesis of ascites formation, the use of vasoconstrictors has been evaluated in the treatment of patients with refractory or recurrent ascites. In two preliminary studies both the acute and 7-day administration of Midodrine, an alfa-1-adrenergic agonist, in nonazotemic cirrhotic patients with ascites improved systemic hemodynamics and sodium excretion [62, 63]. Similarly, in another study, the addition of midodrine corrected the deleterious effects on renal function of octreotide and improved systemic hemodynamics [64]. The first study evaluating its effect on patients with refractory or recurrent ascites was a RCT in which 40 patients were randomized to oral midodrine (7.5 mg every 8 h) plus standard medical therapy (sodium restriction plus diuretics) or to standard medical therapy alone. Midodrine significantly improved systemic hemodynamics without significant complications and was superior for the control of ascites at 3 months, but not at 1 and 6 months after therapy. Moreover, the mortality rate in the standard medical therapy group was significantly higher than that in the midodrine group ($p < 0.046$) [65]. A recent pilot study evaluated the efficacy and safety of midodrine in combination with tolvaptan in 50 cirrhotic patients with refractory or recurrent ascites. Their combination controlled ascites significantly better than standard diuretic treatment alone and more rapidly than midodrine alone [66].

Clonidine, a centrally acting $\alpha2$-agonist and sympatholytic agent, has also been evaluated as an adjunct treatment in patients with cirrhosis and refractory ascites. In two pilot studies, its addition to spironolactone increased natriuresis and body weight loss more efficiently than spironolactone alone in patients with cirrhosis and ascites and activated sympathetic nervous system [67, 68]. Years later, the same group performed a first RCT that included patients with cirrhosis, ascites, and a plasma norepinephrine level of >300 pg/mL. Oral clonidine (0.075 mg b.i.d.) led to an earlier duretic response and was associated with fewer diuretic requirements and complications [69]. A later RCT using the same dose of clonidine for 3 months evaluated its efficacy in 270 patients with refractory ascites. The response rate to the association of clonidine and diuretics was 55–60%. The highest efficacy was obtained in patients who had high serum levels of norepinephine and the presence of two specific polymorphisms of the G-protein and $\alpha2$-adrenergic receptor gene [70]. The efficacy of the combination of clonidine and midrodine was evaluated in a RCT that included 60 patients with refractory and recurrent ascites. Their combination controlled ascites significantly better than standard diuretic treatment alone over a 1-month period, but was not superior to midodrine or clonidine alone [71].

Finally, there is very limited data available with terlipressin. In a small RCT that included 15 patients with nonrefractory ascites and 8 with refractory ascites without HRS, 2 mg of intravenous terlipressin improved renal function and natriuresis in both types of ascites. However, a clinical effect on weight or abdominal girth was not recorded [72]. In a prospective study in which 26 patients with refractory ascites without HRS were treated with maximum diuretic treatment plus albumin and terlipressin, complete and partial response were observed in 62 and 23% of the patients, respectively [73].

With the available evidence, the American Association for the Study of Liver Diseases recommends that the use of oral midodrine should be considered in patients with refractory ascites [3]. On the other hand, the European Association for the Study of the Liver considers that larger RCT with longer follow-up are needed before these drugs can be routinely recommended in the management of these patients [2]. The authors of this chapter are in agreement with this last recommendation.

Figure 1 depicts the pathophysiological rationale for the treatment of patients with ascites and other related complications.

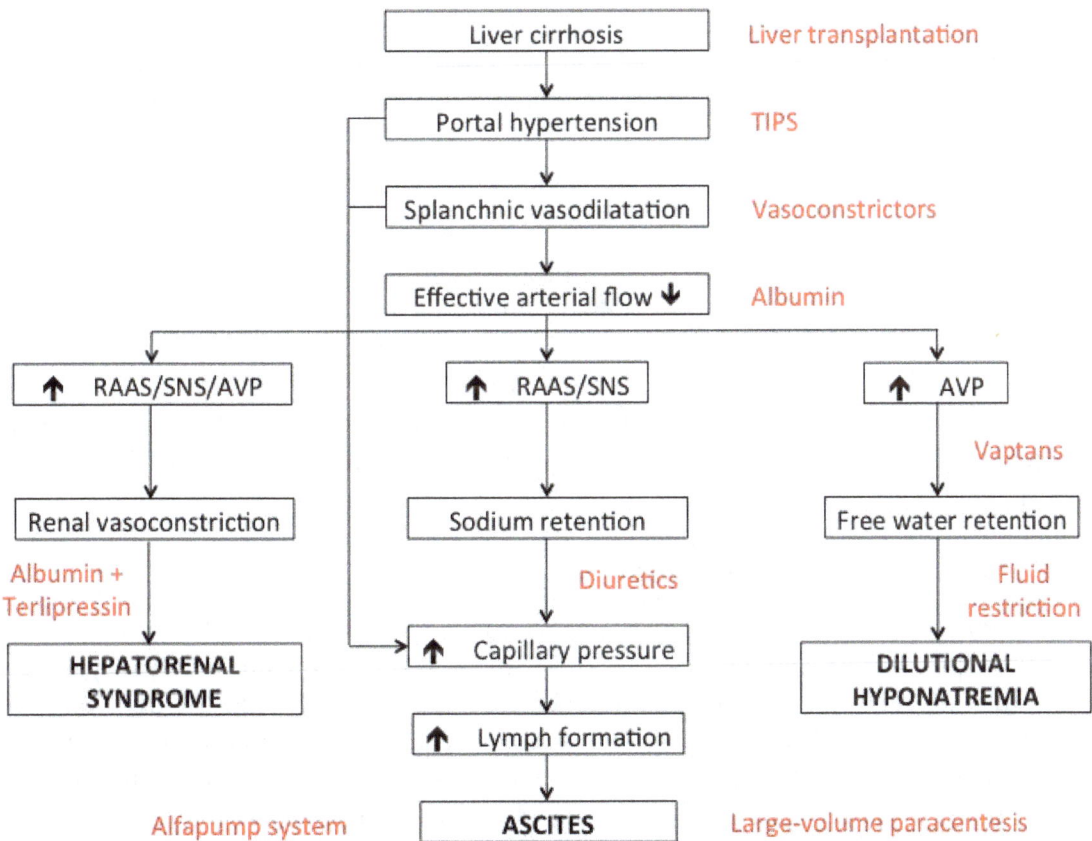

Figure 1. Physiopathology and treatment of patients with ascites and other related complications. Splanchnic vasodilatation driven by portal hypertension leads to an arterial underfilling that is counteracted by the activation of antinatriuretic and vasoconstrictor factors (RAAS, SNS, and AVP) that may lead to development of ascites, dilutional hyponatremia, and hepatorenal syndrome. Current therapies act at different levels of this pathophysiological cascade. Abbreviations: TIPS: transjugular intrahepatic portosystemic shunt; RAAS: renin-angotensin-aldosterone system; sympathetic nervous system; AVP: arginine vasopressin.

5. Spontaneous bacterial peritonitis (SBP)

Compared to general population, patients with cirrhosis have an increased risk of developing bacterial infections and sepsis, for this reason, SBP has a remarkable importance. SBP is a common infection of ascitic fluid developed in patients in the absence of an intra-abdominal genesis of infection. SBP was described for the first-time long time ago, approximately in the 1970s by Harold Conn [74], who pointed out the high in-hospital mortality in patients with this complication. The mechanisms leading to SBP include bacterial translocation, the reduced gut motility giving place to intestinal bacterial overgrowth, altered structure, and function of the intestinal mucosal barrier, and shortage in local immune response systems [75]. Patients with cirrhosis and SBP frequently develop an exaggerated inflammatory response with a severe impairment in renal, cardiovascular, or other organs functions. This syndrome is called acute or chronic liver failure and implies a high rate of hospital mortality [76].

SBP is the most frequent bacterial infection in hospitalized patients with cirrhosis [77]. It occurs in approximately 15–30% of hospitalized patients. Approximately 70% of the episodes of SBP is present when patients are admitted to the hospital, and the rest, 30%, is acquired during hospitalization [78]. The clinical manifestations in patients with SBP are usually symptoms such as abdominal pain, diarrhea, fever, chills, and hepatic encephalopathy, but in approximately 25% of cases of SBP, there are no apparent symptoms. Subclinical manifestations could occur as, for example, deterioration in renal function without other cause or development of tense and refractory ascites in a patient previously responsive to diuretics.

The prognosis in patients with SBP is very poor. The mortality during hospitalization is still remarkably high (20–40%) and is due to other complications that could appear because of the advanced liver disease. The most determinant prognostic factor in patients with SBP is the development of HRS [79]. The development of type-1 HRS and the poor short-term prognosis in these patients mostly depends on the degree of liver and renal impairment at diagnosis of SBP. There are several related-factors to an increased risk of type 1 HRS in patients with SBP; serum bilirubin levels ≥4 mg/dL, serum creatinine levels ≥1 mg/dL, and BUN ≥30 mg/dL [80–83]. In addition, SBP may trigger severe life-threatening complications, as for example, renal impairment, gastrointestinal bleeding, and deterioration of hepatic insufficiency, which are responsible for the associated high mortality.

The importance of an early diagnosis and the use of an adequate treatment are crucial in the survival. As previously mentioned, its diagnosis requires a polymorphonuclear leukocyte count greater than 250 cells/mm^3 [2]. The most common organisms isolated in SBP are *Escherichia coli*, *Klebsiella pneumoniae,* and *Streptococcus pneumoniae* [19]. The organism responsible for the infection is isolated in 60–70% of the cases. The remaining cases without the isolation of the organism are considered to have a culture-negative SBP and are treated in the same way as those with a positive culture. In the diagnostic procedure of SBP, must be a differentiation between SBP and secondary peritonitis. Secondary peritonitis is defined because it follows a primary abdominal infection such as gallbladder infection, diverticulitis, or gut perforation. Patients' general conditions rapidly deteriorates in those with secondary peritonitis, for this reason, the diagnosis must be quick, and can be confirmed by a laboratory workup, showing at least two of the following conditions: low glucose concentration levels in ascitic fluid (<50 mg/mL), ascites lactate dehydrogenase higher than serum lactate dehydrogenase, and finally, ascites concentration of proteins >1.5 g/dL. Other typical characteristics in secondary peritonitis are positive cultures with different bacteria, very high count of neutrophils in blood and ascitic fluid. When these conditions appear, a CT scan is recommended to localize the source of the infection [84, 85].

Current guidelines recommend the onset of the empirical treatment immediately after the diagnosis of the infection, and it should be performed with broad-spectrum antibiotics such as a third-generation cephalosporin [2, 3]. Until the last 10 years, the use of third-generation cephalosporins has been shown to be highly effective in the treatment of SBP. Gram-negative bacteria (particularly enterobacteriaceae) were responsible for the majority of the episodes of SBP [86]. However, the etiology and epidemiology in patients with cirrhosis and SBP have changed in the last years, and the efficacy of the third-generation cephalosporins as well as that of alternative therapies such as amoxicillin-clavulanic or quinolones has decreased [78]. It has been speculated that prophylaxis with norfloxacin and invasive procedures could have caused these changes [87].

Patients with nosocomial SBP have a high incidence of multidrug resistant (MDR) bacteria and have a poor response to third-generation cephalosporin in up to 25–66% of cases [78, 88]. Patients with an ineffective first-line treatment for SBP have been associated with very poor survival [86]. A group of experts suggested in 2014 a modification of the current guidelines in patients with nosocomial SBP by using a broader-spectrum of antibiotics, but it was not until last year, when a randomized controlled trial of 32 patients in Padua compared different antibiotic treatment of nosocomial SBP. Patients were randomized to receive meropenem plus daptomycin vs. cetazidime. After 48 hours of treatment, a paracentesis was performed and if the neutrophil count of the ascitic fluid decreased less than 25% compared to pretreatment value, it was considered a treatment failure. The main outcome was the resolution of SBP after 7 days of treatment. The arm with the combination of meropenem plus daptomycin was markedly more effective than the arm of only the third-generation cephalosporin (87 vs. 25%, respectively) with a p value of <0.001. In the study, 90-day transplant-free survival was also evaluated without significantly different values between both arms of treatment, and the last important issue to be described of the study, in the multivariate analysis of 90-day transplant-free survival. The independent predictive factors or survival were ineffective response to first-line treatment (hazard ratio: 20.6; $p < 0.01$), development of AKI throughout the hospitalization (HR: 23.2; $p < 0.01$), and baseline mean arterial pressure (HR: 0.92; $p < 0.01$) [89].

Different broad-spectrum of antibiotics have been proposed, but carbapenems should be used in order to widely cover the spectrum of Gram-negative MDR bacteria. Regarding Gram-positive bacteria, linezolid, lipo, or glycopeptides should be used, but there are some concerns about the high risk of nephrotoxicity and the high rate of vancomycin-resistant enterococci in patients with cirrhosis and nosocomial infections treated with glycopeptides. Duration of therapy should be a minimum of 5–7 days. In patients who develop renal impairment, it is recommended to use intravenous albumin (1.5 g/kg at diagnosis, followed by 1 g/kg on day 3) along with ceftriaxone [90]. The SBP resolution rate ranges between 70 and 90%. Despite the resolution of the infection, patients recovering from an episode of SBP should be considered as potential candidates for liver transplantation.

In patients who have had one episode of SBP, the recurrence rate within 1 year is 70% [91]. Long-term norfloxacin administration (400 mg/day p.o) decreases the recurrence within the first year after SBP from 68% in the placebo group to 20% in the treated group. Therefore, with these results, all patients with a previous episode of SBP should be treated with norfloxacin indefinitely until liver transplantation, death, or resolution of ascites [90, 92].

Prevention of SBP should always be considered especially in high-risk patients, including those with acute gastrointestinal hemorrhage, low ascitic fluid protein concentration (<10–15 g/L), survivors of a previous episode of SBP, and advanced cirrhosis [2]. A RCT showed that the administration of primary prophylaxis with norfloxacin in patients with low protein ascites (<15 g/L), advanced liver disease (Child Pugh score ≥9, serum bilirubin ≥ 3 mg/dL), or deterioration of kidney function (serum creatinine ≥1.2 mg/dL or serum sodium <130 mEq/L) significantly reduce several complications such as 1 year probability of developing SBP (from 61 to 7%), HRS (from 41 to 28%), and improved 3-month survival (from 62 to 94%) [83]. In addition, Soriano et al. demonstrated that intestinal decontamination with norfloxacin was useful to prevent SBP in hospitalized patients with low ascitic fluid protein levels (23 vs. 0%) [91]. Although prophylaxis strategies are beneficial in several aspects, long-term administration of antibiotics leads to the emergence of MDR bacteria as previously explained. However, due to the problem of antibiotic resistance, clinical judgment must guide the use of antibiotic prophylaxis [93]. Rifaximin has been recently proposed as a possible alternative treatment in prophylaxis of SBP. A case control study published many years ago showed that rifaximin was beneficial in the prevention of SBP in patients with hepatic encephalopathy [94]. Since then two studies have compared the efficacy of rifaximin vs. conventional prophylaxis (i.e., norfloxacin) and have provided contradictory results. In a prospective study including patients with and without previous SBP, rifaximin did not lead to a reduction of SBP occurrence in hospitalized patients with advanced liver disease, despite a greater proportion of patients with previous SBP in the norfloxacin group (89 vs. 15%, $p < 0.001$) [95]. Conversely, in a RCT including 260 patients with ascites and a previous episode of SBP, rifaximin was more effective than norfloxacin in reducing the recurrence of SBP (3.9% vs. 14.1%; $p = 0.04$) and even improved survival (13.7% vs. 24.4%; $p = 0.044$) during an 18 month of follow-up [96].

6. Hyponatremia

Furthermore, ascites is very often complicated by a disability of solute-free water excretion. In this setting, the antinatriuretic pathway involves the oversecretion of arginine vasopressin (AVP) that enhances the function of the vasopressin 2 (V2) receptors in the renal distal collecting tubules, inhibiting solute-free water excretion [97]. In this scenario, the AVP production is increased, and there is a lack of clearance of AVP due to cirrhosis itself. In addition, V2 is excessively bound by AVP, triggering more free water retention in kidney tubules by the creation of more aquaporin-2 channels to retain more water. Therefore, these patients cannot remove enough water and results in worsening serum dilution and hypoosmolarity [98]. All this mechanism gives place to dilutional hyponatremia, which is the commonest form of hyponatremia in patients with cirrhosis.

In patients hospitalized with cirrhosis and ascites, the prevalence of hyponatremia, defined by sodium <135 mEq/L, is about 22%, which rises to 49% if the cut-off point is 130 mEq/L. The presence of hyponatremia implies a poor prognosis. It has been demonstrated that hyponatremia is an independent predictive factor to have an increased morbidity and mortality and has been added to the MELD score (Sodium-MELD) for liver donor allocation in the United States [99]. When there is a decrease of 1 unit of sodium below 135 mEq/L, the mortality risk increases by over 10% in patients who are in the list for liver transplant [100]. In addition, it has been demonstrated that hyponatremia is a common event in patients with cirrhosis that may lead to hepatic encephalopathy, with implies a significant decline in quality of life and increased neurological complications throughout liver transplantation. Several transplant centers require correction of hyponatremia prior to liver transplantation, but there is no standard algorithm.

There are several types of hyponatremia. On the one hand, hypervolemic or dilutional hyponatremia as explained previously, and on the other hand, hypovolemic hyponatremia, which is usually secondary to excessive fluid losses from the kidney (overdiuresis secondary to diuretic treatment) or from gastrointestinal tract due to diarrhea. If there is an evidence of dehydration or prerenal azotemia, the treatment in these patients consists in solving the cause with fluid volume expansion replacement. Otherwise, if there is a hypervolemic hyponatremia in the setting of volume overload, it is much more difficult to correct the hyponatremia and for patients to tolerate properly the correction. The therapy consists mainly in water restriction and the increase of free water renal excretion. Daily dietary fluid restriction is recommended to 1.5 L, particularly when the serum sodium is below 130 mEq/L. The main drawback of this strategy is the poor patient's compliance and low response. Another point in the treatment is the diuretic adjustment or withdrawal if it is required.

A study of 997 patients with cirrhosis and ascites demonstrated that serum sodium is less than or equal to 120 mmol/L in only 1.2% of patients and less than or equal to 125 mmol/L in only 5.7% [101]. Attempts to rapidly correct hyponatremia in this setting with hypertonic saline can lead to more complications than the hyponatremia itself [2]. Fluid restriction (i.e., 1–1.5 L of water per day) is seldom effective in improving hyponatremia, but prevents a further decrease in sodium levels [2, 3].

There are other strategies under investigation such as increasing the effective arterial blood volume with intravenous albumin with or without vasoconstrictors as, for example, midodrine. These studies are nonrandomized, and there is a need of further studies before their incorporation into clinical practice [102]. Another interesting treatment option for dilutional hyponatremia is the use of vaptans. They induce the release of solute-free water into urine and improve hyponatremia in patients with cirrhosis [103, 104]. Vaptans result useful and effective in improving sodium levels in 45–82% of patients with dilutional hyponatremia. However, the effect is short and goes back to baseline hyponatremia after the withdrawal of the drug, and they do not improve survival. The side effects of this drug are dehydration, thirst, AKI, and overcorrection of sodium levels. Experts in the issue recommend the use of vaptans for a short period of time in patients with hyponatremia below 125 mEq/L who are hospitalized waiting for a liver transplant. Although they have been approved by the Food and Drug Administration and the European Medication Agency for the management of hypervolemic hyponatremia, their widespread use in cirrhosis warrants further long-term studies [2].

7. Hepatorenal syndrome (HRS)

Finally, the last important complication related with ascites is the development of a harmful event such as HRS. HRS is a late manifestation of extreme circulatory dysfunction with a marked vasoconstriction of the kidney arteries trying to compensate splanchnic vasodilatation secondary to portal hypertension. HRS usually appears in patients with cirrhosis and advance stage of liver dysfunction, and it is always accompanied by ascites and usually hyponatremia [105].

HRS may appear with or without precipitating factors, and there are several predictive factors for the development of HRS. The development of bacterial infections, particularly SBP, is the most important risk factor for HRS (30%) [106]. Other important causes include infections, hypovolemia, paracentesis, and bleeding and nephrotoxic medication. HRS is a potentially reversible functional renal impairment in patients with cirrhosis. It may be rapidly progressive (type I HRS) or may develop gradually (type II HRS), which is usually associated with refractory ascites [106]. HRS is diagnosed with clinical and analytical data and its definition has been updated recently. Since the first definition of HRS type 1 in 1994, there have been slight changes, the last one being in 2015 in the revised consensus recommendations of the International Club of Ascites (ICA) [93]. This last change has been made adopting the concept of AKI originally developed in general critically ill patients and has removed the high cut-off value of serum creatinine (2.5 mg/dL or 220 μmol/L) to start pharmacological treatment with vasoconstrictors. HRS type 1 is defined when AKI stage 2 or more is fulfilled with the rest of HRS criteria (see **Table 3**) [80]. In this way, vasoconstrictors and albumin can be administrated earlier and thus potentially achieving a better efficacy. Although this new definition could have benefits in the efficacy, there is still a lack of biomarkers to differentiate between HRS and parenchymal kidney disease such as acute tubular necrosis. The adequate differentiation could select patients with a real functional damage to start the correct treatment as soon as possible. Recently, there are several urine biomarkers under study, trying to help in this hard work.

The prognosis of HRS remains poor, with an average median survival time of nearly 3 months. High MELD scores and type 1 HRS are associated with very poor prognosis. Median survival of patients with untreated type 1 HRS is approximately 1 month [107]. Current guidelines from the European Association for the Study of the Liver emphasize the early detection and treatment of HRS and give priority to liver transplantation [2].

- Diagnosis of cirrhosis with the presence of ascites

- Acute kidney injury stage 2 or more following the International Ascites Club—Acute kidney criteria

- No response to the withdrawal of diuretics and albumin expansion for 48 h

- Absence of shock

- Absence of nephrotoxic drugs in the recent days

- Absence of structural kidney damage evaluated with hematuria >50 hematites/camp, proteinuria >500 mg/day, and normal kidney ultrasonography

---

Table 3. Hepatorenal syndrome criteria [93].

7.1. Clinical and pharmacological treatment

7.1.1. Terlipressin and norepinephrine

Diuretics should be removed and albumin expansion (1 g/kg) for 48 hours must be administrated if there is no contraindication. If there is no response and the rest of HRS criteria are fulfilled, these patients should be admitted to an intensive care unit. Fluid balance, arterial pressure, vital signs, and central venous pressure are ideally required to prevent volume overload. Current standard treatment involves the use of vasoconstrictors therapy: Terlipressin (1 mg/4–6 hours intravenous bolus) with albumin (20–40 g/day) should be considered as the first-line treatment, and if not available, norepinephrine is a valid alternative. A recent study demonstrated that the administration of terlipressin in continuous infusion instead of boluses had the same rate of response and less side effects [108]. Seventy-eight patients were randomly assigned to receive either continuous intravenous infusion (2 mg/day) or intravenous boluses (0.5 mg/4 h), and if there was no response, the dose was progressively increased to a final dose of 12 mg/day in both groups. The rate of side effects was lower in the infusion than in the boluses (35.29 vs. 62.16%, respectively, $p < 0.025$). The rate of HRS reversal (total and partial) was not significantly different in both groups (76.47 vs. 64.85%). This standard treatment with vasoconstrictor and albumin is effective in 40–50% approximately, although in the last study explained previously it was about 70%. The recurrence of HRS after stopping the vasoconstrictor is about 40%. There are a few studies assessing independent predictive factors of response to terlipressin, and these studies showed a relationship between the improvement in systemic hemodynamics and the effectiveness of treatment. In a study performed in Barcelona, patients with an increase in mean arterial pressure (MAP) of at least 5 mm Hg at day 3 after the beginning of terlipressin, had a higher rate of response. In addition to the improvement in hemodynamics, the degree of liver dysfunction, evaluated with bilirubin greater than 10 mg/dL, was related to a poor response to terlipressin [109]. Another study performed in United States showed that baseline serum creatinine before the beginning of terlipressin predicted the resolution of HRS, and with this information they suggested that an earlier start of treatment would be more effective [110].

A recent RCT compared norepinephrine with terlipressin and demonstrated that reversal of HRS was similar to terlipressin (43 vs. 39%, respectively). Furthermore, there was no statistical difference in survival in both arms: 39% in norepinephrine group and 48% in terlipressin group ($p = 0.461$) [111]. In addition, a recent meta-analysis of 152 patients suggested that norepinephrine is also an effective option for the treatment of HRS as good as terlipressin, when is used in combination with albumin [112].

7.1.2. Midodrine and octreotide

Other therapeutic option is the combination of midodrine and octreotide plus albumin. This therapeutic option has been used widely in countries where terlipressin is not available. A RCT has demonstrated a worse response rate in patients treated with midodrine and octreotide compared to the arm treated with terlipressin (5 vs. 56%, respectively. $p < 0.001$). Ninety-day survival was also lower in the midodrine and octreotide group (29 vs. 56%, $p < 0.06$) [113].

To summarize all these data, although norepinephrine requires an intensive care unit for its use, it is an effective alternative to terlipressin for the treatment of HRS. On the other side, the combination of midodrine and octreotide is not an effective treatment.

7.1.3. Transjugular intrahepatic portosystemic shunt (TIPS)

Transjugular intrahepatic portosystemic shunt (TIPS) may be considered as a second-line therapy, although there is weak evidence to support its use in this complication [2]. TIPS is usually contraindicated in patients with HRS because the syndrome appears in the setting of advanced liver dysfunction. Few small trials have shown renal function improvement and a decrease in renin, aldosterone, and norepinephrine levels after the TIPS insertion [114, 115]. However, data is not strong enough to recommend its use in clinical practice.

7.1.4. Renal replacement therapy

Renal replacement therapy is recommended in guidelines when everything fails, but implies an even worse prognosis [2, 3, 107]. In clinical practice, it is used in patients awaiting liver transplantation, whose renal function did not respond to vasoconstrictor treatment.

7.1.5. Molecular adsorbent recirculating system (MARS)

Liver support with molecular adsorbent recirculating system (MARS) has been used in studies with small sample size in patients who did not respond to standard treatment and it was not effective in changing systemic hemodynamics and kidney function [116]. Only one trial showed a decrease in serum creatinine and bilirubin levels in the arm treated with MARS in comparison to hemodialysis arm [117].

All these invasive treatments are controversially recommended to use in patients without the possibility of liver transplantation and should only be assessed in patients awaiting liver transplant.

7.2. Prevention of HRS

As previously, HRS can be avoided in several situations. The first situation that HRS could be avoided is in large volume paracentesis (LVP). We must give 6-8g of albumin/liter of ascites removed. This action will prevent worsening of circulatory dysfunction, and second, renal impairment, in addition, it also improves survival [2].

The second situation to prevent HRS is in the scenario of SBP. It could be prevented with primary prophylaxis with norfloxacin. Fernandez et al. showed that norfloxacin administration reduced the development of HRS (28 vs. 41%, $p < 0.001$) and 3-month mortality (94 vs. 62%, $p = 0.003$). In addition, norfloxacin administration reduced the 1-year probability of developing a SBP (7 vs. 61%, $p < 0.001$) compared to placebo [83]. Therefore, primary prophylaxis with norfloxacin has an outstanding impact in the clinical course of patients with cirrhosis, reduces the incidence of SBP, delays de development of HRS, and improves survival. This effect is probably secondary to the reduction of bacterial products in the gut, and hence reducing bacterial translocation.

As explained previously, SBP can trigger a kidney failure, which implies a fatal prognosis. In this situation, the utilization of intravenous albumin infusion may improve the effect on circulatory dysfunction in this setting. The study in the Hospital Clinic of Barcelona showed a better 3-month-survival (41 vs. 22%, $p = 0.03$) and lower incidence of kidney failure in patients treated with albumin. (10 vs. 33%, $p = 0.002$). There are ongoing studies, and others done previously recommending the use of albumin expansion in patients with other infections different from SBP, but there is no enough evidence to recommend it in the current guidelines [118].

Author details

Patricia Huelin, Jose Ignacio Fortea, Javier Crespo and Emilio Fábrega*

*Address all correspondence to: digfge@humv.es

Gastroenterology and Hepatology Department, Marqués de Valdecilla University Hospital, Infection, Immunity and Digestive Pathology Group, Research Institute Marqués de Valdecilla (IDIVAL), Grupo Clínico Vinculado al Centro de Investigación Biomédica en Enfermedades Hepáticas y Digestivas (CIBEREHD), Santander, Spain

References

[1] Gines P, Quintero E, Arroyo V, Teres J, Bruguera M, Rimola A, et al. Compensated cirrhosis: Natural history and prognostic factors. Hepatology. 1987;7(1):122-128. DOI: 10.1002/hep.1840070124

[2] European Association for the Study of the Liver. EASL clinical practice guidelines on the management of ascites, spontaneous bacterial peritonitis, and hepatorenal syndrome in cirrhosis. Journal of Hepatology. 2010;53(3):397-417. DOI: 10.1016/j.jhep.2010.05.004

[3] Runyon BA. Introduction to the revised American Association for the Study of Liver Diseases Practice Guideline management of adult patients with ascites due to cirrhosis 2012. Hepatology. 2013;57(4):1651-1653. DOI: 10.1002/hep.26359

[4] Ripoll C, Groszmann R, Garcia-Tsao G, Grace N, Burroughs A, Planas R, et al. Hepatic venous pressure gradient predicts clinical decompensation in patients with compensated cirrhosis. Gastroenterology. 2007;133(2):481-488. DOI: 10.1053/j.gastro.2007.05.024

[5] Schrier RW, Arroyo V, Bernardi M, Epstein M, Henriksen JH, Rodes J. Peripheral arterial vasodilation hypothesis: A proposal for the initiation of renal sodium and water retention in cirrhosis. Hepatology. 1988;8(5):1151-1157. DOI: 10.1002/hep.1840080532

[6] Fabrega E, Berja A, Garcia-Unzueta MT, Guerra-Ruiz A, Cobo M, Lopez M, et al. Influence of aquaporin-1 gene polymorphism on water retention in liver cirrhosis. Scandinavian Journal of Gastroenterology. 2011;46(10):1267-1274. DOI: 10.3109/00365521.2011.603161

[7]   Tandon P, Garcia-Tsao G. Bacterial infections, sepsis, and multiorgan failure in cirrhosis. Seminars in Liver Disease. 2008;**28**(1):26-42. DOI: 10.1055/s-2008-1040319

[8]   Arroyo V, Gines P, Planas R, Panes J, Rodes J. Management of patients with cirrhosis and ascites. Seminars in Liver Disease. 1986;**6**(4):353-369. DOI: 10.1055/s-2008-1040617

[9]   Cardenas A, Arroyo V. Management of ascites and hepatic hydrothorax. Best Practice & Research Clinical Gastroenterology. 2007;**21**(1):55-75. DOI: 10.1016/j.bpg.2006.07.012

[10] Cattau EL Jr, Benjamin SB, Knuff TE, Castell DO. The accuracy of the physical examination in the diagnosis of suspected ascites. JAMA. 1982;**247**(8):1164-1166. DOI: 10.1001/jama.1982.03320330060027

[11] Pose E, Cardenas A. Translating our current understanding of ascites management into new therapies for patients with cirrhosis and fluid retention. Digestive Diseases. 2017;**35**(4):402-410. DOI: 10.1159/000456595

[12] Northup PG, Caldwell SH. Coagulation in liver disease: A guide for the clinician. Clinical Gastroenterology and Hepatology. 2013;**11**(9):1064-1074. DOI: 10.1016/j.cgh.2013.02.026

[13] Grabau CM, Crago SF, Hoff LK, Simon JA, Melton CA, Ott BJ, et al. Performance standards for therapeutic abdominal paracentesis. Hepatology. 2004;**40**(2):484-488. DOI: 10.1002/hep.20317

[14] Runyon BA, Montano AA, Akriviadis EA, Antillon MR, Irving MA, McHutchison JG. The serum-ascites albumin gradient is superior to the exudate-transudate concept in the differential diagnosis of ascites. Annals of Internal Medicine. 1992;**117**(3):215-220. DOI: 10.7326/0003-4819-117-3-215

[15] Runyon BA, Hoefs JC, Morgan TR. Ascitic fluid analysis in malignancy-related ascites. Hepatology. 1988;**8**(5):1104-1109. DOI: 10.1002/hep.1840080521

[16] Wu SS, Lin OS, Chen YY, Hwang KL, Soon MS, Keeffe EB. Ascitic fluid carcinoembryonic antigen and alkaline phosphatase levels for the differentiation of primary from secondary bacterial peritonitis with intestinal perforation. Journal of Hepatology. 2001;**34**(2):215-221. DOI: 10.1016/S0168-8278(00)00039-8

[17] Moore KP, Wong F, Gines P, Bernardi M, Ochs A, Salerno F, et al. The management of ascites in cirrhosis: Report on the consensus conference of the International Ascites Club. Hepatology. 2003;**38**(1):258-266. DOI: 10.1053/jhep.2003.50315

[18] Bernardi M, Laffi G, Salvagnini M, Azzena G, Bonato S, Marra F, et al. Efficacy and safety of the stepped care medical treatment of ascites in liver cirrhosis: A randomized controlled clinical trial comparing two diets with different sodium content. Liver. 1993;**13**(3):156-162. DOI: 10.1111/j.1600-0676.1993.tb00624.x

[19] Salerno F, Guevara M, Bernardi M, Moreau R, Wong F, Angeli P, et al. Refractory ascites: Pathogenesis, definition and therapy of a severe complication in patients with cirrhosis. Liver International. 2010;**30**(7):937-947. DOI: 10.1111/j.1478-3231.2010.02272.x

[20] El-Bokl MA, Senousy BE, El-Karmouty KZ, Mohammed Iel K, Mohammed SM, Shabana SS, et al. Spot urinary sodium for assessing dietary sodium restriction in cirrhotic ascites. World Journal of Gastroenterology. 2009;**15**(29):3631-3635. DOI: 10.3748/wjg.15.3631

[21] Elia C, Graupera I, Barreto R, Sola E, Moreira R, Huelin P, et al. Severe acute kidney injury associated with non-steroidal anti-inflammatory drugs in cirrhosis: A case-control study. Journal of Hepatology. 2015;**63**(3):593-600. DOI: 10.1016/j.jhep.2015.04.004

[22] Garcia-Tsao G, Abraldes JG, Berzigotti A, Bosch J. Portal hypertensive bleeding in cirrhosis: Risk stratification, diagnosis, and management: 2016 practice guidance by the American Association for the study of liver diseases. Hepatology. 2017;**65**(1):310-335. DOI: 10.1002/hep.28906

[23] Romanelli RG, La Villa G, Barletta G, Vizzutti F, Lanini F, Arena U, et al. Long-term albumin infusion improves survival in patients with cirrhosis and ascites: An unblinded randomized trial. World Journal of Gastroenterology. 2006;**12**(9):1403-1407. DOI: 10.3748/wjg.v12.i9.1403.

[24] EASL Clinical Practice Guidelines: Liver transplantation. Journal of Hepatology. 2016;**64**(2):433-485. DOI: 10.1016/j.jhep.2015.10.006

[25] Lenz K, Buder R, Kapun L, Voglmayr M. Treatment and management of ascites and hepatorenal syndrome: An update. Therapeutic Advances in Gastroenterology. 2015;**8**(2):83-100. DOI: 10.1177/1756283x14564673

[26] Kao HW, Rakov NE, Savage E, Reynolds TB. The effect of large volume paracentesis on plasma volume – a cause of hypovolemia? Hepatology. 1985;**5**(3):403-407. DOI: 10.1002/hep.1840050310

[27] Annamalai A, Wisdom L, Herada M, Nourredin M, Ayoub W, Sundaram V, et al. Management of refractory ascites in cirrhosis: Are we out of date? World Journal of Hepatology. 2016;**8**(28):1182-1193. DOI: 10.4254/wjh.v8.i28.1182

[28] Bernardi M, Caraceni P, Navickis RJ, Wilkes MM. Albumin infusion in patients undergoing large-volume paracentesis: A meta-analysis of randomized trials. Hepatology. 2012;**55**(4):1172-1181. DOI: 10.1002/hep.24786

[29] Alessandria C, Elia C, Mezzabotta L, Risso A, Andrealli A, Spandre M, et al. Prevention of paracentesis-induced circulatory dysfunction in cirrhosis: Standard vs. half albumin doses. A prospective, randomized, unblinded pilot study. Digestive and Liver Disease. 2011;**43**(11):881-886. DOI: 10.1016/j.dld.2011.06.001

[30] Boyer TD, Haskal ZJ. The role of Transjugular Intrahepatic Portosystemic Shunt (TIPS) in the Management of Portal Hypertension: Update 2009. Hepatology. 2010;**51**(1):306. DOI: 10.1002/hep.23383

[31] Gines P, Uriz J, Calahorra B, Garcia-Tsao G, Kamath PS, Del Arbol LR, et al. Transjugular intrahepatic portosystemic shunting versus paracentesis plus albumin for refractory ascites in cirrhosis. Gastroenterology. 2002;**123**(6):1839-1847. DOI: 10.1053/gast.2002.37073

[32] Narahara Y, Kanazawa H, Fukuda T, Matsushita Y, Harimoto H, Kidokoro H, et al. Transjugular intrahepatic portosystemic shunt versus paracentesis plus albumin in patients with refractory ascites who have good hepatic and renal function: A prospective randomized trial. Journal of Gastroenterology. 2011;**46**(1):78-85. DOI: 10.1007/s00535-010-0282-9

[33] Salerno F, Merli M, Riggio O, Cazzaniga M, Valeriano V, Pozzi M, et al. Randomized controlled study of TIPS versus paracentesis plus albumin in cirrhosis with severe ascites. Hepatology. 2004;**40**(3):629-635. DOI: 10.1002/hep.20364

[34] Bureau C, Thabut D, Oberti F, Dharancy S, Carbonell N, Bouvier A, et al. Transjugular intrahepatic portosystemic shunts with covered stents increase transplant-free survival of patients with cirrhosis and recurrent ascites. Gastroenterology. 2017;**152**(1):157-163. DOI: 10.1053/j.gastro.2016.09.016

[35] Lebrec D, Giuily N, Hadengue A, Vilgrain V, Moreau R, Poynard T, et al. Transjugular intrahepatic portosystemic shunts: Comparison with paracentesis in patients with cirrhosis and refractory ascites: A randomized trial. French Group of Clinicians and a Group of Biologists. Journal of Hepatology. 1996;**25**(2):135-144. DOI: 10.1016/S0168-8278(96)80065-1

[36] Rossle M, Ochs A, Gulberg V, Siegerstetter V, Holl J, Deibert P, et al. A comparison of paracentesis and transjugular intrahepatic portosystemic shunting in patients with ascites. The New England Journal of Medicine. 2000;**342**(23):1701-1707. DOI: 10.1056/nejm200006083422303

[37] Sanyal AJ, Genning C, Reddy KR, Wong F, Kowdley KV, Benner K, et al. The North American study for the treatment of refractory ascites. Gastroenterology. 2003;**124**(3):634-641. DOI: 10.1053/gast.2003.50088

[38] Albillos A, Banares R, Gonzalez M, Catalina MV, Molinero LM. A meta-analysis of transjugular intrahepatic portosystemic shunt versus paracentesis for refractory ascites. Journal of Hepatology. 2005;**43**(6):990-996. DOI: 10.1016/j.jhep.2005.06.005

[39] D'Amico G, Luca A, Morabito A, Miraglia R, D'Amico M. Uncovered transjugular intrahepatic portosystemic shunt for refractory ascites: A meta-analysis. Gastroenterology. 2005;**129**(4):1282-1293. DOI: 10.1053/j.gastro.2005.07.031

[40] Deltenre P, Mathurin P, Dharancy S, Moreau R, Bulois P, Henrion J, et al. Transjugular intrahepatic portosystemic shunt in refractory ascites: A meta-analysis. Liver International. 2005;**25**(2):349-356. DOI: 10.1111/j.1478-3231.2005.01095.x

[41] Saab S, Nieto JM, Lewis SK, Runyon BA. TIPS versus paracentesis for cirrhotic patients with refractory ascites. The Cochrane Database of Systematic Reviews. 2006(4):Cd004889. DOI: 10.1002/14651858.CD004889.pub2

[42] Salerno F, Camma C, Enea M, Rossle M, Wong F. Transjugular intrahepatic portosystemic shunt for refractory ascites: A meta-analysis of individual patient data. Gastroenterology. 2007;**133**(3):825-834. DOI: 10.1053/j.gastro.2007.06.020

[43] Bai M, Qi XS, Yang ZP, Yang M, Fan DM, Han GH. TIPS improves liver transplantation-free survival in cirrhotic patients with refractory ascites: An updated meta-analysis. World Journal of Gastroenterology. 2014;**20**(10):2704-2714. DOI: 10.3748/wjg.v20.i10.2704

[44] Rossle M. TIPS: 25 years later. Journal of Hepatology. 2013;**59**(5):1081-1093. DOI: 10.1016/j.jhep.2013.06.014

[45] Fagiuoli S, Bruno R, Debernardi Venon W, Schepis F, Vizzutti F, Toniutto P, et al. Consensus conference on TIPS management: Techniques, indications, contraindications. Digestive and Liver Disease. 2017;**49**(2):121-137. DOI: 10.1016/j.dld.2016.10.011

[46] Smith M, Durham J. Evolving Indications for Tips. Techniques in Vascular and Interventional Radiology. 2016;**19**(1):36-41. DOI: 10.1053/j.tvir.2016.01.004

[47] Stirnimann G, Banz V, Storni F, De Gottardi A. Automated low-flow ascites pump for the treatment of cirrhotic patients with refractory ascites. Therapeutic Advances in Gastroenterology. 2017;**10**(2):283-292. DOI: 10.1177/1756283x16684688

[48] Bureau C, Adebayo D, de Rieu MC, Elkrief L, Valla D, Peck-Radosavljevic M, et al. Alfapump system vs. large volume paracentesis for refractory ascites: A multicenter randomized controlled study. Journal of Hepatology. 2017. In press

[49] Bellot P, Welker MW, Soriano G, von Schaewen M, Appenrodt B, Wiest R, et al. Automated low flow pump system for the treatment of refractory ascites: A multi-center safety and efficacy study. Journal of Hepatology. 2013;**58**(5):922-927. DOI: 10.1016/j.jhep.2012.12.020

[50] Sola E, Sanchez-Cabus S, Rodriguez E, Elia C, Cela R, Moreira R, et al. Effects of alfapump system on kidney and circulatory function in patients with cirrhosis and refractory ascites. Liver Transplantation. 2017;**23**(5):583-593. DOI: 10.1002/lt.24763

[51] Wong F, Gines P, Watson H, Horsmans Y, Angeli P, Gow P, et al. Effects of a selective vasopressin V2 receptor antagonist, satavaptan, on ascites recurrence after paracentesis in patients with cirrhosis. Journal of Hepatology. 2010;**53**(2):283-290. DOI: 10.1016/j.jhep.2010.02.036

[52] Wong F, Watson H, Gerbes A, Vilstrup H, Badalamenti S, Bernardi M, et al. Satavaptan for the management of ascites in cirrhosis: Efficacy and safety across the spectrum of ascites severity. Gut. 2012;**61**(1):108-116. DOI: 10.1136/gutjnl-2011-300157

[53] Sakaida I, Yamashita S, Kobayashi T, Komatsu M, Sakai T, Komorizono Y, et al. Efficacy and safety of a 14-day administration of tolvaptan in the treatment of patients with ascites in hepatic oedema. Journal of International Medical Research. 2013;**41**(3):835-847. DOI: 10.1177/0300060513480089

[54] Zhang X, Wang SZ, Zheng JF, Zhao WM, Li P, Fan CL, et al. Clinical efficacy of tolvaptan for treatment of refractory ascites in liver cirrhosis patients. World Journal of Gastroenterology. 2014;**20**(32):11400-11405. DOI: 10.3748/wjg.v20.i32.11400

[55] Akiyama S, Ikeda K, Sezaki H, Fukushima T, Sorin Y, Kawamura Y, et al. Therapeutic effects of short- and intermediate-term tolvaptan administration for refractory ascites in patients with advanced liver cirrhosis. Hepatology Research. 2015;**45**(11):1062-1070. DOI: 10.1111/hepr.12455

[56] Ohki T, Sato K, Yamada T, Yamagami M, Ito D, Kawanishi K, et al. Efficacy of tolvaptan in patients with refractory ascites in a clinical setting. World Journal of Hepatology. 2015;**7**(12):1685-1693. DOI: 10.4254/wjh.v7.i12.1685

[57] Chishina H, Hagiwara S, Nishida N, Ueshima K, Sakurai T, Ida H, et al. Clinical factors predicting the effect of tolvaptan for refractory ascites in patients with decompensated liver cirrhosis. Digestive Diseases. 2016;34(6):659-664. DOI: 10.1159/000448828

[58] Sakaida I, Kawazoe S, Kajimura K, Saito T, Okuse C, Takaguchi K, et al. Tolvaptan for improvement of hepatic edema: A phase 3, multicenter, randomized, double-blind, placebo-controlled trial. Hepatology Research. 2014;44(1):73-82. DOI: 10.1111/hepr.12098

[59] Okita K, Kawazoe S, Hasebe C, Kajimura K, Kaneko A, Okada M, et al. Dose-finding trial of tolvaptan in liver cirrhosis patients with hepatic edema: A randomized, double-blind, placebo-controlled trial. Hepatology Research. 2014;44(1):83-91. DOI: 10.1111/hepr.12099

[60] Cardenas A, Gines P, Marotta P, Czerwiec F, Oyuang J, Guevara M, et al. Tolvaptan, an oral vasopressin antagonist, in the treatment of hyponatremia in cirrhosis. Journal of Hepatology. 2012;56(3):571-578. DOI: 10.1016/j.jhep.2011.08.020

[61] Torres VE, Chapman AB, Devuyst O, Gansevoort RT, Grantham JJ, Higashihara E, et al. Tolvaptan in patients with autosomal dominant polycystic kidney disease. The New England Journal of Medicine. 2012;367(25):2407-2418. DOI: 10.1056/NEJMoa1205511

[62] Angeli P, Volpin R, Piovan D, Bortoluzzi A, Craighero R, Bottaro S, et al. Acute effects of the oral administration of midodrine, an alpha-adrenergic agonist, on renal hemodynamics and renal function in cirrhotic patients with ascites. Hepatology. 1998;28(4):937-943. DOI: 10.1002/hep.510280407

[63] Kalambokis G, Fotopoulos A, Economou M, Pappas K, Tsianos EV. Effects of a 7-day treatment with midodrine in non-azotemic cirrhotic patients with and without ascites. Journal of Hepatology. 2007;46(2):213-221. DOI: 10.1016/j.jhep.2006.09.012

[64] Kalambokis G, Economou M, Fotopoulos A, Al Bokharhii J, Pappas C, Katsaraki A, et al. The effects of chronic treatment with octreotide versus octreotide plus midodrine on systemic hemodynamics and renal hemodynamics and function in nonazotemic cirrhotic patients with ascites. The American Journal of Gastroenterology. 2005;100(4):879-885. DOI: 10.1111/j.1572-0241.2005.40899.x

[65] Singh V, Dhungana SP, Singh B, Vijayverghia R, Nain CK, Sharma N, et al. Midodrine in patients with cirrhosis and refractory or recurrent ascites: A randomized pilot study. Journal of Hepatology. 2012;56(2):348-354. DOI: 10.1016/j.jhep.2011.04.027

[66] Rai N, Singh B, Singh A, Vijayvergiya R, Sharma N, Bhalla A, et al. Midodrine and tolvaptan in patients with cirrhosis and refractory or recurrent ascites: A randomised pilot study. Liver International. 2017;37(3):406-414. DOI: 10.1111/liv.13250

[67] Lenaerts A, Van Cauter J, Moukaiber H, Meunier JC, Ligny G. Treatment of refractory ascites with clonidine and spironolactone. Gastroentérologie Clinique et Biologique. 1997;21(6-7):524-525. DOI: 10.1016/S1879-8551(16)49558-8

[68] Lenaerts A, Codden T, Van Cauter J, Meunier JC, Henry JP, Ligny G. Interest of the association clonidine-spironolactone in cirrhotic patients with ascites and activation of sympathetic nervous system. Acta Gastro-Enterologica Belgica. 2002;65(1):1-5

[69] Lenaerts A, Codden T, Meunier JC, Henry JP, Ligny G. Effects of clonidine on diuretic response in ascitic patients with cirrhosis and activation of sympathetic nervous system. Hepatology. 2006;**44**(4):844-849. DOI: 10.1002/hep.21355

[70] Yang YY, Lin HC, Lee WP, Chu CJ, Lin MW, Lee FY, et al. Association of the G-protein and alpha2-adrenergic receptor gene and plasma norepinephrine level with clonidine improvement of the effects of diuretics in patients with cirrhosis with refractory ascites: A randomised clinical trial. Gut. 2010;**59**(11):1545-1553. DOI: 10.1136/gut.2010.210732

[71] Singh V, Singh A, Singh B, Vijayvergiya R, Sharma N, Ghai A, et al. Midodrine and clonidine in patients with cirrhosis and refractory or recurrent ascites: A randomized pilot study. The American Journal of Gastroenterology. 2013;**108**(4):560-567. DOI: 10.1038/ajg.2013.9

[72] Krag A, Moller S, Henriksen JH, Holstein-Rathlou NH, Larsen FS, Bendtsen F. Terlipressin improves renal function in patients with cirrhosis and ascites without hepatorenal syndrome. Hepatology. 2007;**46**(6):1863-1871. DOI: 10.1002/hep.21901

[73] Fimiani B, Guardia DD, Puoti C, D'Adamo G, Cioffi O, Pagano A, et al. The use of terlipressin in cirrhotic patients with refractory ascites and normal renal function: A multicentric study. European Journal of Internal Medicine. 2011;**22**(6):587-590. DOI: 10.1016/j.ejim.2011.06.013

[74] Conn HO. Spontaneous peritonitis and bacteremia in laennec's cirrhosis caused by enteric organisms. A relatively common but rarely recognized syndrome. Annals of Internal Medicine. 1964;**60**:568-580. DOI: 10.7326/0003-4819-60-4-568

[75] Berg RD. Bacterial translocation from the gastrointestinal tract. Advances in Experimental Medicine and Biology. 1999;**473**:11-30. DOI: 10.1016/S0966-842X(00)88906-4

[76] Moreau R, Jalan R, Gines P, Pavesi M, Angeli P, Cordoba J, et al. Acute-on-chronic liver failure is a distinct syndrome that develops in patients with acute decompensation of cirrhosis. Gastroenterology. 2013;**144**(7):1426-1437. e1-9. DOI: 10.1053/j.gastro.2013.02.042

[77] Follo A, Llovet JM, Navasa M, Planas R, Forns X, Francitorra A, et al. Renal impairment after spontaneous bacterial peritonitis in cirrhosis: Incidence, clinical course, predictive factors and prognosis. Hepatology. 1994;**20**(6):1495-1501. DOI: 10.1002/hep.1840200619

[78] Fernandez J, Acevedo J, Castro M, Garcia O, de Lope CR, Roca D, et al. Prevalence and risk factors of infections by multiresistant bacteria in cirrhosis: A prospective study. Hepatology. 2012;**55**(5):1551-1561. DOI: 10.1002/hep.25532

[79] Moore KP, Aithal GP. Guidelines on the management of ascites in cirrhosis. Gut. 2006;**55**(Suppl 6):vi1-vi12. DOI: 10.1136/gut.2006.099580

[80] Sort P, Navasa M, Arroyo V, Aldeguer X, Planas R, Ruiz-del-Arbol L, et al. Effect of intravenous albumin on renal impairment and mortality in patients with cirrhosis and spontaneous bacterial peritonitis. The New England Journal of Medicine. 1999;**341**(6):403-409. DOI: 10.1056/nejm199908053410603

[81] Arroyo V, Fernandez J. Management of hepatorenal syndrome in patients with cirrhosis. Nature Reviews Nephrology. 2011;**7**(9):517-526. DOI: 10.1038/nrneph.2011.96

[82] Guarner C, Sola R, Soriano G, Andreu M, Novella MT, Vila MC, et al. Risk of a first community-acquired spontaneous bacterial peritonitis in cirrhotic with low ascitic fluid protein levels. Gastroenterology. 1999;117(2):414-419. DOI: 10.1053/gast.1999.0029900414

[83] Fernandez J, Navasa M, Planas R, Montoliu S, Monfort D, Soriano G, et al. Primary prophylaxis of spontaneous bacterial peritonitis delays hepatorenal syndrome and improves survival in cirrhosis. Gastroenterology. 2007;133(3):818-824. DOI: 10.1053/j.gastro.2007.06.065

[84] Akriviadis EA, Runyon BA. Utility of an algorithm in differentiating spontaneous from secondary bacterial peritonitis. Gastroenterology. 1990;98(1):127-133.

[85] Soriano G, Castellote J, Alvarez C, Girbau A, Gordillo J, Baliellas C, et al. Secondary bacterial peritonitis in cirrhosis: A retrospective study of clinical and analytical characteristics, diagnosis and management. Journal of Hepatology. 2010;52(1):39-44. DOI: 10.1016/j.jhep.2009.10.012

[86] Ariza X, Castellote J, Lora-Tamayo J, Girbau A, Salord S, Rota R, et al. Risk factors for resistance to ceftriaxone and its impact on mortality in community, healthcare and nosocomial spontaneous bacterial peritonitis. Journal of Hepatology. 2012;56(4):825-832. DOI: 10.1016/j.jhep.2011.11.010

[87] Fernandez J, Navasa M, Gomez J, Colmenero J, Vila J, Arroyo V, et al. Bacterial infections in cirrhosis: Epidemiological changes with invasive procedures and norfloxacin prophylaxis. Hepatology. 2002;35(1):140-148. DOI: 10.1053/jhep.2002.30082

[88] Piano S, Romano A, Rosi S, Gatta A, Angeli P. Spontaneous bacterial peritonitis due to carbapenemase-producing *Klebsiella pneumoniae*: The last therapeutic challenge. European Journal of Gastroenterology & Hepatology. 2012;24(10):1234-1237. DOI: 10.1097/MEG.0b013e328355d8a2

[89] Piano S, Fasolato S, Salinas F, Romano A, Tonon M, Morando F, et al. The empirical antibiotic treatment of nosocomial spontaneous bacterial peritonitis: Results of a randomized, controlled clinical trial. Hepatology. 2016;63(4):1299-1309. DOI: 10.1002/hep.27941

[90] Gines P, Rimola A, Planas R, Vargas V, Marco F, Almela M, et al. Norfloxacin prevents spontaneous bacterial peritonitis recurrence in cirrhosis: Results of a double-blind, placebo-controlled trial. Hepatology. 1990;12(4 Pt 1):716-724. DOI: 10.1002/hep.1840120416

[91] Soriano G, Guarner C, Teixido M, Such J, Barrios J, Enriquez J, et al. Selective intestinal decontamination prevents spontaneous bacterial peritonitis. Gastroenterology. 1991;100(2):477-481. DOI: 10.5555/uri:pii:001650859190219B

[92] Jalan R, Fernandez J, Wiest R, Schnabl B, Moreau R, Angeli P, et al. Bacterial infections in cirrhosis: A position statement based on the EASL Special Conference 2013. Journal of Hepatology. 2014;60(6):1310-1324. DOI: 10.1016/j.jhep.2014.01.024

[93] Angeli P, Gines P, Wong F, Bernardi M, Boyer TD, Gerbes A, et al. Diagnosis and management of acute kidney injury in patients with cirrhosis: Revised consensus recommendations of the International Club of Ascites. Gut. 2015;64(4):531-537. DOI: 10.1136/gutjnl-2014-308874

[94] Bass NM, Mullen KD, Sanyal A, Poordad F, Neff G, Leevy CB, et al. Rifaximin treatment in hepatic encephalopathy. The New England Journal of Medicine. 2010;362(12):1071-1081. DOI: 10.1056/NEJMoa0907893

[95] Lutz P, Parcina M, Bekeredjian-Ding I, Nischalke HD, Nattermann J, Sauerbruch T, et al. Impact of rifaximin on the frequency and characteristics of spontaneous bacterial peritonitis in patients with liver cirrhosis and ascites. PLoS One. 2014;9(4):e93909. DOI: 10.1371/journal.pone.0093909

[96] Elfert A, Abo Ali L, Soliman S, Ibrahim S, Abd-Elsalam S. Randomized-controlled trial of rifaximin versus norfloxacin for secondary prophylaxis of spontaneous bacterial peritonitis. European Journal of Gastroenterology & Hepatology. 2016;28(12):1450-1454. DOI: 10.1097/meg.0000000000000724

[97] Gines P, Guevara M. Hyponatremia in cirrhosis: Pathogenesis, clinical significance, and management. Hepatology. 2008;48(3):1002-1010. DOI: 10.1002/hep.22418

[98] Lizaola B, Bonder A, Tapper EB, Mendez-Bocanegra A, Cardenas A. The changing role of sodium management in cirrhosis. Current Treatment Options in Gastroenterology. 2016;14(2):274-284. DOI: 10.1007/s11938-016-0094-y

[99] Biggins SW, Rodriguez HJ, Bacchetti P, Bass NM, Roberts JP, Terrault NA. Serum sodium predicts mortality in patients listed for liver transplantation. Hepatology. 2005;41(1):32-39. DOI: 10.1002/hep.20517

[100] Londono MC, Guevara M, Rimola A, Navasa M, Taura P, Mas A, et al. Hyponatremia impairs early posttransplantation outcome in patients with cirrhosis undergoing liver transplantation. Gastroenterology. 2006;130(4):1135-1143. DOI: 10.1053/j.gastro.2006.02.017

[101] Angeli P, Wong F, Watson H, Gines P. Hyponatremia in cirrhosis: Results of a patient population survey. Hepatology. 2006;44(6):1535-1542. DOI: 10.1002/hep.21412

[102] McCormick PA, Mistry P, Kaye G, Burroughs AK, McIntyre N. Intravenous albumin infusion is an effective therapy for hyponatremia in cirrhotic patients with ascites. Gut. 1990;31(2):204-207. DOI: 10.1136/gut.31.2.204

[103] Schrier RW, Gross P, Gheorghiade M, Berl T, Verbalis JG, Czerwiec FS, et al. Tolvaptan, a selective oral vasopressin V2-receptor antagonist, for hyponatremia. The New England Journal of Medicine. 2006;355(20):2099-2112. DOI: 10.1056/NEJMoa065181

[104] Wong F, Blei AT, Blendis LM, Thuluvath PJ. A vasopressin receptor antagonist (VPA-985) improves serum sodium concentration in patients with hyponatremia: A multi-center, randomized, placebo-controlled trial. Hepatology. 2003;37(1):182-191. DOI: 10.1053/jhep.2003.50021

[105] Gines P, Schrier RW. Renal failure in cirrhosis. The New England Journal of Medicine. 2009;361(13):1279-1290. DOI: 10.1056/NEJMra0809139

[106] Cardenas A, Gines P, Uriz J, Bessa X, Salmeron JM, Mas A, et al. Renal failure after upper gastrointestinal bleeding in cirrhosis: Incidence, clinical course, predictive factors, and short-term prognosis. Hepatology. 2001;34(4 Pt 1):671-676. DOI: 10.1053/jhep.2001.27830

[107] Cavallin M, Piano S, Romano A, Fasolato S, Frigo AC, Benetti G, et al. Terlipressin given by continuous intravenous infusion versus intravenous boluses in the treatment of hepatorenal syndrome: A randomized controlled study. Hepatology. 2016;63(3):983-992. DOI: 10.1002/hep.28396

[108] Martin-Llahi M, Pepin MN, Guevara M, Diaz F, Torre A, Monescillo A, et al. Terlipressin and albumin vs. albumin in patients with cirrhosis and hepatorenal syndrome: A randomized study. Gastroenterology. 2008;134(5):1352-1359. DOI: 10.1053/j.gastro.2008.02.024

[109] Nazar A, Pereira GH, Guevara M, Martin-Llahi M, Pepin MN, Marinelli M, et al. Predictors of response to therapy with terlipressin and albumin in patients with cirrhosis and type 1 hepatorenal syndrome. Hepatology. 2010;51(1):219-226. DOI: 10.1002/hep.23283

[110] Boyer TD, Sanyal AJ, Garcia-Tsao G, Blei A, Carl D, Bexon AS, et al. Predictors of response to terlipressin plus albumin in hepatorenal syndrome (HRS) type 1: Relationship of serum creatinine to hemodynamics. Journal of Hepatology. 2011;55(2):315-321. DOI: 10.1016/j.jhep.2010.11.020

[111] Singh V, Ghosh S, Singh B, Kumar P, Sharma N, Bhalla A, et al. Noradrenaline vs. terlipressin in the treatment of hepatorenal syndrome: A randomized study. Journal of Hepatology. 2012;56(6):1293-1298. DOI: 10.1016/j.jhep.2012.01.012

[112] Nassar Junior AP, Farias AQ, D'Albuquerque LA, Carrilho FJ, Malbouisson LM. Terlipressin versus norepinephrine in the treatment of hepatorenal syndrome: A systematic review and meta-analysis. PLoS One. 2014;9(9):e107466. DOI: 10.1371/journal.pone.0107466

[113] Cavallin M, Kamath PS, Merli M, Fasolato S, Toniutto P, Salerno F, et al. Terlipressin plus albumin versus midodrine and octreotide plus albumin in the treatment of hepatorenal syndrome: A randomized trial. Hepatology. 2015;62(2):567-574. DOI: 10.1002/hep.27709

[114] Guevara M, Gines P, Bandi JC, Gilabert R, Sort P, Jimenez W, et al. Transjugular intrahepatic portosystemic shunt in hepatorenal syndrome: Effects on renal function and vasoactive systems. Hepatology. 1998;28(2):416-422. DOI: 10.1002/hep.510280219

[115] Rossle M, Gerbes AL. TIPS for the treatment of refractory ascites, hepatorenal syndrome and hepatic hydrothorax: A critical update. Gut. 2010;59(7):988-1000. DOI: 10.1136/gut.2009.193227

[116] Lavayssiere L, Kallab S, Cardeau-Desangles I, Nogier MB, Cointault O, Barange K, et al. Impact of molecular adsorbent recirculating system on renal recovery in type-1 hepatorenal syndrome patients with chronic liver failure. Journal of Gastroenterology and Hepatology. 2013;28(6):1019-1024. DOI: 10.1111/jgh.12159

[117] Wong F, Raina N, Richardson R. Molecular adsorbent recirculating system is ineffective in the management of type 1 hepatorenal syndrome in patients with cirrhosis with ascites who have failed vasoconstrictor treatment. Gut. 2010;59(3):381-386. DOI: 10.1136/gut.2008.174615

[118] Guevara M, Terra C, Nazar A, Sola E, Fernandez J, Pavesi M, et al. Albumin for bacterial infections other than spontaneous bacterial peritonitis in cirrhosis. A randomized, controlled study. Journal of Hepatology. 2012;57(4):759-765. DOI: 10.1016/j.jhep.2012.06.013

5

Management of Hepatocellular Carcinoma in the Setting of Liver Cirrhosis

Alexander Giakoustidis and Dimitrios E. Giakoustidis

Abstract

Cirrhosis is an increasing cause of morbidity and mortality in more developed coun tries, being the 14th most common cause of death worldwide. Hepatocellular carcinoma (HCC) consists a significant health issue worldwide, responsible for more than 1 million deaths annually. The incidence and mortality rates vary across different geographical areas. Between 60 and 90% of HCC patients already have liver cirrhosis, attributed mainly to chronic hepatitis B and C, alcohol abuse, and non-alcoholic fatty liver disease (NASH). The surgical management of HCC in the setting of liver cirrhosis with curative intent includes liver resection, ablation or microwave coagulation, and liver transplantation (LT). Liver resection in a cirrhotic liver with HCC is associated with lower survival rates compared with liver transplantation (LT), depending on the diseases' stage but on the contrary liver resection could be potentially offered in a larger population compared to liver transplantation. One of the biggest limitations of liver resection is the risk of tumor recurrence, which is high, and it may exceed 70% 5 years after the procedure. Liver transplantation is considered the best treatment for hepatocellular carcinoma at early stages because it removes the tumor as well as the underlying cirrhotic liver.

Keywords: liver resection, liver transplantation, HCC, cirrhosis, RFA, TACE

1. Introduction

Cirrhosis is an increasing cause of morbidity and mortality in more developed countries, being the 14th most common cause of death worldwide. The natural history of cirrhosis is initially compensated and is asymptomatic progressing into decompensated cirrhosis with portal hypertension and liver dysfunction and in the development of hepatocellular carcinoma (HCC).

Hepatocellular carcinoma consists a significant health issue worldwide, responsible for more than 1 million deaths annually. The incidence and mortality rates vary across different geographical areas [1, 2]. Between 60 and 90% of HCC patients already have liver cirrhosis, attributed mainly to chronic hepatitis B and C, alcohol abuse, and non-alcoholic fatty liver disease (NASH). In the past, HCC was usually diagnosed late during the course of the liver disease, and consequently, the vast majority of patients had a poor prognosis at diagnosis. Survival is poor, and high recurrence rates after treatment were exhibited regardless of treatment. Currently, the implementation of screening programs especially for chronic virus hepatitis, and advances in radiological assessment, leads to an increasing proportion of patients being diagnosed within early stage of HCC. The surgical management of HCC in the setting of liver cirrhosis with curative intent includes liver resection, ablation or microwave coagulation, and liver transplantation (LT).

2. Hepatocellular carcinoma staging

Cancer staging should serve to select the appropriate primary and adjuvant therapy, to estimate the prognosis, and also to assist in the evaluation of the results of treatment and this is also applicable in HCC [3, 4]. The EASL panel of experts recommended the consideration of four-related aspects: tumor stage, degree of liver function impairment, general condition of the patient, and treatment efficacy [5]. In the past, the Okuda classification [6] has been widely applied in HCC patients, and it included parameters related to the liver functional status like albumin, ascites, and bilirubin. The Cancer of the Liver Italian Program (CLIP) score [7] was proposed and validated [8]. It combines four variables that provide a seven-stage classification system and was more discriminatory compared with Okuda stage and TNM. Groups from Asia published different survival rates compromising its external validation [9]. The Barcelona-Clinic Liver Cancer (BCLC) staging system [10] was proposed by the Barcelona group on the basis of the results obtained from cohort and RCT studies. It consists a staging classification that uses variables related to performance status, tumor stage, liver functional status, characteristic of the tumor, vascular invasion, and the presence of portal hypertension (PH). This BCLC classification system has become a widely accepted algorithm for all HCC patients in earlier disease, linking their current status prognosis with treatment recommendations. Recently, a new staging system was proposed from the Hong Kong group [11]. The Hong Kong Liver Cancer (HKLC) used four prognostic factors in the treatment of HCC, the Eastern Cooperative Oncology Group performance status (ECOG PS), Child-Pugh grade, liver tumor status, and presence of extrahepatic vascular invasion/metastasis. Liver tumor status was a composite factor of the size of the largest tumor in the liver, number of tumor nodules, and the presence or absence of intrahepatic vascular invasion. The authors support that the HKLC staging classification has the potential to provide better prognostic classification than BCLC staging and may be more effective in identifying patients suitable for more aggressive treatments, hence yielding a better survival outcome.

3. Liver resection vs. TACE and RFA

Liver resection when it is feasible, in a cirrhotic liver with HCC, is associated with lower survival rates compared with liver transplantation (LT), varying from 35 to 62% at 3 years and from 17 to 50% at 5 years, depending on the diseases' stage but on the contrary liver resection could be potentially offered in a larger population compared to liver transplantation. One of the biggest limitations of liver resection is the risk of tumor recurrence, which is high, and it may exceed 70% 5 years after the procedure. Hepatic resection tends to be applicable only in patients with cirrhosis that is classified as Child-Pugh class A or B and with mild portal hypertension. The application of palliative therapies like radiofrequency ablation (RFA), microwave coagulation (MC) and transarterial chemoembolization (TACE) is frequently limited by impaired hepatocellular function, severe portal hypertension, or multiple tumor nodules.

Huang et al. [12] in a large randomized trial of 230 patients within the Milan criteria (BCLC stage A) compared surgical resection and radiofrequency ablation for HCC patients indicating a favorable outcome for surgically treated patients. Wang et al. in their meta-analysis evaluated three randomized and 25 nonrandomized trials, and they confirmed the long-term superiority of surgical treatment [13]. In another meta-analysis by Kapitanov et al. and taking into account the limited available literature and prospective studies, they concluded that liver resection shows significantly improved long-term survival compared to TACE in cirrhotic patients with BCLC stage A and B HCC. T. Utsunomiya et al. conducted a large prospective multicenter trial and demonstrated clear superiority for hepatic resection when compared to TACE and RFA for patients with Child-Pugh stage A and B liver cirrhosis and stage II HCC (JIS scores 1 and 2) [14]. Peng et al. [15] showed that even for patients with portal venous tumor, thrombus liver resection improves long-term survival compared to TACE as long as tumor thrombosis was confined to the liver. This effect vanished in the presence of extensive tumor thrombosis into the portal venous confluence and the superior mesenteric vein. Zhong et al. [16] demonstrate clear superiority for hepatic resection versus TACE in terms of patient survival. They analyzed an impressive total number of 1259 of patients with the vast majority of cases being hepatitis-B positive. Limitations of the study were a rather heterogeneous patient collective and a mean patient age and tumor size being both greater in the TACE group. For this reason, matched-pair analysis was performed between TACE and resection patients with identical demographics confirming the positive overall results for surgically treated patients.

Laparoscopic liver resection (LLR) consists a contemporary surgical approach in the management of hepatocellular carcinoma with or without liver cirrhosis. The indications for LLR have changed substantially since its introduction. In the beginning, it was limited to benign diseases, while gaining increased knowledge and experience of the procedure, its indications have expanded to malignant diseases, including HCC and colorectal liver metastasis [17]. However, laparoscopy has been limitedly used for liver resection due to the risk of air embolism and the difficulty of parenchymal dissection and bleeding control [18]. Therefore, LLR has been frequently performed for tumors superficially located in the anterolateral segments

[19]. Liver cirrhosis consists a substantial risk factor for developing postoperative complications following hepatectomy. Severe blood loss or prolonged ascites after major hepatectomy, especially by open surgery, can occur by interruption of collateral circulation in the parietal wall and surrounding ligamentsin patients with liver cirrhosis [20] and may prolong the postoperative hospital stay or induce hepatic failure in some patients. However, LLR may minimize the reduction in collateral and lymphatic flow caused by laparotomy and mobilization [21, 22]. The benefits of LLR in liver cirrhosis include enhanced recovery, less postoperative pain, and potentially less postoperative complications. Other important advantages of LLR in patients with liver cirrhosis are the lower incidences of postoperative liver failure and ascites due to minimal invasiveness of LLR, which helps to preserve collateral circulation. Therefore, laparoscopic hepatectomy may be a good option in patients with cirrhosis [23].

4. Down-staging and bridge therapies

4.1. TACE

Down-staging in HCC patients includes but not limited to TACE, radiofrequency ablation (RFA), percutaneous ethanol injection (PEI), microwave coagulation (MC), resection, and radiation [24]. The objective of down-staging is to decrease the tumor size and/or number of nodules in those patients that initially are presenting with tumors beyond the acceptable criteria for liver transplantation in different centers. The response to different DS treatment has to be based on radiological measurement of tumor characteristics. The EASL HCC guidelines suggested, and this was also endorsed by the AASLD guideline, that assessment of tumor response should consider only the area of viable tumor [25], defined by arterial enhancement on a radiological contrast study modified response evaluation criteria in solid tumors (mRECIST).

Prospective studies showed that survival after liver transplantation in patients with large tumor burden successfully treated by down-staging was similar to survival in patients who initially met the criteria for transplantation [26]. There is currently no well-defined upper limit for size and number of lesions as eligibility criteria for down-staging, although the presence of vascular invasion and extrahepatic disease is generally considered absolute contraindications.

The role of DS has been ambiguous concerning the overall and recurrence-free survival post-transplantation. In the case that complete tumor necrosis with locoregional therapy is achieved, this is associated with better survival. A multicenter case-control study compared matched patients with TACE (100) and without TACE (100) [27] showed that survival rates 5 years after OLT were similar 59.3% versus 59.4%, respectively. In addition, there were fewer recurrences in the TACE group although this was not statistically significant. Moreover, the waiting times were short, and the median number of TACE procedures was only 1, and this may impact negatively the detection of any advantage for TACE.

Comparisons of the dropout rates of treated and untreated patients are limited with the existing data. Yao et al. from the UCSF analyzed 70 patients a proportion of them having pretransplant therapy either TACE or ablation, and this was associated with a significantly lower risk of dropout. Disadvantage of the study was that the population was heterogeneous regarding the disease stage, and the criteria for treatment were influenced by external factors [28]. Another study from Toronto including 74 patients identified a difference in tumor-related dropout that became apparent only after 300 days [29].

Drug-eluting beads loaded with chemotherapy agents are delivered into the tumor through the feeding artery. Chemotherapy agents are released gradually, so systemic side effects are reduced, and tumor drug delivery is enhanced. The PRECISION study compared conventional TACE with DEB for the treatment of 212 patients with Child-Pugh A or B cirrhosis and unresectable HCC [30]. Subpopulation analysis revealed that patients with Child-Pugh B cirrhosis or bilobar tumor disease showed a better response to DEB. In addition, the overall DEB was better tolerated than conventional TACE. While it appears that DEB might be better tolerated than conventional TACE, more extensive data are needed.

4.2. RFA

The use of RFA as a bridge to transplantation in HCC patients is also applicable. It has been reported complete tumor necrosis at pathological evaluation of the explanted liver in 47–75% of cases, with a mean value of 58% [31–35]. Different rates of complete necrosis ranges have been observed between 50 and 78% in HCCs up to 3 cm and between 13 and 43% in larger neoplasms, respectively [31–33]. Furthermore, in two studies, a tumor size larger than 3 cm was the only risk factor found for HCC recurrence after treatment [31–33]. Analysis of the largest available series of HCC patients awaiting LT regarding RFA-related complications showed the safety of the procedure. From five large series, we could see that the mean rate of post-ablation major complications was below 5% [31–36], and in addition, the risk of tumor seeding at the level of the abdomen wall appears to be low.

4.3. Liver resection

Belghiti [37] proposed that resection can be used as an alternative treatment option for HCC or before LT as "down-staging" procedure. Liver resection can be used as a primary therapy in patients with HCC and well-preserved liver function, with LT reserved as a "salvage" therapy for patients who developed recurrence or liver failure. Moreover, resection can be used as an initial therapy in order to select patients whose explants pathology would be favorable for LT. Resection could also be used as a "bridge" therapy for patients who have been already enlisted for LT. Whether resection or LT should be the treatment of choice for small HCC in patients with preserved liver function is a hot issue and still in debate. Long-term overall survival after resection or transplantation appears comparable in a well-selected population with HCC within the Milano criteria [37–39]. LT has the advantage of increased disease-free survival compared with liver resection, but its use is limited by shortage of liver organs. It has been proposed by the group of Belgiti but also from other groups that resection as the first-line treatment for patients with small HCC with preserved liver function, followed by salvage transplantation only for recurrence or liver failure, would feasible in a large proportion of HCC patients [37–39].

Considering emergency LT after resection as center, policy would require a strict selection of the candidate with clear and strong indicators of irreversible postoperative liver insufficiency. Patients with liver failure due to massive necrosis of the remnant liver or those with uncontrollable bleeding are easy to be identified, but it is unclear and very difficult to ascertain the irreversibility of liver insufficiency in all settings. A significant increase in international normalized ratio (INR) and serum bilirubin within the first postoperative days is a common characteristic of extended resection making identification and selection of patients in need for early liver transplantation tricky. It is documented that, in the absence of any treatable complication, the lack of significant improvement on postoperative day 5 may lead to strongly considering rescue transplantation [40].

Poon et al. [38] proposed liver resection for HCC lesions in selected patients eligible for LT and to reserve LT for those who develop recurrence or deterioration of liver function. This approach, which proposes resection as a bridge treatment to prevent tumor progression during the waiting period, looks attractive but has not been studied well, especially with prospective studies and needs external validation of published data from the various transplant centers. As major concern from transplant surgeons is that prior liver resection especially if done in no-specialized centers could complicate the operative transplant procedure, increase the risk of postoperative complications, and finally compromise results and impair the survival advantage of transplantation over resection alone.

5. Liver transplantation

Liver transplantation is considered the best treatment for hepatocellular carcinoma at early stages because it removes the tumor as well as the underlying cirrhotic liver. However, as a result of organ shortage, it is anticipated that transplantation to HCC patients will be performed with an expected five-year post-transplantation survival of greater than 50%, and, in most programs, an expected five-year post-transplantation survival similar to survival achieved after liver transplantation for benign liver diseases (i.e., 70%).

In 1996, Mazzaferro et al. [41] conducted a prospective cohort study defining restrictive selection criteria (Milan Criteria (MC)) that led to improved survival for transplant patients compared with any other previous experience with transplantation for HCC. Adopting the MC demonstrated a five-year survival of 70% after LT [41]. The survival outcome of MC is comparable to LT in benign diseases and given that this excellent outcome MC has been established from most liver societies (EASL and AASLD guidelines) as the golden standard in selecting HCC patients for liver transplant [42, 43].

In 2001, Yao et al. from University of California San Francisco (UCSF) [44] demonstrated a tumor recurrence rate of little more than 10% and survival rates exceeding 70% in T1, T2 and T3 tumors. The new criteria included solitary tumors smaller or equal to 6.5 cm in size or three or fewer tumors with the largest diameter not exceeding 4.5 cm and the total tumor diameter being less or equal to 8 cm and became known as the UCSF criteria.

Alternative criteria have been proposed by other centers. These include criteria from the Asan Medical Center in Korea [45], from Hangzhou, China [46], the University Clinic of Navarra in Spain [47], Kyoto, Japan [48]. All use different criteria in terms of number of nodules and size and in addition try to implement some biological criteria like α-FP, protein induced by vitamin K absence II (PIVKA II) and other. Unfortunately, none of these criteria have been externally validated in order to get wider acceptance.

In 2009, the Metroticket was introduced by Mazzafero et al. [49]. The Metroticket introduced the logic that the further you expand HCC staging criteria for LT, this would impact negatively the outcome in terms of higher recurrence rates and poorer overall survival. This model potential could be a simple predictive model for estimating the survival of patients undergoing LT with tumors exciding the Milan criteria in number and size of the tumors.

High α-fetoprotein (AFP) levels are predictive of poor prognosis in non-transplant patients, and AFP levels greater than 1000 ng/mL have been associated with a high risk of recurrence in the University of California, San Francisco (UCSF), experience [44] after liver transplantation.

AFP value is proposed as a good indicator in selecting HCC patients for LT [50, 51]. In the non-transplant patients, an elevated AFP is a marker of advanced disease. It has been proposed that an increase in AFP levels might be an indicator of tumor aggressiveness including differentiation degree and vascular invasion and, consequently, lead to a higher risk of tumor recurrence. Toso et al. [52] analyzed adult recipients in the Scientific Registry of Transplant Recipients. In the multivariate analysis, it was shown that high AFP levels and TTV >115 cm^3 were associated with poor long-term survival.

Duvoux et al. [53] in a French multicenter study showed that AFP levels strongly correlated with the pathologic features of HCC. Based on the analysis of 453 explanted livers, they found that increased AFP levels were associated with vascular invasion and loss of differentiation.

Living Donor Liver Transplantation (LDLT) consists of an alternative option to Deceased Donor Liver Transplantation (DDLT). Special consideration regarding LDLT for HCC is required, since patients for LDLT are not dependent of the cadaveric donor pool, but bring their "own" liver graft. It is important to stress that the application of strict eligibility criteria similar the one required with cadaveric grafts for patients with HCC might not be necessary. However, survival benefit to the recipient should be substantial, and the risk to the donor must be incorporated into the centers policy, since it is clearly unethical to expose a donor to a significant risk of morbidity or mortality. Generally, similar criteria apply to patients undergoing DDLT or LDLT. For patients subjected to either DDLT or LDLT for HCC within MC, similar outcomes have been documented [54, 55]. Asian groups have proposed different policies concerning different criteria for LDLT in the setting of HCC. The Tokyo group applies the 5–5 rule (number of tumors not exceeding 5 and maximum tumor diameter not exceeding 5 cm); the Kyoto group the 10–5 rule (number of tumors not exceeding 10; each tumor not exceeding 5 cm) in combination with the biological tumor marker PIVKA (or DCP) (not exceeding 400 mAu/ml), and finally, the Seoul group adopts an intermediate policy with limiting the number of tumors not exceeding 6 and the maximum tumor diameter not exceeding 5 cm. All three groups obtained around 85% 3–5 years disease free survival (DFS) survival rates.

In the West, LDLT is often stretched in patients who do not strictly meet the Milan criteria for MELD exception points and have tumors with a probable worse prognosis. Updated re-analyzed data of the A2ALL cohorts concluded that "differences in tumor characteristics and management of HCC in patients who received LDLT likely accounted for the higher HCC recurrence rates observed in their LDLT group."

Systematic review analysis by Grant et al. [56] suggests that DFS is worse after LDLT compared with DDLT for HCC. Decreased DFS may eventually translate to decreased OS, and it is advisable that the increased risk of recurrence should be communicated to all potential donors and recipients who are considering LDLT for HCC.

Author details

Alexander Giakoustidis[1] and Dimitrios E. Giakoustidis[2]*

*Address all correspondence to: dgiak@auth.gr

1 Department of HPB Surgery, Royal London Hospital, London, UK

2 Division of Transplant Surgery, Department of Surgery, School of Health Sciences, Aristotle University of Thessaloniki, Thessaloniki, Greece

References

[1] Fattovich G, Stroffolini T, Zagni I, Donato F. Hepatocellular carcinoma in cirrhosis: Incidence and risk factors. Gastroenterology. 2004;**127**:S35-S50.

[2] Sangiovanni A, Del Ninno E, Fasani P, De Fazio C, Ronchi G, Romeo R, et al. Increased survival of cirrhotic patients with a hepatocellular carcinoma detected during surveillance. Gastroenterology. 2004;**126**:1005-1014.

[3] Fleming I. AJCC/TNM cancer staging, present and future. Journal of Clinical Oncology. 2001;**77**:233-236.

[4] Pons F, Varela M, Llovet JM. Staging systems in hepatocellular carcinoma. HPB. 2005;**7**: 35-41.

[5] Bruix J, Sherman M, Llovet JM, Beaugrand M, Lencioni R, Christensen E, et al. Clinical management of hepatocellular carcinoma. Conclusions of the Barcelona-2000 EASL Conference. Journal of Hepatology. 2001;**35**:421-430.

[6] Okuda K, Ohtsuki T, Obata H, Tomimatsu M, Okazaki N, Haregawwa H, et al. Natural history of hepatocellular carcinoma and prognosis in relation to treatment. Cancer. 1985;**56**:918-928.

[7] CLIP. Prospective validation of the CLIP score: A new prognostic system for patients with cirrhosis and hepatocellular carcinoma. Hepatology. 2000;**31**:840-845.

[8] Levy I, Sherman M. Staging of hepatocellular carcinoma: Assessment of the CLIP, Okuda and Child-Pugh staging systems in a cohort of 257 patients in Toronto. Gut. 2002;**50**:881-885.

[9] Ueno S, Tanabe G, Sako K, Hiwaki T, Hokotate H, Fukukura Y, et al. Discrimination value of the new western prognostic system (CLIP score) for hepatocellular carcinoma in 662 Japanese patients. Hepatology. 2001;**34**:529-534.

[10] Llovet JM, Bru C, Bruix J. Prognosis of hepatocellular carcinoma: The BCLC staging classification. Seminars in Liver Disease. 1999;**19**:329-338.

[11] Yau T, Tang VYF, Yao TJ, Fan ST, Lo CM, Poon RTP. Development of Hong Kong liver cancer staging system with treatment stratification for patients with hepatocellular carcinoma. Gastroenterology. 2014;**146**:1691-1700.

[12] Huang J, Yan L, Cheng Z, et al. A randomized trial comparing radiofrequency ablation and surgical resection for HCC conforming to the Milan criteria. Annals of Surgery. 2010;**252**(6):903-912.

[13] Wang J-H, Wang C-C, Hung C-H, Chen C-L, Lu S-N. Survival comparison between surgical resection and radiofrequency ablation for patients in BCLC very early/early stage hepatocellular carcinoma. Journal of Hepatology. 2012;**56**(2):412-418.

[14] Utsunomiya T, Shimada M, Kudo M, et al. Nationwide study of 4741 patients with non-B non-C hepatocellular carcinoma with special reference to the therapeutic impact. Annals of Surgery. 2014;**259**(2):336-345.

[15] Peng Z-W, Guo R-P, Zhang Y-J, Lin X-J, Chen M-S, Lau WY. Hepatic resection versus transcatheter arterial chemoembolization for the treatment of hepatocellular carcinoma with portal vein tumor thrombus. Cancer. 2012;**118**(19):4725-4736.

[16] Zhong JH, Peng NF, You XM, Ma L, Li LQ. Hepatic resection is superior to transarterial chemoembolization for treating intermediate-stage hepatocellular carcinoma. Liver International. 2016; 31. doi: 10.1111/liv.13290

[17] Koffron A, Geller D, Gamblin TC, Abecassis M. Laparoscopic liver surgery: Shifting the management of liver tumors. Hepatology. 2006;**44**:1694-1700.

[18] Buell JF, Thomas MJ, Doty TC, Gersin KS, Merchen TD, Gupta M, Rudich SM, Woodle ES. An initial experience and evolution of laparoscopic hepatic resectional surgery. Surgery. 2004;**136**:804-811.

[19] Cherqui D, Husson E, Hammoud R, Malassagne B, Stéphan F, Bensaid S, Rotman N, Fagniez PL. Laparoscopic liver resections: A feasibility study in 30 patients. Annals of Surgery. 2000;**232**:753-762.

[20] Kanazawa A, Tsukamoto T, Shimizu S, Kodai S, Yamazoe S, Yamamoto S, Kubo S. Impact of laparoscopic liver resection for hepatocellular carcinoma with F4-liver cirrhosis. Surgical Endoscopy. 2013;**27**:2592-2597.

[21] Nguyen KT, Gamblin TC, Geller DA. World review of laparoscopic liver resection—2,804 patients. Annals of Surgery. 2009;**250**:831-841.

[22] Belli G, Limongelli P, Fantini C, D'Agostino A, Cioffi L, Belli A, Russo G. Laparoscopic and open treatment of hepatocellular carcinoma in patients with cirrhosis. British Journal of Surgery. 2009;**96**:1041-1048.

[23] Morise Z, Kawabe N, Kawase J, Tomishige H, Nagata H, Ohshima H, Arakawa S, Yoshida R, Isetani M. Pure laparoscopic hepatectomy for hepatocellular carcinoma with chronic liver disease. World Journal of Hepatology. 2013;**5**:487-495.

[24] Barakat O, Wood RP, Ozaki CF, Ankoma-Sey V, Galati J, Skolkin M, et al. Morphological features of advanced hepatocellular carcinoma as a predictor of downstaging and liver transplantation: An intention-to-treat analysis. Liver Transplantation. 2010;**16**:289-299.

[25] Lencioni R, Llover JM. Modified RECIST (mRECIST) assessment for hepatocellular carcinoma. Seminars in Liver Disease. 2010;**30**:52-60.

[26] Ravaioli M, Grazi GL, Piscaglia F, Trevisani F, Cescon M, Ercolani G, et al. Liver transplantation for hepatocellular carcinoma: Results of down-staging in patients initially outside the Milan selection criteria. American Journal of Transplantation. 2008;**8**:2547-2557.

[27] Decaens T, Roudot-Thoraval F, Bresson-Hadni S, Meyer C, Gugenheim J, Durand F, et al. Impact of pretransplantation transarterial chemoembolization on survival and recurrence after liver transplantation for hepatocellular carcinoma. Liver Transplantation. 2005;**11**:767-775.

[28] Yao FY, Bass NM, Nikolai B, Merriman R, Davern TJ, Kerlan R, et al. A follow-up analysis of the pattern and predictors of dropout from the waiting list for liver transplantation in patients with hepatocellular carcinoma: Implications for the current organ allocation policy. Liver Transplantation. 2003;**9**:684-692.

[29] Cheow PC, Al-Alwan A, Kachura J, Ho CS, Grant D, Cattral M, et al. Ablation of hepatoma as a bridge to liver transplantation reduces drop-out from prolonged waiting time [abstract]. Hepatology. 2005;**42**(suppl 1):333A.

[30] Lammer J, Malagari K, Vogl T, Pilleul F, Denys A, Watkinson A, Pitton M, Sergent G, Pfammatter T, Terraz S, Benhamou Y, Avajon Y, Gruenberger T, Pomoni M, Langenberger H, Schuchmann M, Dumortier J, Mueller C, Chevallier P, Lencioni R; PRECISION V Investigators. Prospective randomized study of doxorubicin-eluting-bead embolization in the treatment of hepatocellular carcinoma: Results of the PRECISION V study. Cardiovascular and Interventional Radiology. 2010;**33**:41-52.

[31] Mazzaferro V, Battiston C, Perrone S, Pulvirenti A, Regalia E, Romito R, Sarli D, Schiavo M, Garbagnati F, Marchianò A, Spreafico C, Camerini T, Mariani L, Miceli R, Andreola S. Radiofrequency ablation of small hepatocellular carcinoma in cirrhotic patients awaiting liver transplantation: A prospective study. Annals of Surgery. 2004;**240**:900-909. PMID: 15492574. DOI: 10.1097/01.sla.0000143301.56154.95

[32] Lu DS, Yu NC, Raman SS, Lassman C, Tong MJ, Britten C, Durazo F, Saab S, Han S, Finn R, Hiatt JR, Busuttil RW. Percutaneous radiofrequency ablation of hepatocellular carcinoma as a bridge to liver transplantation. Hepatology. 2005;**41**:1130-1137. PMID: 15841454. DOI: 10.1002/hep.20688

[33] Pompili M, Mirante VG, Rondinara G, Fassati LR, Piscaglia F, Agnes S, Covino M, Ravaioli M, Fagiuoli S, Gasbarrini G, Rapaccini GL. Percutaneous ablation procedures in cirrhotic patients with hepatocellular carcinoma submitted to liver transplantation: Assessment of efficacy at explant analysis and of safety for tumor recurrence. Liver Transplantation. 2005;**11**:1117-1126. PMID: 16123960. DOI: 10.1002/lt.20469

[34] Brillet PY, Paradis V, Brancatelli G, Rangheard AS, Consigny Y, Plessier A, Durand F, Belghiti J, Sommacale D, Vilgrain V. Percutaneous radiofrequency ablation for hepatocellular carcinoma before liver transplantation: A prospective study with histopathologic comparison. American Journal of Roentgenology. 2006;**186**:S296–S305. PMID: 16632691. DOI: 10.2214/AJR.04.1927

[35] Rodríguez-Sanjuán JC, González F, Juanco C, Herrera LA, López-Bautista M, González-Noriega M, García-Somacarrera E, Figols J, Gómez-Fleitas M, Silván M. Radiological and pathological assessment of hepatocellular carcinoma response to radiofrequency. A study on removed liver after transplantation. World Journal of Surgery. 2008;**32**:1489-1494. PMID: 18373117. DOI: 10.1007/s00268-008-9559-z

[36] DuBay DA, Sandroussi C, Kachura JR, Ho CS, Beecroft JR, Vollmer CM, Ghanekar A, Guba M, Cattral MS, McGilvray ID, Grant DR, Greig PD. Radiofrequency ablation of hepatocellular carcinoma as a bridge to liver transplantation. HPB (Oxford) 2011;**13**:24-32. PMID: 21159100. DOI: 10.1111/j.1477-2574.2010.00228.x

[37] Belghiti J. Resection and liver transplantation for HCC. Journal of Gastroenterology. 2009;**44**:132-135.

[38] Poon RT, Fan ST, Lo CM, Liu CL, Wong J. Long-term survival and pattern of recurrence after resection of small hepatocellular carcinoma in patients with preserved liver function: Implications for a strategy of salvage transplantation. Annals of Surgery. 2002;**235**:373-382.

[39] Cha CH, Ruo L, Fong Y, Jarnagin WR, Shia J, Blumgart LH, DeMatteo RP. Resection of hepatocellular carcinoma in patients otherwise eligible for transplantation. Annals of Surgery. 2003;**238**:315-321.

[40] Balzan S, Belghiti J, Farges O, Ogata S, Sauvanet A, Delefosse D, et al. The "50-50 Criteria" on postoperative day 5: An accurate predictor of liver failure and death after hepatectomy. Annals of Surgery. 2005;**242**:824-829.

[41] Mazzaferro V, Regalia E, Doci R, Andreola S, Pulvirenti A, Bozzetti F, Montalto F, Ammatuna M, Morabito A, Gennari L. Liver transplantation for the treatment of small hepatocellular carcinomas in patients with cirrhosis. The New England Journal of Medicine. 1996;**334**:693-699.

[42] EASL–EORTC Clinical Practice Guidelines: Management of hepatocellular carcinoma. Journal of Hepatology. 2012;**56**:908-943.

[43] Bruix J, Sherman M. AASLD practice guideline management of hepatocellular carcinoma: An update. Hepatology. 2011;**53**:1020-1022.

[44] Yao FY, Ferrell L, Bass NM, et al. Liver transplantation for hepatocellular carcinoma: Expansion of the tumor size limits does not adversely impact survival. Hepatology. 2001;**33**:1394-1403.

[45] Lee SG, Hwang S, Moon DB, Ahn CS, Kim KH, Sung KB, Ko GY, Park KM, Ha TY, Song GW. Expanded indication criteria of living donor liver transplantation for hepatocellular carcinoma at one large-volume center. Liver Transplantation. 2008;**14**:935-945.

[46] Zheng SS, et al. Liver transplantation for hepatocellular carcinoma: Hangzhou experiences. Transplantation. 2008;**85**:1726-1732.

[47] Herrero JI, Sangro B, Pardo F, Quiroga J, Iñarrairaegui M, Rotellar F, Montiel C, Alegre F, Prieto J. Liver transplantation in patients with hepatocellular carcinoma across Milan criteria. Liver Transplantation. 2008;**14**:272-278.

[48] Takada Y, Ito T, Ueda M, Sakamoto S, Haga H, Maetani Y, et al. Living donor liver transplantation for patients with HCC exceeding the Milan criteria: A proposal of expanded criteria. Digestive Diseases. 2007;**25**:299-302.

[49] Mazzaferro V, Llovet JM, Miceli R, Bhoori S, Schiavo M, Mariani L, Camerini T, Roayaie S, Schwartz ME, Grazi GL, Adam R, Neuhaus P, Salizzoni M, Bruix J, Forner A, De Carlis L, Cillo U, Burroughs AK, Troisi R, Rossi M, Gerunda GE, Lerut J, Belghiti J, Boin I, Gugenheim J, Rochling F, Van Hoek B, Majno P. Predicting survival after liver transplantation in patients with hepatocellular carcinoma beyond the Milan criteria: A retrospective, exploratory analysis. Lancet Oncology. 2009;**10**:35-43.

[50] Chevret S, Trinchet JC, Mathieu D, et al. A new prognostic classification for predicting survival in patients with hepatocellular carcinoma. Groupe d'Etude et de Traitement du Carcinome Hepatocellulaire. Journal of Hepatology. 1999;**31**:133-141.

[51] Farinati F, Rinaldi M, Gianni S, et al. How should patients with hepatocellular carcinoma be staged? Validation of a new prognostic system. Cancer. 2000;**89**:2266-2273.

[52] Toso C, Asthana S, Bigam DL, Shapiro MJ, Kneteman NM. Reassessing selection criteria prior to liver transplantation for hepatocellular carcinoma utilizing the scientific registry of transplant recipients database. Hepatology. 2009;**49**:832-838.

[53] Duvoux C, Roudot-Thoraval F, Decaens T, Pessione F, Badran H, Piardi T, Francoz C, Compagnon P, Vanlemmens C, Dumortier J, Dharancy S, Gugenheim J, Bernard PH, Adam R, Radenne S, Muscari F, Conti F, Hardwigsen J, Pageaux GP, Chazouillères O, Salame E, Hilleret MN, Lebray P, Abergel A, Debette-Gratien M, Kluger MD, Mallat A, Azoulay D, Cherqui D; Liver Transplantation French Study Group. Liver transplantation for hepatocellular carcinoma: A model including α-fetoprotein improves the performance of Milan criteria. Gastroenterology. 2012;**143**:986-994.

[54] Hwang S, Lee SG, Joh JW, Suh KS, Kim DG. Liver transplantation for adult patients with hepatocellular carcinoma in Korea: Comparison between cadaveric donor and living donor liver transplantations. Liver Transplantation. 2005;**11**:1265-1272.

[55] Di Sandro S, Slim AO, Giacomoni A, et al. Living donor liver transplantation for hepato-cellular carcinoma: Long-term results compared with deceased donor liver transplanta-tion. Transplantation Proceedings. 2009;**41**:1283-1285.

[56] Grant RC, Sandhu L, Dixon PR, Greig PD, Grant DR, McGilvray ID. Living vs. deceased donor liver transplantation for hepatocellular carcinoma: A systematic review and meta-analysis. Clinical Transplantation. 2013;**27**:140-147.

6

Cirrhotic Ascites: Pathophysiological Changes and Clinical Implications

Abdulrahman Bendahmash, Hussien Elsiesy and
Waleed K. Al-hamoudi

Abstract

Liver cirrhosis is associated with a wide range of systemic and pulmonary vascular abnormalities. Cardiac dysfunction also occurs in patients with advanced liver disease (cirrhotic cardiomyopathy). The circulation in cirrhosis is hyperdynamic, which is typically characterized by hypotension resulting from the associated vasodilatation and reflex tachycardia. The circulatory dysfunction in cirrhosis is the proposed pathophysiological mechanism leading to sodium and water retention in patients with liver cirrhosis. Hyperdynamic circulation is triggered by increased intrahepatic resistance due to cirrhosis, leading to a progressive increase in portal venous pressure. As portal hypertension worsens, local production of vasodilators increases due to endothelial activation, leading to splanchnic and systemic arterial vasodilation. Nitric oxide (NO) is considered one of the most important vasodilator molecules in the splanchnic and systemic circulation. The reduction in the effective arterial blood volume results in diminished renal arterial blood flow and subsequently triggers the rennin-angiotensin-aldosterone system (RAAS), antidiuretic hormones (ADHs) and sympathetic nervous system (SNS), leading to renal artery vasoconstriction. All these changes lead to sodium retention and volume expansion, manifested as ascites and peripheral edema. Furthermore, disease progression is associated with various degrees of renal dysfunction.

Keywords: cirrhosis, portal hypertension, hyperdynamic circulation, ascites

1. Introduction

Liver cirrhosis is associated with a wide range of systemic and pulmonary vascular abnormalities. Cardiac dysfunction has also been described in patients with advanced liver disease (cirrhotic cardiomyopathy) [1–4]. The circulation in cirrhosis has been described as being hyperdynamic, which is typically characterized by hypotension resulting from the associated vasodilatation and reflex tachycardia. These cardiovascular abnormalities play a major role in the pathogenesis of multiple life-threatening complications, including ascites, spontaneous bacterial peritonitis, hepatorenal syndrome (HRS), esophageal varices and pulmonary related complications [5, 6]. The hyperdynamic circulation is triggered by increased intrahepatic resistance due to cirrhosis, leading to a progressive increase in portal venous pressure [7, 8]. As portal hypertension worsens, there is an increased local production of vasodilators due to endothelial activation, leading to splanchnic and systemic arterial vasodilation. Nitric oxide (NO) is thought to be one of the most important vasodilator molecules in the splanchnic and systemic circulation. NO is overproduced in cirrhosis; measured serum levels are significantly elevated in both cirrhotic patients and in animal models [9–11]. The reduction in the effective arterial blood volume results in diminished renal arterial blood flow and subsequently triggers the rennin-angiotensin-aldosterone system (RAAS), antidiuretic hormone (ADH) and sympathetic nervous system (SNS), leading to renal artery vasoconstriction. All these changes lead to sodium retention and volume expansion, manifested as ascites and peripheral edema. Furthermore, advanced liver disease is usually associated with various degrees of renal dysfunction. In cirrhotic patients with hepatorenal syndrome (HRS), renal plasma flow and glomerular filtration rate (GFR) are significantly diminished and may reach levels similar to those seen in patients with advanced renal disease [12, 13]. Sodium retention usually occurs in association with the inability to excrete a normal water load, resulting in increased total body water and dilutional hyponatremia [14, 15]. However, unlike the situation of end-stage renal disease, no significant histological abnormality is present within the kidneys of patients with HRS, and the process is reversible after liver transplantation (LT) [16]. The aim of this chapter is to discuss the impact of portal hypertension on the cardiovascular system in cirrhosis, with special emphasis on the pathogenesis of ascites.

2. Ascites

The peritoneum is a serous membrane made up of visceral and parietal layers. The parietal peritoneum lines the coelomic cavity, and the visceral layer of the peritoneum lines the surface of organs. The peritoneal cavity is an empty space between the visceral and parietal layers of the peritoneum. The potential space of the peritoneal cavity is normally not visible on imaging as it contains only a small amount of fluid (approximately 100 mL). The fluid is mostly water with electrolytes, antibodies, white blood cells, albumin, glucose and other biochemicals [17]. Its main function is to reduce the friction between the abdominal organs as they move around during digestion. The word ascites is derived from the Greek word "askos," which means a bag or sack and is defined as pathological fluid accumulation within the peritoneal cavity. Ascites is a frequent complication of cirrhosis and portal hypertension because of the increase of the sinusoidal hydrostatic pressure. Cirrhosis accounts for over 75% of episodes of ascites, with all other causes accounting for less than 25% (**Table 1**) [18]. Ascites has been associated with increased morbidity and mortality, with liver transplant-free mortality rates ranging from 15 to 20% at 1 year to nearly 50–60% at 5 years from the time of diagnosis [19, 20].

Causes of ascites
Portal hypertension
Infection
Heart failure
Malignancy and hematological disorders
Connective tissue disease
Pancreatic disease
Nephrotic syndrome
Severe malnutrition
Congenital causes

Table 1. Causes of ascites.

3. The heart (cirrhotic cardiomyopathy)

In 1953, Kowalski and Abelmann described an abnormal circulatory pattern in a group of cirrhotic patients. The examined the circulation in 22 alcoholic cirrhotic patients and concluded that these patients had a large stroke volume, prolonged Q-T interval and reduced peripheral vascular resistance. They were some of the first researchers to question the impact of liver disease on the heart [21]. These findings were then confirmed in multiple experimental models of portal hypertension and in patients with cirrhosis. Initially, it was thought that these circulatory manifestations were secondary to alcoholic-related malnutrition; however, future studies confirmed the same circulatory dysregulation in cirrhotic patients with various underlying etiologies [1–4]. In the absence of known cardiac disease, the diagnostic criteria for cirrhotic cardiomyopathy rest on the presence of an attenuated systolic or diastolic response to stressful stimuli and are supported by the presence of structural or histological changes in cardiac chambers, electrophysiological abnormalities and elevation in serum markers suggestive of cardiac stress [22]. In addition to abnormal systolic dysfunction, cirrhotic patients also clearly demonstrate abnormal diastolic dysfunction, especially in patients with ascites, and it has been shown that paracentesis can improve diastolic dysfunction. Left ventricular (LV) diastolic dysfunction manifests as impaired LV relaxation secondary to LV wall stiffness, which results in the increase in filling pressure. Glenn et al. investigated the role of passive tension regulators—titin and collagen—in the pathogenesis of cirrhotic diastolic dysfunction. They showed that alterations in titin modulation, PKA levels, and collagen configuration contributed to the pathogenesis of this condition [23]. Velocity of blood flow from the left atrium to the left ventricle during early (E wave) and late (A wave) phases of diastole can help in assessing diastolic function. A low E/A ratio indicates a non-compliant ventricle [24]. This finding was also confirmed in other studies [25, 26]. Multiple factors affecting cardiac cell function have been implicated in the pathogenesis of cirrhotic cardiomyopathy, including: (a) Down regulation of β-adrenergic receptors, which negatively impacts cardiac contractility [27]; (b) Reduction in the cardiac cell membrane fluidity, which impairs the function of membrane-bound ion channels, alters control of vascular tone and reduces the β-adrenoceptor function [28, 29]; (c) Reduced muscarinic receptor activity, which has a negative inotropic effect on the heart [30]; (d) Augmented nitric oxide activity, which negatively impacts cardiac contractility [31, 32]; (e) Carbon monoxide (CO) and endocannabinoid activity negatively impacts cardiac contractility in cirrhotic patients [33–35]. Multiple other studies have demonstrated significant structural cardiac abnormalities in all cardiac chambers of cirrhotic patients [36].

4. Systemic and splanchnic circulation

Portosystemic collaterals are formed secondary to cirrhosis-induced portal hypertension, which allows gut-derived humoral substances to directly enter systemic circulation without detoxification by the liver. Arterial vasodilatation in portal hypertension results from the predominant production of various vasodilators [37]. NO is thought to be the major vasodilator molecule in cirrhotic patients. The intrahepatic microcirculation is altered significantly in liver cirrhosis, secondary to both architectural and vasoactive humoral changes, resulting in an increase in vasoactive molecules associated with a decrease in intrahepatic NO production [38, 39]. On the other hand, multiple studies have documented an elevated serum level of NO in the systemic and splanchnic circulation in both cirrhotic patients and in animal models [40–43]. NO is an endothelial-derived relaxing factor that leads to systemic arterial vasodilatation. Three isoforms of NO synthase (NOS) have been described: endothelial (eNOS), inducible (iNOS), and neuronal (nNOS). However, the leading isoform contributing to these vascular changes remains obscure [44]. Ferguson and colleagues were the first group to use a highly selective iNOS inhibitor to evaluate the role iNOS in the regulation of vascular tone in patients with ascites. Forearm blood flow was measured in eight patients with ascites and was compared with eight matched healthy volunteers, during intrabrachial infusion of 1400 W (0.1–1 µmol/min), NG-monomethyl-L-arginine (L-NMMA, a non-selective NOS inhibitor; 2–8 µmol), and norepinephrine. They showed that iNOS inhibitor causes systemic vasoconstriction in patients with ascites only. This supports the role of iNOS in the circulatory changes associated with cirrhosis [45]. One major factor that plays an important role in promoting NO production is the altered intestinal permeability in patients with advanced liver disease. As a result various endotoxins cross the intestine to the systemic circulation and stimulate the production of NO [46, 47]. TNF-α is also considered to be a NO inducers. Inhibition of TNF-α production resulted in improvement in the hyperdynamic circulation in various animal model studies [48, 49]. Endocannabinoids have also been implicated in the peripheral vasodilatation of cirrhosis. Activation of endothelial cannabinoid receptors by the endogenously produced endocannabinoids causes pronounced vasodilatation in cirrhotic rats [50, 51]. Interestingly, multiple studies have shown a potentially important role of the central nervous system (CNS) in the pathogenesis of the portal hypertension-induced hyperdynamic circulation. The cardiovascular system is controlled by neural influences that include the central nervous system (CNS) and peripheral afferent and efferent nerves. Portal hypertension activates receptors in the mesenteric area; the signals are relayed to central

Pathogenic mechanisms	Cardiovascular effect
Down regulation of β-adrenergic receptors	Decreases cardiac contractility
Reduction in the cardiac cell membrane fluidity	Alters control of vascular tone and reduces the β-adrenoceptor function
Reduced muscarinic receptor activity	Negative inotropic effect on the heart
Augmented nitric oxide activity	Decreases cardiac contractility
Carbon monoxide	Decreases cardiac contractility
Endocannabinoid activity	Decreases cardiac contractility
Portosystemic collaterals	This allows gut-derived humoral substances to directly enter the systemic circulation augmenting the hyperdynamic circulation
Systemic nitric oxide	Systemic vasodilatation
Central nervous system-gut-axis	Denervation prevents the development of hyperdynamic circulation and ascites formation
Activation of renin-angiotensin aldosterone system, sympathetic nervous system and nonosmotic release of antidiuretic hormone	Restores the normal hemodynamics in the setting of a hyperdynamic circulation through sodium and water retention

Table 2. Pathogenic mechanisms of cardiovascular disturbance in cirrhotic patients.

cardiovascular-regulatory nuclei via afferent nerves. These nuclei then process the inputs and send out signals to the cardiovascular system through efferent pathways, leading to cardiovascular changes [52]. Li and colleagues demonstrated that neonatal capsaicin denervation in rats prevented the development of hyperdynamic circulation and renal dysfunction as well as ascites formation in cirrhosis. These results indicate that intact primary afferent innervation is necessary for the development of hyperdynamic circulation and ascites formation [53]. A recent study revealed reversal of the cirrhosis associated vascular dysregulation after afferent denervation in an animal model. Portal vein ligation in cirrhotic rats activates a marker protein in the brain stem indicating CNS activation. Furthermore, blocking CNS Fos expression in cirrhotic rats resulted in eliminating the development of the hyperdynamic circulation [54]. The various potential pathogenic mechanisms leading to cardiovascular disturbance and fluid retention are summarized in **Table 2**.

5. The lymphatic system

The lymphatic vascular system plays a critical role in ascites formation [55]. Lymphatic vessels remove fluid from the interstitial fluid from various parts of the body and drain it into the blood stream. In healthy adult individuals, the lymphatic system returns as much as eight liters of interstitial fluid with 20–30 g of protein per liter to venous circulation every day. Any disturbance to this process leads to fluid accumulation, manifested as edema and ascites [55–58]. As with systemic and splanchnic circulation, the lymphatic system is also influenced by nitric oxide, leading to vasodilatation [59]. The development of portal hypertension in cirrhosis is associated with an increase in portal lymph flow. Normally, the liver produces a large amount of lymph, which is estimated to be over 25% of the lymph flowing through the thoracic duct. Barrowman and colleagues demonstrated an increase in lymph flows from the intestine and liver in cirrhotic animals by threefold and 30-fold, respectively, over values obtained from control animals. They also demonstrated a good correlation between intestinal and liver lymph flows and portal venous pressure [60]. In portal hypertension, compensatory lymphangiogenic response may initially help to reduce the high portal pressure. Oikawa and colleagues used a morphometric analysis to examine portal hypertensive-associated changes in lymph vessels and branches of the portal vein, with use of immunohistochemical staining for alpha smooth muscle actin, and quantitated these changes using an image analysis system. They obtained wedge liver biopsies from 10 patients with advanced portal hypertension and 10 control samples from patients with gastric carcinoma without liver disease. They showed that the proliferation of lymph vessels were higher in portal hypertension samples compared to the control samples. On the other hand, the number of portal vein branches in portal hypertension samples was not different from control samples. They concluded that these alterations in portal hypertension may result in a decrease in portal flow associated with an increase in lymph flow resulting in a reduction of the high portal vein pressure in idiopathic portal hypertension [61]. With worsening liver fibrosis and ongoing portal hypertension, the lymphatic system fails, resulting in buildup of interstitial fluids and ascites formation [55].

6. Renal response

The systemic vasodilation in patients with cirrhosis leads to under filling of arterial vascular space and that leads to systemic hypotension. Consequently, baroreceptor-mediated activation of the renin-angiotensin-aldosterone system (RAAS) and sympathetic nervous system (SNS) and nonosmotic release of antidiuretic hormone (ADH) occur to restore normal hemodynamics. This leads to fluid and sodium retention (**Figure 1**). Sodium retention is the most common abnormality of renal function in patients with cirrhosis and ascites [12, 62, 63]. The total amount of sodium retained in patients with cirrhosis is dependent on sodium intake, non-renal sodium losses and sodium excreted in the urine. Minimizing sodium intake in cirrhotic patients may help control ascites. With ongoing hemodynamic disturbance in cirrhosis, the equation tips toward sodium retention. Associated with this is an increase in splanchnic permeability that, aided by the changes in oncotic pressure, combines to lead to ascites formation [63]. In the initial phases of the disease, this is compensated by an increase in lymph return. In fact, the thoracic duct lymph flow, which in normal conditions is lower than 1 liter per day, may increase by several folds. When lymph formation overcomes lymph drainage, this also results in ascites formation. As a result, renal vasoconstriction persists and results in various degrees of renal impairment. The extreme effect would result in severe renal failure with elevation of blood urea nitrogen and serum-creatinine concentration. The associated hyponatremia in portal hypertensive ascites carries a bad prognostic value and has been linked to mortality [64].

Refractory ascites refers to ascites that cannot be resolved by dietary sodium restriction and diuretic treatment. The severity of renal sodium retention increases with the progression of

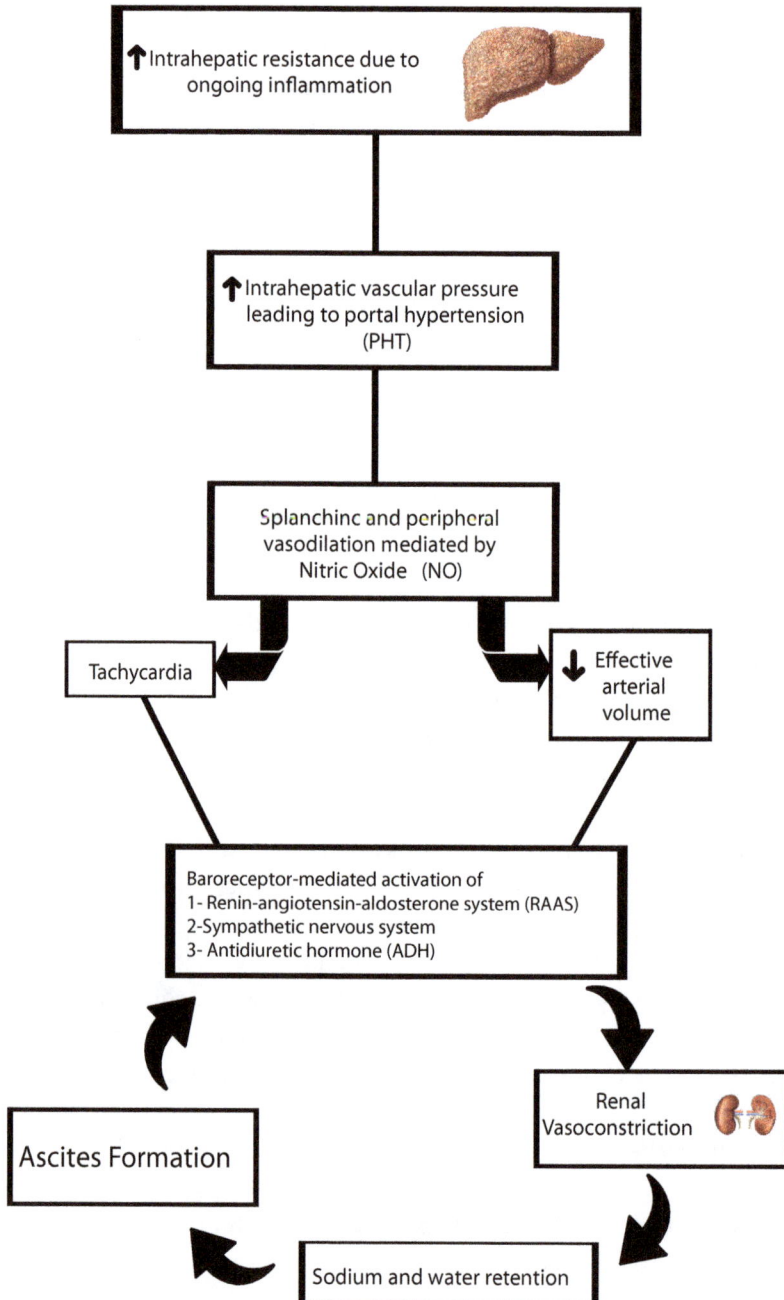

Figure 1. The cascade of changes leading to ascites formation.

the underlying liver disease and associated portal and systemic hemodynamic disturbance. The ongoing activation of the various neurohumoral pathways leads to aggressive renal reabsorption of sodium and water. Activation of the neurhormonal pathway also leads to a reduction in the glomerular filtration rate (GFR) and subsequently leads to a decline in the renal function. The enhanced sodium reabsorption at the proximal convoluted tubule leads to a significant reduction in the sodium reaching the distal segments of the nephron. This explains the failure of loop diuretics and antimineralocorticoid in treating these patients as they work predominantly at the distal segments of the nephron. Thus, renal sodium retention mainly occurs proximally to the site of action of both antimineralocorticoid and loop diuretics, and this can explain why diuretic treatment becomes unsuccessful in some patients. Furthermore, when cirrhosis progresses and the arterial vasodilation becomes more marked, the heart can no longer keep pace with the marked systemic vasodilatation. This results in an increase in the production of endogenous vasoactive compounds, which further increases sodium and water retention as a result of this physiological response to the relative arterial underfilling [63, 64]. This increased sodium and water retention contributes to increasing ascites, and in many cases, to the development of refractory ascites and type 2 HRS. Kraq and colleagues investigated the relation between cardiac and renal function in patients with cirrhosis and ascites and the impact of cardiac systolic function on survival. Cardiac function was investigated by gated myocardial perfusion imaging for assessment of cardiac index and cardiac volumes. Renal function was assessed by determination of GFR and renal blood flow, and the patients were followed up for 12 months. They demonstrated that patients with a low CI had a lower GFR and a higher creatinine level. The number of patients who developed type 1 HRS within 3 months was significantly higher in the group with low CI than that in the group with high CI. They also showed that patients with the lowest CI had significantly poorer survival at 3, 9, and 12 months than did those with a higher CI [65].

7. Clinical implications

This circulatory dysfunction in cirrhosis is the proposed pathophysiological mechanism leading to sodium and water retention in patients with liver cirrhosis. Treatment aimed at reversing this pathophysiological process would likely result in improving the outcome. Albumin has been used in clinical trials as a volume expander and, when given with a vasoconstrictor, has been shown to improve renal function in the setting of cirrhotic ascites. Martín-Llahí and colleagues randomized 46 patients with cirrhosis and HRS to receive terlipressin, a vasopressin analog, and albumin (n = 23) or albumin alone (n = 23) for a maximum of 15 days. They monitored renal function closely during the study period. Improvement of renal function occurred in 10 patients (43.5%) treated with terlipressin and albumin compared with that in two patients (8.7%) treated with albumin alone (P = .017) [66]. Similarly, Guevara and colleagues treated 16 patients with HRS with a combination of ornipressin, a potent vasoconstrictor agent, and albumin to improve the cardiovascular dysfunction. The combined treatment was administered for either 3 or 15 days (eight patients each). The shorter treatment duration was associated with normalization of the overactivity of renin-angiotensin and sympathetic nervous systems, a marked increase in atrial-natriuretic peptide levels, and only a slight improvement in renal function. However, when treatment was administered for 15 days outcome was significantly better. Renal function improved dramatically manifested by normalization of serum creatinine associated with an increase in the GFR and a persistent suppression in the activity of vasoconstrictor systems [67]. In another study, Ortega and colleagues showed that terlipressin therapy reverses HRS, and the effect was augmented when coupled with albumin [68]. Patel and colleagues assessed the efficacy of midodrine and octreotide as a therapeutic approach to increasing urinary electrolyte-free water clearance in advanced cirrhosis. Patients were treated with albumin, midodrine and octreotide within the first 24 h. Urinary electrolyte-free water clearance and serum sodium concentration were assessed before and 72 h after treatment. The assessments showed a statistically significant increase in serum sodium concentration and urinary electrolyte-free water clearance with the use of midodrine and octreotide in the treatment of cirrhosis-associated hyponatremia [69]. These studies demonstrate the importance of targeting circulatory dysfunction in end-stage liver disease. A more challenging aspect in managing these patients is the associated cirrhotic cardiomyopathy. The development of HRS in the setting of advanced liver disease is associated with a drop in the cardiac output, emphasizing the additional role of cirrhotic cardiomyopathy in the pathogenesis of hepatorenal dysfunction [65]. Other reports suggested a possible role of cirrhotic cardiomyopathy in spontaneous bacterial peritonitis [70].

Transjugular intrahepatic portosystemic shunts (TIPS) have been commonly used to treat refractory ascites. Following TIPS insertion, a sudden increase in the preload results in further hemodynamic disturbance, and therefore, careful cardiovascular evaluation prior to the procedure is a necessity [71, 72]. The preexisting subclinical diastolic dysfunction becomes clinically obvious with the sudden increase in the right atrial and pulmonary circulation, leading to heart failure. In a recent study, Ascha and colleagues investigated if echocardiographic and hemodynamic changes at the time of TIPS can provide any prognostic information. After evaluating 418 patients, they showed that a change in the right atrial (RA) pressure after TIPS predicted long-term mortality [73]. Others showed a possible impact of intra-procedural RA pressure on early post-TIPS mortality [74]. Other studies suggested that an E/A ratio of ≤1 was predictive of slow ascites clearance and mortality post-TIPS insertion [75, 76].

Liver transplantation results in correction of portal hypertension and reversal of all the pathophysiological mechanisms that lead to hyperdynamic circulation [77]. We studied the hemodynamics in the immediate post-transplant period and compared patients with alcoholic vs. viral cirrhosis. Within the first 24 h, there was a significant decrease in HR and increase in MAP; the extent of the change was similar in both groups. The central venous pressure (CVP), pulmonary capillary wedge pressure (PCWP), and systemic vascular resistance index (SVRI) increased, and changes were more pronounced in the viral group [78]. Navasa and colleagues assessed systemic hemodynamics and plasma levels of aldosterone, glucagon and plasma renin in 12 patients with advanced cirrhosis before and 2 weeks and 2 months after LT. Elevated aldosterone, plasma renin and glucagon levels decreased to near-normal values 2 weeks after transplantation. This decrease was associated with reversal of the associated splanchnic and systemic vasodilation and restoration of normal hemodynamics [79]. Following LT, the rapid reversal of systemic vasodilatation and the associated increase in blood pressure exposes the previously subclinical cirrhotic cardiomyopathy. Cardiovascular complications are a major cause of postoperative morbidity and mortality after liver transplantation [80]. Fouad and colleagues reviewed 197 liver transplant recipients for post-liver transplant-related cardiac complications. Eighty-two patients suffered one or more cardiac complications within 6 months after LT. Pulmonary edema was the most common complication, occurring in 61 patients; other complications included heart failure (7 patients), arrhythmia (13 patients), pulmonary hypertension (7 patients), pericardial effusion (2 patients), and cardiac thrombus formation (1 patient). In their study, cardiac causes were the leading cause of death (23.8% of all mortality) [81].

LT induces significant cardiovascular stress. Predicting the development of postoperative cardiac complications is very difficult. Two-dimensional and dobutamine stress echocardiography were utilized to predict the development of adverse cardiac events following liver transplantation, and both had a low predictive value [82]. More recently, a study utilizing dobutamine stress perfusion, which provides an assessment of both regional systolic and diastolic function as well as microvascular perfusion, revealed a better prediction of post-transplant cardiac outcome [83]. Management at the time of liver transplantation should involve careful fluid management. Immediate postoperative care should include continuous cardiac and hemodynamic monitoring and early detection of any potential arrhythmia or any other cardiac complication.

Author details

Abdulrahman Bendahmash[1], Hussien Elsiesy[2,3] and Waleed K. Al-hamoudi[2,4*]

*Address all correspondence to: walhamoudi@gmail.com

1 Department of Pediatrics, King Faisal Specialist Hospital & Research Center, Riyadh, Saudi Arabia

2 Department of Liver Transplantation, King Faisal Specialist Hospital & Research Center, Riyadh, Saudi Arabia

3 Department of Medicine, Alfaisal University, Riyadh, Saudi Arabia

4 Department of Medicine, College of Medicine, King Saud University, Riyadh, Saudi Arabia

References

[1] Ma Z, Lee SS. Cirrhotic cardiomyopathy: Getting to the heart of the matter. Hepatology. 1996;**24**:451-459

[2] Møller S, Henriksen JH. Cirrhotic cardiomyopathy: A pathophysiological review of circulatory dysfunction in liver disease. Heart. 2002;**87**:9-15

[3] Al Hamoudi W, Lee SS. Cirrhotic cardiomyopathy. Annals of Hepatology. 2006 Jul-Sep; **5**(3):132-139

[4]   Al-Hamoudi WK. Cardiovascular changes in cirrhosis: Pathogenesis and clinical impli-cations. Saudi Journal of Gastroenterology. 2010 Jul-Sep;**16**(3):145-153

[5]   Salerno F, Gerbes A, Wong F, et al. Diagnosis, prevention and treatment of hepatorenal syndrome in cirrhosis. Gut. 2007;**56**:1310-1318

[6]   Arroyo V, Gines P, Gerbes AL, et al. Definition and diagnostic criteria of refractory ascites and hepatorenal syndrome in cirrhosis. International ascites Club Hepatology. 1996;**23**:164-176

[7]   Gines P, Fernandez-Esparrach G, Arroyo V, et al. Pathogenesis of ascites in cirrhosis. Seminars in Liver Disease. 1997;**17**:175-189

[8]   Arroyo V, Badalamenti S, Gines P. Pathogenesis of ascites in cirrhosis. Minerva Medica. 1987;**78**:645-650

[9]   Chang SW, Ohara N. Chronic biliary obstruction induces pulmonary intravascular phagocytosis and endotoxin sensitivity in rats. The Journal of Clinical Investigation. 1994;**94**:2009-2019

[10] Carter EP, Hartsfield CL, Miyazono M, Jakkula M, Morris KG Jr, McMurtry IF. Regulation of heme oxygenase-1 by nitric oxide during hepatopulmonary syndrome. American Journal of Physiology. Lung Cellular and Molecular Physiology. 2002;**283**:L346-L353

[11] Sztrymf B, Rabiller A, Nunes H, Savale L, Lebrec D, Le Pape A, et al. Prevention of hepa-topulmonary syndrome and hyperdynamic state by pentoxifylline in cirrhotic rats. The European Respiratory Journal. 2004;**23**:752-758

[12] Jalan R, Forrest EH, Redhead DN, et al. Reduction in renal blood flow following acute increase in the portal pressure: Evidence for the existence of a hepatorenal reflex in man? Gut. 1997;**40**:664-670

[13] Ming Z, Smyth DD, Lautt WW. Decreases in portal flow trigger a hepatorenal reflex to inhibit renal sodium and water excretion in rats: Role of adenosine. Hepatology. 2002;**35**:167-175

[14] Arroyo V, Claria J, Salo J, Jimnez W. Antidiuretic hormone and the pathogenesis of water retention in cirrhosis with ascites. Seminars in Liver Disease. 1994;**14**:44-58

[15] McCullough AJ, Mullen KD, Kalhan SC. Measurements of total body and extracellular water in cirrhotic patients with and without ascites. Hepatology. 1991;**14**:1102-1111

[16] Mindikoglu AL, Pappas SC. New developments in Hepatorenal syndrome. Clinical Gastroenterology and Hepatology. 2017 Jun 7; pii: S1542-3565(17)30672-9 [Epub ahead of print]

[17] Pannu H, Oliphant M. The subperitoneal space and peritoneal cavity: Basic concepts. Abdominal Imaging. 2015;**40**(7):2710-2722

[18] Reynolds TB. Ascites. Clinics in Liver Disease. 2000;**4**:151-168

[19] Planas R, Montoliu S, Ballesté B, et al. Natural history of patients hospitalized for management of cirrhotic ascites. Clinical Gastroenterology and Hepatology. 2006;4:1385-1394

[20] Heuman DM, Abou-Assi SG, Habib A, et al. Persistent ascites and low serum sodium identify patients with cirrhosis and low MELD scores who are at high risk for early death. Hepatology. 2004;40:802-810

[21] Kowalski HJ, Abelmann WH. The cardiac output at rest in Laennec's cirrhosis. The Journal of Clinical Investigation. 1953 Oct;32(10):1025-1033

[22] Yang YY, Lin HC. The heart: Pathophysiology and clinical implications of cirrhotic cardiomyopathy. Journal of the Chinese Medical Association. 2012;75:619-623

[23] Glenn TK, Honar H, Liu H, ter Keurs HE, Lee SS. Role of cardiac myofilament proteins titin and collagen in the pathogenesis of diastolic dysfunction in cirrhotic rats. Journal of Hepatology. 2011;55:1249-1255

[24] Lee RF, Glenn TK, Lee SS. Cardiac dysfunction in cirrhosis. Best Practice & Research. Clinical Gastroenterology. 2007;21:125-140

[25] Finucci G, Desideri A, Sacerdoti D, et al. Left ventricular diastolic function in liver cirrhosis. Scandinavian Journal of Gastroenterology. 1996;31(3):279-284

[26] Pozzi M, Carugo S, Boari G, et al. Evidence of functional and structural cardiac abnormalities in cirrhotic patients with and without ascites. Hepatology. 1997;26(5):1131-1137

[27] Lee SS, Marty J, Mantz J, Samain E, Braillon A, Lebrec D. Desensitization of myocardial β-adrenergic receptors in cirrhotic rats. Hepatology. 1990;12:481-485

[28] Ma Z, Lee SS, Meddings JB. Effects of altered cardiac membrane fluidity on beta -adrenergic receptor signalling in rats with cirrhoticcardiomyopathy. Journal of Hepatology. 1997;26:904-912

[29] Le Grimellec C, Friedlander G, el Yandouzi EH, Zlatkine P, Giocondi MC. Membrane fluidity and transport properties in epithelia. Kidney International 1992;42:825-836.

[30] Jaue DN, Ma Z, Lee SS. Cardiac muscarinic receptor function in rats with cirrhotic cardiomyopathy. Hepatology. 1997;25:1361-1365

[31] Balligand JL, Kelly RA, Marsden PA, Smith TW, Michel T. Control of cardiac muscle cell function by an endogenous nitric oxide signaling system. Proceedings of the National Academy of Sciences of the United States of America. 1993;90:347-351

[32] Liu H, Ma Z, Lee SS. Contribution of nitric oxide to the pathogenesis of cirrhotic cardiomyopathy in bile duct-ligated rats. Gastroenterology. 2000;118:937-944

[33] Liu H, Song D, Lee SS. Role of heme oxygenase - carbon monoxide pathway in pathogenesis of cirrhotic cardiomyopathy in the rat. American Journal of Physiology. Gastrointestinal and Liver Physiology. 2001;280:G68-G74

[34] Bonz A, Laser M, Küllmer S, Kniesch S, Babin-Ebell J, Popp V, et al. Cannabinoids acting on CB1 receptors decrease contractile performance in human atrial muscle. Journal of Cardiovascular Pharmacology. 2003;**41**:657-664

[35] Ford WR, Honan SA, White R, Hiley CR. Evidence of a novel site mediating anandamide-induced negative inotropic and coronary vasodilatator responses in rat isolated hearts. British Journal of Pharmacology. 2002;**135**:1191-1198

[36] Alqahtani SA, Fouad TR, Lee SS. Cirrhotic cardiomyopathy. Seminars in Liver Disease. 2008;**28**:59-69

[37] Kim MY, Baik SK, Lee SS. Hemodynamic alterations in cirrhosis and portal hypertension. The Korean Journal of Hepatology. 2010 Dec;**16**(4):347-352

[38] Sanyal AJ, Bosch J, Blei A, Arroyo V. Portal hypertension and its complications. Gastroenterology. 2008;**134**:1715-1728

[39] Hendrickson H, Chatterjee S, Cao S, Morales Ruiz M, Sessa WC, Shah V. Influence of caveolin on constitutively activated recombinant eNOS: Insights into eNOS dysfunction in BDL rat liver. American Journal of Physiology. Gastrointestinal and Liver Physiology. 2003;**285**:652-660

[40] Wiest R, Shah V, Sessa WC, Groszmann RJ. NO overproduction by eNOS precedes hyperdynamic splanchnic circulation in portal hypertensive rats. The American Journal of Physiology. 1999;**276**:G1043-G1051

[41] Vallance P, Moncada S. Hyperdynamic circulation in cirrhosis: A role for nitric oxide? Lancet. 1991;**337**:776-778

[42] Genesca J, Gonzalez A, Segura R, Catalan R, Marti R, Varela E, Cadelina G, Martinez M, Lopez Talavera JC, Esteban R, Groszmann RJ, Guardia J. Interleukin-6, nitric oxide, and the clinical and hemodynamic alterations of patients with liver cirrhosis. The American Journal of Gastroenterology. 1999;**94**:169-177

[43] Hori N, Wiest R, Groszmann RJ. Enhanced release of nitric oxide in response to changes in flow and shear stress in the superior mesenteric arteries of portal hypertensive rats. Hepatology. 1998;**28**:1467-1473

[44] Martell M, Coll M, Ezkurdia N, Raurell I, Genescà J. Physiopathology of splanchnic vasodilation in portal hypertension. World Journal of Hepatology. 2010 Jun 27;**2**(6):208-220

[45] Ferguson JW, Dover AR, Chia S, Cruden NL, Hayes PC, Newby DE. Inducible nitric oxide synthase activity contributes to the regulation of peripheral vascular tone in patients with cirrhosis and ascites. Gut. 2006;**55**:542-546

[46] Bode C, Kugler V, Bode JC. Endotoxemia in patients with alcoholic and non-alcoholic cirrhosis and in subjects with no evidence of chronic liver disease following acute alcohol excess. Journal of Hepatology. 1987;**4**:8-14

[47] García-Tsao G. Bacterial translocation: Cause or consequence of decompensation in cirrhosis? Journal of Hepatology. 2001;**34**:150-155

[48]   Lopez-Talavera JC, Merrill WW, Groszmann RJ. Tumor necrosis factor alpha: A major contributor to the hyperdynamic circulation in prehepatic portal-hypertensive rats. Gastroenterology. 1995;**108**:761-767

[49] Lopez-Talavera JC, Cadelina G, Olchowski J, Merrill W, Groszmann RJ. Thalidomide inhibits tumor necrosis factor alpha, decreases nitric oxide synthesis, and ameliorates the hyperdynamic circulatory syndrome in portal-hypertensive rats. Hepatology. 1996;**23**:1616-1621

[50] Moezi L, Gaskari SA, Lee SS. Endocannabinoids and liver disease. V. Endocannabinoids as mediators of vascular and cardiac abnormalities in cirrhosis. American Journal of Physiology. Gastrointestinal and Liver Physiology. 2008;**295**:G649-G653

[51] Bátkai S, Járai Z, Wagner JA, Goparaju SK, Varga K, Liu J, et al. Endocannabinoids acting at vascular CB1 receptors mediate the vasodilated state in advanced liver cirrhosis. Nature Medicine. 2001;**7**:827-832

[52] Song D, Liu H, Sharkey KA, Lee SS. Hyperdynamic circulation in portalhypertensive rats is dependent on central c-fos gene expression. Hepatology. 2002;**35**:159-166

[53] Li Y, Song D, Zhang Y, Lee SS. Effect of neonatal capsaicin treatment on haemodynamics and renal function in cirrhotic rats. Gut. 2003;**52**:293-299

[54] Liu H, Schuelert N, McDougall JJ, Lee SS. Central neural activation of hyperdynamic circulation in portal hypertensive rats depends on vagal afferent nerves. Gut. 2008;**57**:966-973

[55] Chung C, Iwakiri Y. The lymphatic vascular system in liver diseases: Its role in ascites formation. Clinical and Molecular Hepatology. 2013 Jun;**19**(2):99-104

[56] Harvey NL, Oliver G. Choose your fate: Artery, vein or lymphatic vessel? Current Opinion in Genetics & Development. 2004;**14**:499-505

[57] Oliver G, Alitalo K. The lymphatic vasculature: Recent progress and paradigms. Annual Review of Cell and Developmental Biology. 2005;**21**:457-483

[58] Tammela T, Alitalo K. Lymphangiogenesis: Molecular mechanisms and future promise. Cell. 2010;**140**:460-476

[59] Hagendoorn J, Padera TP, Kashiwagi S, Isaka N, Noda F, Lin MI, et al. Endothelial nitric oxide synthase regulates microlymphatic flow via collecting lymphatics. Circulation Research. 2004;**95**:204-209

[60] Barrowman JA, Granger DN. Effects of experimental cirrhosis on splanchnic microvascular fluid and solute exchange in the rat. Gastroenterology. 1984;**87**:165-172

[61] Oikawa H, Masuda T, Sato S, Yashima A, Suzuki K, Sato S, et al. Changes in lymph vessels and portal veins in the portal tract of patients with idiopathic portal hypertension: A morphometric study. Hepatology. 1998;**27**:1607-1610

[62] DiBona GF, Sawin LL. Hepatorenal baroreflex in cirrhotic rats. The American Journal of Physiology. 1995;**269**:29-33

[63] Fortune B, Cardenas A. Ascites, refractory ascites and hyponatremia in cirrhosis. Gastroenterology report (Oxford). 2017 May;**5**(2):104-112

[64] Salerno F, Guevara M, Bernardi M, Moreau R, Wong F, Angeli P, Garcia-Tsao G, Lee SS. Refractory ascites: Pathogenesis, definition and therapy of a severe complication in patients with cirrhosis. Liver International. 2010 Aug;**30**(7):937-947

[65] Krag A, Bendtsen F, Henriksen JH, et al. Low cardiac output predicts development of hepatorenal syndrome and survival in patients with cirrhosis and ascites. Gut. 2010;**59**:105-110

[66] Martín-Llahí M, Pépin MN, Guevara M, Díaz F, Torre A, Monescillo A, Soriano G, Terra C, Fábrega E, Arroyo V, Rodés J, Ginès P, TAHRS Investigators. Terlipressin and albumin vs albumin in patients with cirrhosis and hepatorenal syndrome: A randomized study. Gastroenterology. 2008 May;**134**(5):1352-1359

[67] Guevara M, Ginès P, Fernández-Esparrach G, Sort P, Salmerón JM, Jiménez W, Arroyo V, Rodés J. Reversibility of hepatorenal syndrome by prolonged administration of ornipressin and plasma volume expansion. Hepatology. 1998 Jan;**27**(1):35-41

[68] Ortega R, Ginès P, Uriz J, Cárdenas A, Calahorra B, De Las Heras D, Guevara M, Bataller R, Jiménez W, Arroyo V, Rodés J. Terlipressin therapy with and without albumin for patients with hepatorenal syndrome: Results of a prospective, nonrandomized study. Hepatology. 2002 Oct;**36**(4 Pt 1):941-948

[69] Patel S, Nguyen DS, Rastogi A, Nguyen MK, Nguyen MK. Treatment of cirrhosis-associated Hyponatremia with Midodrine and Octreotide. Frontiers in Medicine (Lausanne). 2017 Mar 14;**4**:17

[70] Lee SS. Cardiac dysfunction in spontaneous bacterial peritonitis: A manifestation of cirrhotic cardiomyopathy? Hepatology. 2003 Nov;**38**(5):1089-1091

[71] Azoulay D, Castaing D, Dennison A, Martino W, Eyraud D, Bismuth H. Transjugular intrahepatic portosystemic shunt worsen the hyperdynamic circulatory state of the cirrhotic patient: Preliminary report of a prospective study. Hepatology. 1994;**19**:129-132

[72] Rodríguez-Laiz JM, Bañares R, Echenagusia A, Casado M, Camuñez F, Pérez-Roldán F, et al. Effects of transjugular intrahepatic portasystemic shunt (TIPS) on splanchnic and systemic hemodynamics, and hepatic function in patients with portal hypertension. Preliminary results. Digestive Diseases and Sciences. 1995;**40**:2121-2127

[73] Ascha M, Abuqayyas S, Hanouneh I, Alkukhun L, Sands M, Dweik RA, Tonelli AR. Predictors of mortality after transjugular portosystemic shunt. World Journal of Hepatology. 2016 Apr 18;**8**(11):520-529

[74] Parvinian A, Bui JT, Knuttinen MG, Minocha J, Gaba RC. Right atrial pressure may impact early survival of patients undergoing transjugular intrahepatic portosystemic shunt creation. Annals of Hepatology. 2014 Jul-Aug;**13**(4):411-419

[75] Rabie RN, Cazzaniga M, Salerno F, Wong F. The use of E/A ratio as a predictor of outcome in cirrhotic patients treated with transjugular intrahepatic portosystemic shunt. The American Journal of Gastroenterology. 2009;**104**:2458-2466

[76] Cazzaniga M, Salerno F, Pagnozzi G, Dionigi E, Visentin S, Cirello I, et al. Diastolic dysfunction is associated with poor survival in cirrhotic patients with transjugular intrahepatic portosystemic shunt. Gut. 2007;**56**:869-875

[77] Liu H, Lee SS. What happens to cirrhotic cardiomyopathy after liver transplantation? Hepatology. 2005 Nov;**42**(5):1203-1205

[78] Al-Hamoudi WK, Alqahtani S, Tandon P, Ma M, Lee SS. Hemodynamics in the immediate post-transplantation period in alcoholic and viral cirrhosis. World Journal of Gastroenterology. 2010 Feb 7;**16**(5):608-612

[79] Navasa M, Feu F, García-Pagán JC, Jiménez W, Llach J, Rimola A, et al. Hemodynamic and humoral changes after liver transplantation in patients with cirrhosis. Hepatology. 1993;**17**:355-360

[80] Liu H, Jayakumar S, Traboulsi M, Lee SS. Cirrhotic cardiomyopathy: Implications for liver transplantation. Liver Transplantation. 2017 Jun;**23**(6):826-835

[81] Fouad TR, Abdel-Razek WM, Burak KW, Bain VG, Lee SS. Prediction of cardiac complications after liver transplantation. Transplantation. 2009;**87**:763-770

[82] Donovan CL, Marcovitz PA, Punch JD, Bach DS, Brown KA, Lucey MR, et al. Two-dimensional and dobutamine stress echocardiography in the preoperative assessment of patients with end-stage liver disease prior to orthotopic liver transplantation. Transplantation. 1996;**61**:1180-1188

[83] Baibhav B, Mahabir CA, Xie F, Shostrom VK, McCashland TM, Porter TR. Predictive value of Dobutamine stress perfusion echocardiography in contemporary end-stage liver disease. Journal of the American Heart Association. 2017 Feb 20;**6**(2). pii: e005102. [Epub ahead of print]

7

Hemodynamic Optimization Strategies in Anesthesia Care for Liver Transplantation

Alexander A. Vitin, Dana Tomescu and
Leonard Azamfirei

Abstract

In this chapter, aspects of hemodynamic regulation in the end-stage liver disease (ESLD) patient, factors, contributing to the hemodynamic profile, coagulation-related problems, blood products transfusion tactics and problems, and hemodynamic optimization strategies during different stages of liver transplantation procedure—specifically what, when, and how to correct, with special attention to vasoactive agents use, will be discussed.

Keywords: liver transplantation, anesthesia, hemodynamic optimization, vasoactive agents, transfusion management

1. Introduction

Inseparable part of liver transplantation procedure, anesthesia, and perioperative care for the liver transplant recipient has made a remarkable progress during last decades, becoming a clinical specialty with well-defined goals, requirements, and approaches. Today, with a rapid expansion of liver transplant programs worldwide and growing numbers of liver transplant procedures performed, many aspects of anesthesia care, complicated and risky in the relatively recent past, have become routine and safe. And yet some problems remain unresolved, still posing a challenge for anesthesiologist in the field. Despite incessant and plentiful research, investigating literally every imaginable aspect and angle of the anesthesia and perioperative care for liver transplant recipient, and myriad of publications coming out every year, no consensus has been reached so far as for the best choice of anesthesia induction and maintenance, intraoperative hemodynamics management, fluid and blood products transfusion, patient's monitoring, and more. One of the most important time- and effort-consuming aspects of anesthesia care, expanding well beyond proper intraoperative time onto the first long hours of ICU stay, is patient's hemodynamic management. Its multicomponent nature, sometimes a very short time resolution in the decision-making process, poorly predictable course of patients reactions, overall instability with rapid, oftentimes detrimental and life-threatening changes makes management of patient's hemodynamics an extremely challenging and complicating task.

2. Factors contributing to hemodynamic profile of the ESLD patient

Typical hemodynamic pattern of end-stage liver disease (ESLD) patients includes high cardiac output (CO)/cardiac index (CI)—hyperdynamic circulation pattern, with normal-to-low mean blood pressure, variable central venous pressure (CVP), along with general arterial and venous vasodilatation due to substantially decreased systemic vascular resistance (SVR). The hyperdynamic circulation is thought to be a compensatory change, induced by splanchnic and peripheral vasodilatation, reducing the effective blood volume. This, and also decreased perfusion pressures, leads to a diminished renal blood flow in cirrhotic patients, which in turn stimulates the renin-angiotensin-aldosterone system and antidiuretic hormone production, resulting in renal artery vasoconstriction, sodium retention, and volume expansion. Worsening liver disease results in progressive vasodilatation, making the hyperdynamic circulation and renal artery vasoconstriction more pronounced [1].

Arterial vascular tone is regulated by complex interactions of different vasoactive substances, namely catecholamines and NO complex. In ESLD patients, sensitivity of β-adrenoreceptors is relatively decreased, causing cardiovascular response to endogenic catecholamines substantially attenuated [2]. Plasma-free norepinephrine and epinephrine levels are significantly higher. Fraction of epinephrine, contributing to total catecholamines, increased up to 50% (normal: about 17%). Dopamine concentration is unchanged [3].

In recent years, nitric oxide (NO) has been recognized as the most important vasodilator of the splanchnic and systemic circulation. Cytokines, especially TNF-α, are considered to be NO inducers. Endothelial NO synthase has been found as a main source of the vascular NO overproduction in the splanchnic arterial circulation [4–6].

Augmented intrahepatic vascular resistance due to sinusoidal constriction is considered the major cause of portal hypertension. Hepatic stellate cells (HSC) provide a basis for control of sinusoidal vascular tone and an arrangement for sinusoidal constriction and hepatic blood flow (HBF) reduction. The dynamic part of hepatic resistance is caused by active contraction/relaxation of HSC. Portocaval collaterals divert up to 80% of blood flow away from liver [7].

Cardiomyopathy plays a substantial role in the hemodynamic profile and cardiovascular compensation mechanisms in a cirrhotic patient. The characteristic features of cirrhotic cardiomyopathy include an attenuated systolic or diastolic response to stress stimuli, structural and histological changes of myocardium, electrophysiological abnormalities, and increased concentrations of serum markers, suggestive of cardiac stress. The impaired cardiovascular responsiveness in cirrhosis is likely related to a combination of factors that include among other reasons, β-adrenergic receptor dysfunction and reduction of β-adrenergic receptor density in cirrhotic patients. Recently, it has been found that, in cirrhotic patients, the control of vascular tone by Ca^{++} and K^+ channels is altered. The calcium channel dysfunction, leading to decreased cardiomyocyte contractility, was demonstrated in an animal model study [2, 8–10].

Albeit commonly overlooked, many of these pathogenic mechanisms resulted in RV overload with gradual dilatation and impaired contractile function, leading to elevated mean pulmonary artery pressure (MPAP). Despite characteristically increased resting CO, ventricular contractile response is, actually, substantially attenuated. Cardiomyopathy may contribute to portopulmonary hypertension.

However, overt severe Congestive Heart Failure (CHF) is rare. Increased intra-abdominal pressure (ascites) contributes to both portal and PA hypertension [11].

Pulmonary vascular changes in cirrhosis are often quite substantial. They include portopulmonary hypertension (POPH) syndrome, which entails development of pulmonary hypertension in a cirrhotic patient with portal hypertension, and also hepatopulmonary syndrome, which is, essentially, increased pathological shunting and V/Q mismatch due to development of the arteriovenous malformations in the lung, resulting in hypoxemia. Portopulmonary hypertension is less prevalent than hepatopulmonary syndrome with an estimated prevalence of about 5%.

POPH is best defined as pulmonary arterial hypertension (PAH). Necessary conditions include presence of portal hypertension and absence of other secondary causes of PH, such as valvular disease, chronic thromboembolism, collagen vascular disease, or exposure to certain drugs or toxins. Current diagnostic criteria include the presence of portal hypertension (either inferred from the presence of splenomegaly, thrombocytopenia, portosystemic shunts, esophageal varices or portal vein abnormalities, or confirmed by hemodynamic measurements), but not necessarily the presence of cirrhosis; and hemodynamic parameters, specifically MPAP >25 mmHg at rest, >30 mmHg with exercise/stress, PCWP<15 mmHg, PVR>120 dynes/s/cm^5, and transpulmonary gradient >10 mmHg [12–16].

A most common suggested mechanism for POPH maintains that the increased blood flow (high cardiac output) in chronic liver disease causes pulmonary vascular wall shear stress, which can trigger the dysregulation of numerous vasoactive substances. The presence of portosystemic shunts may lead to the shunting of vasoactive substances from the splanchnic to the pulmonary circulation, causing deleterious effects in the pulmonary vasculature [17, 18].

The severity of hepatopulmonary syndrome is classified according to the degree of arterial hypoxemia, specifically mild (PaO_2 of 60–80 mm Hg), moderate (50–60 mm Hg), and severe (<50 mm Hg). Intrapulmonary vascular dilation leads to increased V/Q mismatching plus a degree of intrapulmonary shunting of deoxygenated, mixed venous blood. Both these mechanisms cause systemic arterial hypoxemia [19–22]. Impairment of hypoxic pulmonary vasoconstriction means that gravitational effects on pulmonary blood flow are poorly tolerated. Many authors observed at least partial resolution of the hepatopulmonary syndrome following liver transplant [23, 24].

A common complication of liver disease and portal hypertension is the accumulation of ascites, whereas the presence of significant ascites sometimes compromises respiratory function mostly by creating the restrictive pattern of lung mechanics, a more significant complication is the presence of fluid in the thorax, termed hepatic hydrothorax. Hydrothorax may exacerbate the restriction pattern even further, sometimes leading to atelectasis development, with associated V/Q mismatch and intrapulmonary shunt that adds to already pre-existing hypoxemia, and also to increase of PA pressure.

3. Hemodynamic changes during orthotopic liver transplant surgery

3.1. Anesthesia-related factors

From the days, when the first successful liver transplantation surgery was performed to this day, anesthesiologists all over the world, despite plenty of ongoing and already published research works in the field, have not yet arrived at a consensus, let alone adopted unified guidelines or protocols of the anesthetic technique for liver transplantation surgery.

Since anesthesia-related systemic hemodynamic changes are well described elsewhere, the only aspect of these effects, specifically an impact of anesthesia factors and adjuvant drugs on hepatic blood flow (HBF) and oxygen delivery, needs to be discussed here. The degree to which the hemodynamic changes, caused by anesthetic agents, take place in patients with advanced liver disease, depends on the patient's particular hemodynamics, volume status and compensation pattern, nature of the surgical procedure, and many other factors. Patients with cirrhosis may be more sensitive to hepatic hypoperfusion, and may be more susceptible to liver injury (such as administration of a hepatotoxic drug, rapid blood loss).

It has been shown that practically all general anesthesia techniques, regardless of drug combinations, in the absence of surgical stimulation, reduce the HBF by about 30%. It appears that the systemic arterial blood pressure is a main determinant of hepatic blood as the hepatic artery exhibits almost no autoregulatory capacity [25]. Commonly used IV induction anesthetic agent, etomidate, along with maintaining well the systemic hemodynamic parameters at baseline levels, only moderately reduces the HBF in a dose-dependent manner, and causes the increase in hepatic arterial resistance (by 40%).

Propofol, however, has shown an ability to preserve baseline levels of the HBF, as long as systemic hemodynamic changes were insignificant [26].

Use of isoflurane and sevoflurane for anesthesia maintenance, albeit being associated with minimal-to-moderate global reduction of HBF, has not been found to be associated with any significant influence on arterial hepatic blood flow or oxygen transport and extraction ratio in the liver. Short-action opioids, fentanyl in particular, has shown no discernible effect on HBF [27–31].

Other potential perioperative causes of a reduction of HBF include mechanical ventilation, positive end-expiratory pressure, systemic hypotension due to hypovolemia, hemorrhage, etc., and hypoxemia. Beta (β)-blockers, alpha (α)-agonists, H_2 blockers, hypocapnia, alkalosis, and hypoglycemia have been found to be associated with moderate HBF reduction.

Dopamine (3 mcg/kg/min), epinephrine (from 0.01 mcg/kg/min), hypercapnia, acidosis, and hypoxemia, however, are among the factors that actually can increase HBF [32, 33].

With a substantial variety of anesthetic techniques currently in use and with full awareness of ESLD hemodynamic profile specifics and patient-to-patient variety in that respect, it appears to be reasonable to set hemodynamic goals (i.e., hemodynamic parameters to possibly maintain) for anesthesia care for liver transplant. These should include mean arterial pressure (MAP) around 75–85 mmHg, Heart rate (HR): <100/min, Central venous pressure (CVP): <20 mmHg, Mean Pulmonary Artery Pressure (MPAP): <25 mmHg, CO/CI: >4 L/min/>2 L/min m^2, Systemic Vascular Resistance (SVR): >500 dynes/s/cm^{-5}, and mixed venous SvO2: >75%.

3.2. Surgery-related factors

The course of liver transplantation surgery includes four stages. During preanhepatic, or dissection phase, the diseased liver is being dissected and prepared for removal. Portal vein clamping, followed by hepatic artery and IVC clamp, heralds the start of anhepatic phase, during which part of the diseased liver is being removed from the body and being replaced by the donor's organ. Vascular anastomoses are being performed, followed by organ reperfusion phase, the shortest one with most significant hemodynamic impact. After venous blood flow restoration in the transplanted organ, postreperfusion phase include common hepatic arterial anastomosis, cholecyctectomy, and bile duct reconstruction.

During preanhepatic (dissection) phase, laparotomy, often followed by ascites evacuation, causes drop of intra-abdominal pressure, with rapid splanchnic volume increase (i.e., mesenteric blood pooling) ensued. Ongoing blood loss at this stage may be very substantial, due to abundance of venous collaterals in cases with longstanding portal hypertension, and also in cases of re-do transplants, or cases with significant adhesions after previous surgeries. Decrease of venous return, ongoing blood loss, fluid shift, and developing acidosis further contribute to CO/CI and mean arterial blood pressure (MABP) decrease.

Portal cross clamp, which portends the anhepatic stage start, causes variable (20–30% of baseline) degree of venous return decrease. However, in cases of well-developed portocaval collaterals (longstanding portal hypertension), this loss of preclamp venous return may be less significant, around 15–20%, and generally well tolerated. IVC complete cross-clamp oftentimes leads to a more substantial and poorly tolerated (approximately 50%) decrease of venous return, whereas IVC partial clamp causes variable, about 25–50%, decrease of venous return [34, 35]. ESLD patients have very limited ability, if any, to compensate for the rapid decrease in venous return with systemic vasoconstriction due to inherent low SVR. Veno-venous bypass (VVB) may present a possible solution to compensate for decreased venous return. Hemodynamic instability following test clamping of IVC is the most common indication for initiating VVB [36]. It has been suggested [37] that hypotension (30% decrease in MAP) or a decrease in cardiac index (50%) during a 5-min test period of hepatic vascular occlusion can be used to identify the group of patients who require VVB. Other indications of the VVB include presence of pulmonary hypertension, impaired ventricular function from previous myocardial infarction, ischemic heart disease, and cardiomyopathy [38]. In patients with pulmonary hypertension, excessive fluid loading to compensate for hemodynamic changes during anhepatic phase may result in acute right ventricular dysfunction. Patients with cardiomyopathy have impaired left ventricular function, and consequently a limited ability to generate adequate CO in the face of the increase in SVR during the anhepatic phase. These patients, too, may benefit from ameliorative effect of the preload associated with VVB. Some centers use VVB in patients with impaired renal function (i.e., hepato-renal syndrome) in order to prevent further kidneys damage during the anhepatic phase and to reduce the need for postoperative renal support. Among the advantages of VVB, some researchers listed the ability to reduce hemodynamic instability during anhepatic phase. It is useful in patients with pulmonary hypertension and cardiomyopathy who tolerate anhepatic period poorly. VVB has been shown to maintain intraoperative renal function [39, 40]. It also helps to maintain cerebral perfusion pressure in patients with acute fulminant failure by avoiding rapid swings in blood pressure, and, at least theoretically, may reduce blood loss [41]. However, VVB is not devoid of certain disadvantages. It does not guarantee normal perfusion of abdominal organs and lower limbs, since venous return never could be maintained at prebypass levels. The pump could only provide up to 2 L/min output (most commonly, only 1.5–1.8 L/min), which is, however comparable with low-to-normal levels of CO, cannot ensure the normal or even near-normal level of preload [42]. There is neither evidence of general(patient- and organ survival) outcome improvement, nor that it's use reduces or prevents the occurrence of postoperative renal failure [43]. VVB may exacerbate coagulation problems and cause excessive bleeding by inducing hemolysis, platelet depletion.

Graft reperfusion causes major hemodynamic changes along with possible substantial end-organ injury. These may include direct myocardial injury, resulting in tachy/bradyarrhythmias and cardiac arrest, profound vasoplegia, acute interstitial pulmonary oedema, leading to further RV overload/acute insufficiency, raise of pulmonary artery pressure (PAP) and CVP. Blood loss, hemodilution, hypovolemia, temperature drop, and rapidly developing lactic acidosis contribute to decreased sensitivity to catecholamines and efficiency of vasopressors. All these factors lead to rapid drop of SVR, resulting in a decrease of MABP with or without CO/CI decrease. Postreperfusion syndrome (PRS) was defined as a more than 30% decrease of MABP from that in the anhepatic stage, longer than for 1 min during the first 5 min after reperfusion of the liver graft [44–46].

In the postreperfusion period, the major factors of hemodynamic instability include ongoing blood loss, exacerbated by consumption coagulopathy in the face of very limited or almost nonexisting production of coagulation factors by the liver graft. Hypocalcemia, resulting from the effects of citrate-containing blood conservation solution, associated with transfusion of large amounts of RBC, exacerbates reduction of myocardial contractility caused by recent reperfusion. Acidemia, mostly due to lactic acidosis, substantially decreases efficacy of vaso-active agents.

4. Blood loss and coagulopathy management

4.1. Blood loss estimation and prediction factors

Blood loss during OLT is a well-known major factor of morbidity/mortality and overall hemodynamic instability, varying from just hundreds of ml up to dozens of liters. Predisposing factors for major blood loss may include pre-existing + ongoing consumption and dilution coagulopathy (i.e., preoperative prothrombin time (PT), International normalized ratio (INR) and platelets numbers, factor V levels, etc.), MELD score >25, severe portal hypertension, "hostile abdomen" —postlaparotomy, re-do orthotopic liver transplant (OLT), long ischemia times, aged/marginal quality donor organ, donor-recipient organ size discrepancy, long, traumatic liver dissection, and surgeon-related factors.

Substantial number of studies reported no statistically significant correlations between blood loss and most of aforementioned parameters, particularly in respect to MELD score [47] and INR [48].

To date, blood loss and associated massive blood transfusion during OLTs remain difficult to predict [49]. Intraoperative blood salvage technique provides at least some way for blood loss estimation, with considerable approximation. Correspondent guidelines, based on calculations of hematocrit during blood loss (25–30%) and that of returned red blood cells by Cell-Saver (approximately 55–65% depending on Cell-Saver model), have been developed. Authors calculated estimated blood loss by multiplying the total volume of Cell-Saver returned RBCs by factor 3.4–4.0 [50, 51].

4.2. Coagulopathy: mechanisms and assessment

Of all the aforementioned factors, coagulopathy presents by far the most important and potentially most correctable problem, contributing to overall blood loss and, therefore, hemodynamic instability. Bleeding during OLT is multifactorial due both to surgical trauma and to coagulation defects. Coagulation defect in ESLD patients include impaired coagulation factor synthesis, dysfunction of coagulation factors, increased consumption, and fibrinolysis. Commonly, the levels of factor VII and protein C decrease first, followed by reductions in factors V, II, and X levels [52]. Platelet function is also affected by liver disease, and thrombocytopenia is common. Predisposing factors include hypersplenism secondary to portal hypertension, decreased thrombopoietin synthesis, immune complex-associated platelet clearance, and reticuloendothelial destruction [53].

During the dissection phase of the transplant, excessive bleeding is related to the technical difficulties during the liver dissection, and presence of portal hypertension, with large dilated collaterals [54].

During the anhepatic phase, coagulation factor synthesis is practically nonexistent, and ongoing factors consumption exacerbate the bleeding.

Right after graft reperfusion, profound coagulation abnormalities are very common. Factors that contribute to excessive bleeding in postreperfusion period include platelet entrapment in the sinusoids of the donor liver, a global reduction of all coagulation factors (mainly due to increased consumption, and partially due to hemodilution), and decreased level of antifibrinolytic factors [55, 56].

Method of thromboelastography (TEG) allows a rapid graphic assessment of the functional clotting status and degree of fibrinolysis. In various studies, the amount of RBCs and fresh frozen plasma (FFP) usage has been significantly reduced when TEG monitoring that was compared to the conventional "clinician-directed" transfusion management [57, 58]. Although the usefulness of TEG in complex coagulation defects has been questioned [59], recent studies have shown, that the use of TEG can reduce the number of blood products transfused [58].

4.3. Hemotransfusion requirements and strategies

Blood transfusion therapy remains a critical component of anesthetic management and peri-operative care in OLT. Multiple studies have shown a large variability in the use of blood products among different centers and among individual anesthesiologists within the same center [60]. The decision of when to transfuse RBCs, remains debatable. Some authors recommend keeping the hematocrit between 30 and 35%; others think it advisable and acceptable to maintain it between 26 and 28% [61, 62]. The modern trends have shown a substantial change from a transfusion of 10–20 units to 0–5.

The standard indication for fresh frozen plasma (FFP) infusion is coagulation defect treatment. FFP is expected to improve complex coagulation disorders in case of severe bleeding as it contains all coagulation factors and inhibitors. However, Freeman et al. [62] maintain that FFP administration is not essential during OLT, and that platelets and fibrinogen concentrates may be given when platelet count and fibrinogen level fall below 50,000 mm^3 and 1 g/L. In some centers, the trigger point is INR lower than two, which remains controversial. It has been shown that TE-guided coagulation defect management generally lowers the FFP amount. There is currently no consensus on the volume of FFP or rate of infusion required; in common practice, 10–15 mL/kg are usually administered. Because of the lack of universally accepted guidelines, the amount and timing of FFP administration during OLT are still guided by experienced clinical judgment, local practices, and coagulation tests (including TEG).

Although there is no consensus regarding the appropriate threshold value [64], platelet concentrates are frequently administered during OLT to address "oozing" on the operation field that likely could be attributed to the lack clot formation ability. Inter-center indications for platelet transfusion vary, but it seems that the current trend is to administer platelet transfusions pretty much regardless of the absolute PLT count.

It has been shown in many studies that the massive use of blood products during OLT is associated with increase in morbidity and mortality [65, 66]. It has been demonstrated that the intraoperative transfusion of red blood cells (RBCs) is associated with increase of postoperative mortality, specifically reduce survival rates at six months (63.8 vs. 83.3%) and at 5 years (34.5 vs. 49.2%), thus became a major prediction factor of mortality [59, 67, 68]. Higher intraoperative RBC transfusion requirements are associated with higher reintervention rates. Patients, who undergo reintervention, have three times higher mortality than those who do not have reinterventions [69, 70]. All blood products (RBCs, fresh frozen plasma (FFP), and platelets) have been shown to be negatively associated with graft survival at 1 and 5 years by univariate analysis [71]. Recent studies show that FFP and platelet transfusions are linked to the development of ALI/ARDS [71]. Pereboom et al. demonstrated, that platelet transfusion during OLTx is associated with increased postoperative mortality due to transfusion-related acute lung injury (TRALI)/ARDS [63]. Intraoperative platelet transfusions have been identified as a strong independent risk factor for patient survival after OLT in addition to RBCs [72]. Studies have demonstrated that platelets are involved in the pathogenesis of reperfusion injury of the liver graft by inducing endothelial cell apoptosis. This effect is independent of ischemia-related endothelial cell injury [73].

4.4. Ways of blood loss reduction

Ways of blood loss reduction include surgical techniques such as Piggy-back technique with IVC preservation—partial Inferior vena cava (IVC) clamp, and anesthesia management options, such as maintaining the low CVP, minimal hemodilution with limited crystalloids infusion, and vasoactive agents use. Discussion of surgical techniques is beyond the scope of this review; however, anesthetic management options and techniques, intended to reduce blood loss during OLT are in the focus of discussion.

4.4.1. Fluid management and "low CVP" paradigm

Balanced fluid administration and maintaining relative hypovolemia have been advocated by many authors. A low CVP has been recommended to minimize blood loss during dissection stage of the liver transplantation. Massicotte et al. [74, 75] reported that maintaining a low CVP before the anhepatic phase was an efficient technique to decrease blood loss and transfusion rate. However, low CVP is associated with increased risk of complications, such as tissue hypoperfusion, development of lactic acidosis and renal failure, and also significant morbidity and mortality [76]. As it has been observed, increase in serum creatinine level, indications for dialysis, and 30-days mortality were higher in group of liver transplant patients, where CVP has been kept at low levels (around 3–5 smH_2O), in order to avoid venous congestion of the graft. However, no supportive evidence has been found for decreasing CVP and effective circulating blood volume during OLT levels, currently accepted in some centers for liver resection [77]. Due to the lack of adequately powered, randomized, prospective controlled trials further investigations are needed to determine which patients would benefit from restrictive volume management in the intraoperative period of OLT.

4.4.2. Blood salvage technique during OLT

The use of intraoperative blood salvage and autologous blood transfusion has been for a long time an important method to reduce the need for allogeneic blood and the associated complications [78]. It has been demonstrated, that, for systematic use of Cell Saver salvaged blood in 75 OLT cases, retransfusion volume was enough and adequate in 65% of the cases [79].

The resultant hematocrit after Cell Saver processing ranges between 50 and 80% [80]. The safety of cell-salvaging procedure has been widely demonstrated [81]. Use of intraoperative autologous transfusion resulted in conservation of RBCs and reduction in exposure to homologous blood and blood components [82, 83]. Use of Cell Saver during OLT made it possible to recover up to 50% of blood loss [84]. Substantial reduction in FFP and a lesser reduction in platelet requirement have also been seen.

Nonetheless, blood-salvaging techniques during OLT are still being considered as controversial. Some studies have reported relatively higher blood loss, increased incidence of fibrinolysis, and cost rise [85, 86].The increased blood loss in recipients, receiving Cell Saver blood has been attributed to the release of fibrinolytic compounds from blood cells in the collected blood and/or from the transplanted liver [87]. These findings, however, have not dissuaded the anesthesiologists from using Cell Saver during OLTs; in fact, this method is gaining wider popularity, and becoming almost a standard of care in many centers around the world.

5. Vasoactive agents applied pharmacology and use in hemodynamic management during OLT

Hemodynamic instability during OLT due to blood loss, graft reperfusion, and postreperfusion vascular tone adjustment, substantial fluid shift oftentimes necessitates the use of vasoactive agents. Different vasopressors, such as dopamine, dobutamine, epinephrine, norepinephrine, phenylephrine, vasopressin, and, more recently, terlipressin and octreotide have been used for hemodynamic optimization and end-organ perfusion improvement during OLTs for decades [88, 89].

Norepinephrine and phenylephrine have a universal vasoconstrictor effect due to α-receptor stimulation, thus effectively increasing systemic vascular resistance, while decreasing cardiac index, peripheral and portal blood flow [90–93]. However, norepinephrine in higher doses causes severe peripheral vasospasm and promotes metabolic (lactic) acidosis [88]. Phenylephrine increases SVR and MPAP, while it decreases CO/CI, peripheral, and portal BF [93], and does not affect portal VP during the dissection phase. CVP is often increased and does not seem to reflect cardiac filling [94].

Epinephrine and norepinephrine decrease liver and kidney tissue perfusion, thereby reducing lactate clearance, promote lactic acidosis, cause temporary alterations of hepatic macro- and microcirculation (return to baseline 2 h after onset of infusion). Dose-dependent progressive decline of hepatic macro- (33–75% reduction) and microcirculation (39–58% reduction) was found in transplanted livers. Norepinephrine has a direct constrictor effect on liver sinusoids, thereby reducing hepatic blood volume/flow and aggravating portal hypertension, and demonstrates effects similar to those of vasopressin effects on CO/CI and SVR [95], does not increase HBF, hepatic DO2 or VO2, and does not improve the hepatic lactate extraction ratio [96]. Vasopressin increases SVR, decreases MPAP; normalizes CO/CI, and potentially, CVP; maintains mean BP; decreases portal pressure, HBF, and systemic blood flow (SBF); improves impaired renal function; enhances diuresis, and thus improves Na balance and lactate elimination; enhances platelet aggregation; and increases levels of Profactor VIII and von Willebrand factor, and does not promote lactic acidosis. Its use after reperfusion, albeit having been shown beneficial by many authors, remains controversial, mainly due to splanchnic flow restriction effect with potential impairment of portal flow to the graft. Vasopressin has been demonstrated to have a dose-dependent vasoconstrictor effect on the peripheral vasculature with substantial SVR increases, while having little effect on heart rate, systemic arterial blood pressure, and CI in normotensive patients [97]. The ability of vasopressin to selectively constrict splanchnic vasculature, and thus decrease portal blood flow, is thought to constitute a physiological basis for variceal bleeding control by a higher vasopressin (0.4 U/min) dose [98, 99]. Vasopressin decreases portal vein pressure and flow in the native liver during liver transplantation [100]. Authors' own study has shown that use of low-dose vasopressin (0.04 U/min) infusion in an attempt to reduce blood loss seems to be a promising and a feasible technique. Vasopressin decreases portal vein pressure and blood flow in the native liver, as do terlipressin and octreotide [101]. A low-dose vasopressin (0.04 U/min) infusion apparently exerts only a minimal effect on the general hemodynamics. Low-dose vasopressin infusion is proved to be safe: to date, no cases of liver graft damage have been documented. To the contrary, cases where a high-dose of vasopressin (0.8 U) bolus, followed by a vasopressin infusion (4U/h) to attenuate refractory hypotension secondary to graft reperfusion, was used without causing any identifiable liver graft damage, have been reported [102]. Vasopressin has been shown to have a stimulation effect on lactate production by liver cells and adipose tissue in the septic model [103], and to be able to decrease blood loss during pre- and anhepatic phases of OLT (namely, EBL before graft reperfusion has been decreased by 50.2% [104] **Figure 1**)

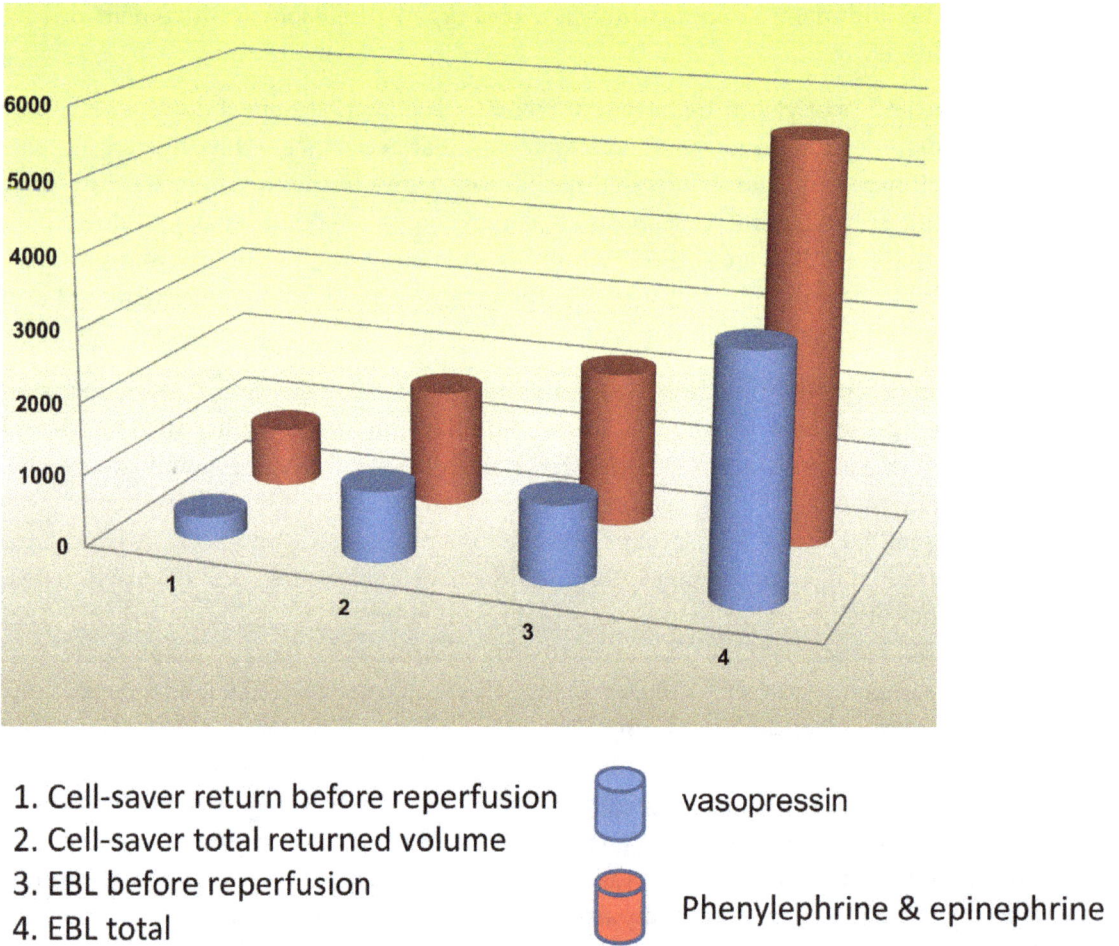

1. Cell-saver return before reperfusion   vasopressin
2. Cell-saver total returned volume
3. EBL before reperfusion
4. EBL total   Phenylephrine & epinephrine

Figure 1. Blood loss decrease in pre-reperfusion stages of OLT: comparison of low-dose vasopressin and phenylephrine infusions.

5.1. Suggested algorithm of vasoactive agents used during anesthesia for OLT

Phenylephrine, epinephrine, norepinephrine, dopamine, and vasopressin are commonly used during different stages of OLT. The task of attaining hemodynamic stability sometimes dictates concomitant use of two or more vasoactive agents (**Figure 2**).

Intraoperative use of dopamine, 3 mcg/kg/min in OLT is intended to preserve and protect the adequate renal function, especially in cases of hepatorenal syndrome [105]. Higher rates of dopamine infusion, 5–10 to 20 mcg/kg/min, increase cardiac output and SVR. However, gaining CO/CI increase at the expense of tachycardia and, potentially, some rhythm disturbances makes dopamine a less desirable agent.

Early in the perunhepatic (dissection) stage of the surgery, phenylephrine infusion may be started, along with already running dopamine and low-dose vasopressin. Due to phenylephrine's almost purely α-mimetic activity, its use actually addresses the low SVR problem, a main culprit for low MABP in majority of cases, provided that volume status correction and maintenance is being performed properly. In the majority of cases, phenylephrine infusion continues throughout the case. Providers in the other centers prefer and advocate early norepinephrine-only infusion be started, while others combine these agents [106].

Anhepatic stage often presents a challenge in terms of maintaining of hemodynamic stability. Rapid decrease in venous return; therefore, potential drop of CO, exacerbated by significant blood loss, usually necessitates more aggressive approach. Along with increase of norepinephrine (and phenylephrine, if its infusion is running along with the former), epinephrine may be added, with the purpose of using its β-stimulation activity. In preparation graft reperfusion,

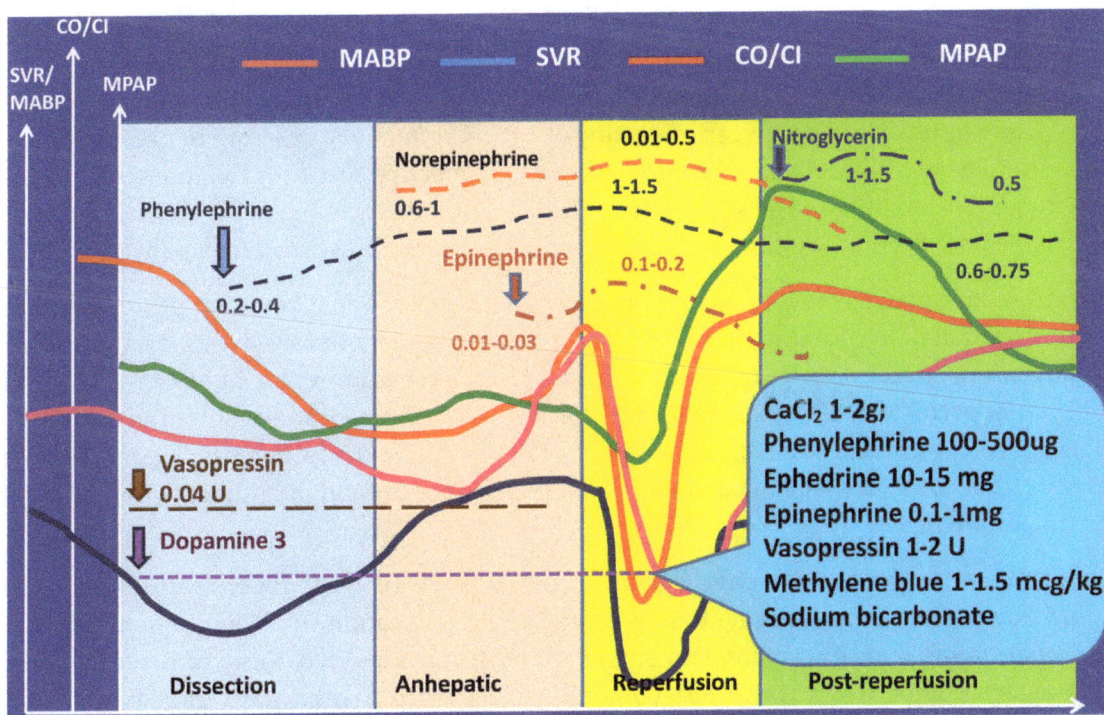

Figure 2. Use of different vasoactive agents throughout the whole of the OLT procedure.

some authors actually recommend "pretreatment" [107] with epinephrine and phenylephrine combination for postreperfusion syndrome prevention.

Graft reperfusion and postreperfusion syndrome presents a most significant challenge for hemodynamic management. Many different techniques and drug combinations has been tested and recommended for rapid hemodynamic recovery after liver graft reperfusion. Along with vasoactive agents and their combinations that are already in use by the time of a graft reperfusion, other agents has been successfully used (Figure 1). Vasopressin in small boluses, 1–2 U, may be highly efficient in opposing the significant and rapid decrease of SVR, and calcium chloride, up to 100 mg, may enhance inotropic effects of epinephrine [108]. Another agent, namely Methylene Blue, 2 mg/kg, has been reported as very efficient and "last resort" drug for prolonged and profound hypotension, refractory to treatment with other vasoactive drugs [109].

The presence of significant metabolic, mainly lactic, acidosis is a well-known cause of decreased vasoactive agent's efficiency [110]. To overcome hyporesponsiveness to vasopressors, sodium bicarbonate infusion may be necessary. THAM infusion provides a fast and efficient way of acidosis reversal and returning pH closer to the physiological range [111].

In certain cases, shortly after even seemingly uneventful graft reperfusion, PAP and CVP start to rise and graft congestion ensues. Reasons for this pulmonary pressure surge include postreperfusion left ventricle diastolic dysfunction as a result of direct myocardial injury, caused by free oxygen radicals containing metabolic substances, relative overload due to rapid transfusion of substantial amounts of blood products, interstitial pulmonary edema with PVR increase, and more. Graft congestion causes substantial perfusion and oxygen delivery impairment in the newly transplanted liver, that delays normal function restoration, specifically restart of coagulation components synthesis, which, in turn, exacerbates and prolongs the coagulation deficit. To address this problem, infusion rates of vasoactive drugs should be adjusted to the best possible balance of MAP and PAP, blood products transfusion rate (but not necessarily volume) should be decreased, diuretics (Furosemide) may be administered, and infusion of nitroglycerin, starting at 1 mcg/kg/min, may be commenced, as blood pressure tolerates. Nitroglycerin has proved to be an effective agent for treatment of pulmonary hypertension. It has been shown that nitroglycerin infusion resulted in pulmonary vascular resistance decrease by 43%, and mean pulmonary artery pressure decrease by 19% [112].

Hemodynamic management of postreperfusion stage of liver transplantation procedure consists of continuation of vasoactive agents infusion and usually involves a gradual decrease of infusion rates and also weaning from most aggressive vasopressors, like epinephrine. In substantial percentage of the cases, despite the adequate volume status restoration and coagulation defect complete reversal, the necessity for vasoactive drugs persists. Hemodynamic optimization continues well beyond the actual end of the surgery, oftentimes for a few days in critical care units.

Choice and dosage of vasoactive agents at every stage of OLT depend and should be guided by hemodynamic parameters. We suggest the allocation to all the patient population undergoing liver transplantation surgery, in three groups, according to hemodynamic parameters: compensated (MAP 80–100 mmHg, SVR > 600 dynes/s/cm^5), subcompensated (MAP 60–70 mmHg, SVR 300–600 dynes/s/cm^5), and decompensated (MAP <50 mmHg, SVR <200–250 dynes/s/cm^5)

Suggested algorithm of vasoactive agents use and dosage is summarized in **Table 1**.

OLT stage	Hemodynamics					
	MAP 80–100, SVR>600		MAP 60–70, SVR 300–600		MAP<50, SVR <200–250	
	Agent	Dose	Agent	Dose	Agent	Dose
Dissection	Dop	3	Dop	3	Dop	5–10
	Phen	0.2–0.4	Phen	0.4–0.6	Phen	0.6–1.0
	Vas	0.04	Vas	0.04	Vas	0.04–0.08
					NE	0.01–0.03
An-hepatic	Dop	3	Dop	3	Dop	5–10
	Phen	0.2–0.4	Phen	0.4–0.8	Phen	0.8–1.2
	Vas	0.04	NE	0.01–0.03	NE	0.04–0.08
			Vas	0.04	Epi	0.01–0.03
					Vas	0.04–0.08
Reperfusion	Dop	3–5	Dop	3–5	Dop	3–5
	Phen	0.2–0.6	Phen	0.6–0.8	Phen	0.8–1.2
	Ca	500	NE	0.04–0.08	NE	0.06–0.1
			Epi	0.02–0.04	Epi	0.04–0.08
			Ca	1000	Vas	3–5
			Vas	1–2	Ca	1000–2000
					MB	1–1.5
					Bic	50–100
Post-reperfusion	Dop	3	Dop	3	Dop	3–5
	Phen	0.02–0.06	Phen	0.4–0.8	Phen	6–1.0
			NE	0.02–0.04	NE	0.08–0.1
					Epi	0.02–0.04

Dop—dopamine; Phen—phenylephrine; NE—norepinephrine; Epi—epinehrine, all dosage in mcg/kg/min; Vas—vasopressin, units/min; Ca—calcium chloride, mg; MB—Methylene Blue, mg/kg; Bic—sodium bicarbonate, mEq.

Table 1. Algorithm of vasoactive agents use and dosage during OLT.

6. Conclusion

Hemodynamic optimization during liver transplant surgery presents very complex, challenging, sometimes formidable task, many aspects of which remain unclear, thus warrant further research. A wide variety of anesthetic techniques and standards, institutional policies, hemodynamic triggers for vasoactive agents use and transfusion thresholds, arriving at the even nation-wide consensus, let alone worldwide, remain extremely difficult, if not mere a unrealistic task. Nonetheless, introduction of comprehensive guidelines, based on most common clinical practices and realities of perioperative hemodynamic management appears to be not only conceivable but rather timely and a necessary enterprise. Once introduced, such guidelines may lay the ground for successful and safe intra and perioperative practices and also provide support for much-needed research efforts in this complicated area of transplant anesthesia practice.

Author details

Alexander A. Vitin[1]*, Dana Tomescu[2] and Leonard Azamfirei[3]

*Address all correspondence to: vitin@uw.edu

1 Department of Anesthesiology, University of Washington, Seattle, WA, USA

2 Department of Anesthesia and Intensive Care "Carol Davila", University of Medicine and Pharmacy, Fundeni Clinical Institute, Bucharest, Romania

3 University of Medicine and Pharmacy Tîrgu Mureș, Tîrgu Mureș, Romania

References

[1] Groszmann RJ. Hyperdynamic circulation of liver disease 40 years later: Pathophysiology and clinical consequences. Hepatology. 1994;**20**:1359-1363

[2] Lee SS, Marty J, Mantz J, Samain E, Braillon A, Lebrec D. Desensitization of myocardial β-adrenergic receptors in cirrhotic rats. Hepatology. 1990;**12**:481-485

[3] Gaudin C, Braillon A, Selz F, Cuche JL, Lebrec D. Free and conjugated catecholamines in patients with cirrhosis. Journal of Laboratory and Clinical Medicine. 1990 May;**115**(5):589-592

[4] Chang SW, Ohara N. Chronic biliary obstruction induces pulmonary intravascular phagocytosis and endotoxin sensitivity in rats. Journal of Clinical Investigation. 1994;**94**:2009-2019.

[5] Carter EP, Hartsfield CL, Miyazono M, Jakkula M, Morris KG Jr, McMurtry IF. Regulation of heme oxygenase-1 by nitric oxide during hepatopulmonary syndrome. American Journal of Physiology—Lung Cellular and Molecular Physiology. 2002;**283**:L346-L353

[6] Sztrymf B, Rabiller A, Nunes H, Savale L, Lebrec D, Le Pape A, et al. Prevention of hepatopulmonary syndrome and hyperdynamic state by pentoxifylline in cirrhotic rats. European Respiratory Journal. 2004;**23**:752-758

[7] Miyao M, Kotani H, Ishida T, Kawai C, Manabe S, Abiru H, Tamaki K. Pivotal role of liver sinusoidal endothelial cells in NAFLD/NASH progression. Laboratory Investigation. 2015;95(10):1130-1144. DOI: 10.1038/labinvest.2015.95

[8] Bayley TJ, Segel N, Bishop JM. The circulatory changes in patients with cirrhosis of the liver at rest and during exercise. Clinical Science. 1964;26:227-235

[9] Limas CJ, Guiha NH, Lekagul O, Cohn JN. Impaired left ventricular function in alcoholic cirrhosis with ascites. Circulation. 1974;49:755-760

[10] Inglés AC, Hernandez I, García-Estañ J, Quesada T, Carbonell LF. Limited cardiac preload reserve in conscious cirrhotic rats. American Journal of Physiology. 1991;260: H1912-H1917

[11] Møller S, Henriksen JH. Cirrhotic cardiomyopathy: A pathophysiological review of circulatory dysfunction in liver disease. Heart. 2002;87:9-15

[12] Porres-Aguilar M, Altamirano JT, Torre-Delgadillo A, Charlton M, Duarte-Rojo A. Portopulmonary hypertension and hepatopulmonary syndrome: A clinician-oriented overview. European Respiratory Review. 2012:21:223-233

[13] Porres-Aguilar M, Zuckerman MJ, Figueroa-Casas JB, et al. Portopulmonary hypertension: State-of-the-art. Annals of Hepatology. 2008;7:321-330

[14] Golbin JM, Krowka MJ. Portopulmonary hypertension. Clinics in Chest Medicine. 2007;28:203-218.

[15] Savale L, O'Callaghan DS, Magnier R, et al. Current management approaches to portopulmonary hypertension. International Journal of Clinical Practice. Supplement. 2011;169:11-18

[16] Simonneau G, Robbins IM, Beghetti M, et al. Updated clinical classification of pulmonary hypertension. Journal of the American College of Cardiology. 2009;54(Suppl. 1):S43-S54

[17] Benjaminov FS, Prentice M, Sniderman KW, et al. Portopulmonary hypertension in decompensated cirrhosis with refractory ascites. Gut. 2003;52:1355-1362

[18] Neuhofer W, Gülberg V, Gerbes AL. Endothelin and endothelin receptor antagonism in portopulmonary hypertension. European Journal of Clinical Investigation. 2006;36(Suppl. 3):54-61

[19] Kochar R, Nevah Rubin MI, Fallon MB. Pulmonary complications of cirrhosis. Current Gastroenterology Reports. 2011;13:34-39

[20] Vachiéry F, Moreau R, Hadengue A, et al. Hypoxemia in patients with cirrhosis: Relationship with liver failure and hemodynamic alterations. Journal of Hepatology. 1997;27:492-495

[21] Schenk P, Fuhrmann V, Madl C, et al. Hepatopulmonary syndrome: Prevalence and predictive value of various cut offs for arterial oxygenation and their clinical consequences. Gut. 2002;51:853-859

[22] Rodríguez-Roisin R, Agustí AG, Roca J. The hepatopulmonary syndrome: New name, old complexities. Thorax. 1992;**47**:897-902

[23] Rodriguez-Roisin R, Krowka MJ. Hepatopulmonary syndrome—A liver-induced lung vascular disorder. New England Journal of Medicine. 2008;**29**:2378-2387

[24] Krowka MJ, Porayko MK, Plevak DJ, et al. Hepatopulmonary syndrome with progressive hypoxemia as an indication for liver transplantation: Case reports and literature review. Mayo Clinic Proceedings. 1997;**72**:44-53

[25] Gelman SI. Disturbances in hepatic blood flow during anesthesia and surgery. Archives of Surgery. 1976 Aug;**111**:881-893

[26] Thompson I, Fitch W, Hughes RL, Campbell D, Watson R. Effects of certain IV anesthetics on liver blood flow and hepatic oxygen consumption Br. J. Anaesth. 1986;**58**:69-80

[27] Haberer JP, Schoeffler P, Couderc E, Duvaldestin P. Fentanyl pharmacokinetics in anaesthetized patients with cirrhosis. British Journal of Anaesthesia. 1982;**54**:1267-1270

[28] Zaleski L, Abello D, Gold MI. Desflurane versus isoflurane in patients with chronic hepatic and renal disease. Anesthesia and Analgesia. 1993;**76**:353-356

[29] Meierhenrich R, Gauss A, Muhling B, Bracht, Radermacher P, Georgieff M, Wagner F. The effect of propofol and desflurane anaesthesia on human hepatic blood flow: A pilot study. Anaesthesia. 2010:**65**:1085-1093

[30] Carmichael FJL. Effects of temperature and propofol on hepatic blood flow. Anesthesia and Analgesia. 1996;**82**:426-439

[31] Dalal A, Lang J D Jr. Anesthetic considerations for patients with liver disease. In: Hepatic Surgery. INTECH, chapter 3, pp. 61-80. http://dx.doi.org/10.5772/54222 Chapter from the book Hepatic Surgery

[32] Hannaman M. Hevesi Z. Anesthesia care for liver transplantation. Transplantation Reviews. 2011;**25**:36-43

[33] Fonouni H, Mehrabi A, Soleimani M, Müller SA, Büchler MW, Schmidt J. The need for venovenous bypass in liver transplantation. HPB: The Official Journal of the International Hepato Pancreato Biliary Association. 2008;**10**(3):196-203

[34] Mehrabi A, Fonouni H, Müller SA, Schmidt J.Langenbecks. Current concepts in transplant surgery: Liver transplantation today. Archives of Surgery. 2008 May;**393**(3):245-260

[35] Reddy K, Mallett S, Peachey T. Venovenous bypass in orthotopic liver transplantation: Time for a rethink? Liver Transplantation. 2005 July;**11**(7):741-749

[36] Veroli P, el Hage C, Ecoffey C. Does adult liver transplantation without venovenous bypass result in renal failure? Anesthesia and Analgesia. 1992;**75**:489-494

[37] Beltran J, Taura P, Grande L, Garcia-Valdecasas JC, Rimola A, Cugat E. Venovenous bypass and liver transplantation. Anesthesia and Analgesia 1993;**77**:642

[38] Johnson MW, Powelson JA, Auchincloss H Jr, Delmonico FL, Cosimi AB. Selective use of veno-venous bypass in orthotopic liver transplantation. Clinical Transplantation. 1996;**10**:181-185

[39] Corti A, Degasperi A, Colussi S, Mazza E, Amici O, Cristalli A, et al. Evaluation of renal function during orthotopic liver transplantation. Minerva Anestesiologica. 1997;**63**:221-228

[40] Shaw BW Jr, Martin DJ, Marquez JM, Kang YG, Bugbee AC Jr, Iwatsuki S, et al. Venous bypass in clinical liver transplantation. Annals of Surgery. 1984;**200**:524-534

[41] Cheema SP, Hughes A, Webster NR, Bellamy MC. Cardiac function during orthotopic liver transplantation with venovenous bypass. Anaesthesia. 1995;**50**:776-778

[42] Schwarz B, Pomaroli A, Hoermann C, Margreiter R, Mair P. Liver Transplantation without venovenous bypass: Morbidity and mortality in patients with greater than 50% reduction in cardiac output after vena cava clamping. Journal of Cardiothoracic and Vascular Anesthesia. 2001;**15**:460-462

[43] Paugam-Burtz C, Kavafyan J, Merckx P, Dahmani S, Sommacale D, Ramsay M, Belghiti J, Mantz J. Postreperfusion syndrome during liver transplantation for cirrhosis: Outcome and predictors. Liver Transplantation. 2009 May;**15**(5):522-529

[44] Aggarwal S, Kang Y, Freeman JA, Fortunato FL, Pinsky MR. Postreperfusion syndrome: Cardiovascular collapse following hepatic reperfusion during liver transplantation. Transplantation Proceedings. 1987;**19**:54-55

[45] Aggarwal S, Kang Y, Freeman J, DeWolf AM, Begliomini B. Is there a post-reperfusion syndrome? Transplantation Proceedings. 1989;**21**:3497-3499

[46] Massicotte L, Beaulieu D, Roy JD, Marleau D, Vandenbroucke F, et al. MELD score and blood product requirements during liver transplantation: No link. Transplantation. 2009 Jun 15;**87**(11):1689-94. DOI: 10.1097/TP.0b013e3181a5e5f1

[47] Findlay JY, Rettke SR. Poor prediction of blood transfusion requirements in adult liver transplantations from preoperative variables. Clinical Anesthesia. 2000:**12**: 319-323

[48] Steib A, Freys G, Lehmann C, Meyer C, Mahoudeau G. Intaoperative blood losses and transfusion requirements during adult liver transplantation remain difficult to predict. Canadian Journal of Anesthesia. 2001;**48**:1075-1079

[49] Schorn MN. Measurement of blood loss: Review of the literature. Journal of Midwifery & Women's Health. 2010;**55**:20-27

[50] Drummond JC, Petrovitch CT. Intraoperative blood salvage: Fluid replacement calculations. Anesthesia and Analgesia. 2005;**100**:645-649

[51] Feltracco P, Brezzi ML, Barbieri S, Galligioni H, Milevoj M, Carollo C, Ori C. Blood loss, predictors of bleeding, transfusion practice and strategies of blood cell salvaging during liver transplantation. World Journal of Hepatology. 2013 Jan 27:**5**(1):1-15

[52] Kerr R, Newsome P, Germain L, Thomson E, Dawson P, Stirling D, Ludlam CA. Effects of acute liver injury on blood coagulation. Journal of Thrombosis and Haemostasis. 2003;**1**:754-759

[53] Yost CS, Niemann CU. Miller's Anesthesia. Anesthesia for Abdominal Organ Transplantation. 7th ed. Philadelphia: Churchill Livingstone Elsevier; 2010. pp. 2155-2184

[54] Ramos E, Dalmau A, Sabate A, Lama C, Llado L, Figueras J, Jaurrieta E. Intraoperative red blood cell transfusion in liver transplantation: Influence on patient outcome, prediction of requirements, and measures to reduce them. Liver Transplantation. 2003;**9**:1320-1327

[55] Mangus RS, Kinsella SB, Nobari MM, Fridell JA, Vianna RM, Ward ES, Nobari R, Tector AJ. Predictors of blood product use in orthotopic liver transplantation using the piggyback hepatectomy technique. Transplantation Proceedings. 2007;**39**:3207-3213

[56] Wang SC, Shieh JF, Chang KY, Chu YC, Liu CS, Loong CC, Chan KH, Mandell S, Tsou MY. Thromboelastography-guided transfusion decreases intraoperative blood transfusion during orthotopic liver transplantation: Randomized clinical trial. Transplantation Proceedings. 2010;**42**:2590-2593

[57] Roullet S, Pillot J, Freyburger G, Biais M, Quinart A, Rault A, Revel P, Sztark F. Rotation thromboelastometry detects thrombocytopenia and hypofibrinogenaemia during orthotopic liver transplantation. British Journal of Anaesthesia. 2010;**104**:422-428

[58] Wegner J, Popovsky MA. Clinical utility of thromboelastography: One size does not fit all. Seminars in Thrombosis and Hemostasis. 2010;**36**:699-706

[59] Ozier Y, Pessione F, Samain E, Courtois F. Institutional variability in transfusion practice for liver transplantation. Anesthesia and Analgesia. 2003;**97**:671-679

[60] Klink JR. Liver transplantation: Anesthesia. In: Klink JR, Lindop MJ, editors. Anesthesia and Intensive Care for Organ Transplantation. London: Chapman and Hall; 1998. pp. 169-199.

[61] Kang Yg, Gasior TA. Blood coagulation during liver, kidney, pancreas, and lung transplantation. In: Spiess BD, Counts RB, Gould SA, editors. Perioperative Transfusion Medicine. Baltimore, MD: Williams and Wilkins; 1998. pp. 471-492

[62] Freeman JW, Williamson LM, Llewelyn C, Fisher N, Allain JP, Bellamy M, Baglin TP, Klinc J, Ala FA, Smith N, et al. A randomized trial of solvent/detergent and standard fresh frozen plasma in the treatment of the coagulopathy seen during Orthotopic Liver Transplantation. Vox Sanguinis. 1998;**74**(Suppl 1):225-229

[63] Pereboom IT, de Boer MT, Haagsma EB, Hendriks HG, Lisman T, Porte RJ. Platelet transfusion during liver transplantation is associated with increased postoperative mortality due to acute lung injury. Anesthesia and Analgesia. 2009;**108**:1083-1091

[64] Palomo Sanchez JC, Jimenez C, Moreno Gonzalez E, Garcia I, Palma F, Loinaz C, Gonzalez Ghamorro A. Effects of intraoperative blood transfusion on postoperative complications and survival after orthotopic liver transplantation. Hepato-Gastroenterology. 1998;**45**:1026-1033

[65] Liu LL, Niemann CU. Intraoperative management of liver transplant patients. Transplantation Reviews (Orlando, Fla.). 2011;**25**:124-129

[66] Butler P, Israel L, Nusbacher J, Jenkins DE, Starzl TE. Blood transfusion in liver transplantation. Transfusion. 1985;**25**:120-123

[67] Farrar RP, Hanto DW, Flye MW, Chaplin H. Blood component use in orthotopic liver transplantation. Transfusion. 1988;**28**:474-478

[68] Murthy TVSP. Transfusion support in liver transplantation. Indian Journal of Anaesthesia. 2007;**51**:13-19. Available from: http: //www.ijaweb.org/text.asp?2007/51/1/13/61108

[69] Yost CS, Niemann CU. Length of stay has been widely demonstrated to increase with RBC transfusion. In: Miller's Anesthesia. Anesthesia for Abdominal Organ Transplantation. 7th ed. Philadelphia: Churchill Livingstone Elsevier; 2010. p. 2155-2184

[70] Khan H, Belsher J, Yilmaz M, Afessa B, Winters JL, Moore SB, Hubmayr RD, Gajic O. Fresh-frozen plasma and platelet transfusions are associated with development of acute lung injury in critically ill medical patients. Chest. 2007;**131**:1308-1314

[71] de Boer MT, Christensen MC, Asmussen M, van der Hilst CS, Hendriks HG, Slooff MJ, Porte RJ. The impact of intraoperative transfusion of platelets and red blood cells on survival after liver transplantation. Anesthesia and Analgesia. 2008;**106**:32-44

[72] Sindram D, Porte RJ, Hoffman MR, Bentley RC, Clavien PA. Platelets induce sinusoidal endothelial cell apoptosis upon reperfusion of the cold ischemic rat liver. Gastroenterology. 2000;**118**:183-191

[73] Massicotte L, Lenis S, Thibeault L, Sassine MP, Seal RF, Roy A. Effect of low central venous pressure and phlebotomy on blood product transfusion requirements during liver transplantations. Liver Transplantation. 2006;**12**:117-123

[74] Massicotte L, Beaulieu D, Thibeault L. Con: Low central venous pressure during liver transplantation. Journal of Cardiothoracic and Vascular Anesthesia. 2008;**22**:315-317

[75] Schroeder RA, Collins BH, Tuttle-Newhall E, Robertson K, Plotkin J, Johnson LB, Kuo PC. Intraoperative fluid management during orthotopic liver transplantation. Journal of Cardiothoracic and Vascular Anesthesia. 2004;**18**:438-441

[76] Schroeder RA, Kuo PC. Pro: Low central venous pressure during liver transplantation—not too low. Journal of Cardiothoracic and Vascular Anesthesia. 2008;**22**:311-314

[77] Ashworth A, Klein AA. Cell salvage as part of a blood conservation strategy in anaesthesia. British Journal of Anaesthesia. 2010;**105**:401-416

[78] Massicotte L, Thibeault L, Beaulieu D, Roy JD, Roy A. Evaluation of cell salvage autotransfusion utility during liver transplantation. HPB: The Official Journal of the International Hepato Pancreato Biliary Association. 2007;**9**:52-57

[79] Massicotte L, Lenis S, Thibeault L, Sassine MP, Seal RF, Roy A. Reduction of blood product transfusions during liver transplantation. Canadian Journal of Anaesthesia. 2005;**52**:545-546

[80] Cardone D, Klein AA. Perioperative blood conservation. European Journal of Anaesthesiology. 2009;**26**:722-729

[81] Carless PA, Henry DA, Moxey AJ, O'connell DL, Brown T, Fergusson DA. Cell salvage for minimising perioperative allogeneic blood transfusion. Cochrane Database of Systematic Reviews. 2006 Oct 18;(4):CD001888.

[82] Williamson KR, Taswell HF, Rettke SR, Krom RA. Intraoperative autologous transfusion: Its role in orthotopic liver transplantation. Mayo Clinic Proceedings. 1989;**64**:340-345

[83] Sankarankutty AK, Teixeira AC, Souza FF, Mente ED, Oliveira GR, Almeida RC, Andrade CM, Origuella EA, Silva Ode C. Impact of blood salvage during liver transplantation on reduction in transfusion requirements. Acta Cirúrgica Brasileira. 2006;**21**(Suppl 1):44-47

[84] Lutz JT, Valentín-Gamazo C, Görlinger K, Malagó M, Peters J. Blood-transfusion requirements and blood salvage in donors undergoing right hepatectomy for living related liver transplantation. Anesthesia and Analgesia. 2003;**96**:351-355

[85] Kemper RR, Menitove JE, Hanto DW. Cost analysis of intraoperative blood salvage during orthotopic liver transplantation. Liver Transplantation and Surgery. 1997;**3**:513-517

[86] Brajtbord D, Paulsen AW, Ramsay MA, Swygert TH, Valek TR, Ramon VJ, Johnson DD, Parks RI, Pyron JT, Walling PT. Potential problems with autotransfusion during hepatic transplantation. Transplantation Proceedings. 1989;**21**:2347-2348

[87] Zhang LP, Li M, Yang L. Effects of different vasopressors in patients undergoing orthotopic liver transplantation. Chinese Medical Journal. 2005;**118**:1952-1958

[88] Vater Y, Levy A, Martay K, Hunter C, Weinbroum AA. Adjuvant drugs for end-stage liver failure and transplantation. Medical Science Monitor. 2004;**10**:RA77-RA88

[89] Dünster MW, Mayr AJ, Ulmer H, Knotzer H, Sumann G, et al. Arginine vasopressin in advanced vasodilatory shock. A prospective, randomized, controlled study. Circulation. 2003;**107**:2313-2319

[90] Guerin JP, Levrant J, Samat-Long C, Leverve X, Grimaud D, et al. Effects of dopamine and norepinephrine on systemic and hepatosplanchnic hemodynamics, oxygen exchange, and energy balance in vasoplegic septic patients. Shock. 2005;**23**:18-24

[91] Guzman JA, Rosado AE, Kruse JA. Vasopressin vs. norepinephrine in endotoxic shock: Systemic, renal, and splanchnic hemodynamic and oxygen transport effects. Journal of Applied Physiology. 2003;**95**:803-809

[92] Gregory JS, Bonfiglio MF, Dasta JF, Reilley TE, Townsend MC, et al. Experience with phenylephrine as a component of the pharmacological support of septic shock. Critical Care Medicine. 1991;**19**:1395-1400

[93] Massicotte L, Perrault MA, Denault AY, Klinck JR, Beaulieu D, Roy JD, Thibeault L, Roy A, McCormack M, Karakiewicz P. Effects of phlebotomy and phenylephrine infusion on portal venous pressure and systemic hemodynamics during liver transplantation. Transplantation. 2010 Apr 27;**89**(8):920-927

[94] Reilly FD, McCuskey RS, Cilento EV. Hepatic microvascular regulatory mechanisms. I. Adrenergic mechanisms. Microvascular Research. 1981 Jan;21(1):103-116

[95] Regueira T, Bänziger B, Djafarzadeh S, Brandt S, Gorrasi J, Takala J, Lepper PM, Jakob SM. Norepinephrine to increase blood pressure in endotoxaemic pigs is associated with improved hepatic mitochondrial respiration. Critical Care. 2008;12(4):R88

[96] Martikainen TJ, Tenhunen JJ, Uusaro A, Ruokonen E. The effects of vasopressin on systemic and splanchnic hemodynamics and metabolism in endotoxin shock. Anesthesia and Analgesia. 2003;97:1756-1763

[97] Mandell MS, Tsou MY. The development of perioperative practices for liver transplantation: Advances and current trends. Journal of the Chinese Medical Association. 2008;71:433-441

[98] Di Giantomasso D, Morimatsu H, Bellomo R, May CN. Effect of low dose vasopressin infusion on vital organ flow in the conscious normal and septic sheep. Anaesthesia and Intensive Care. 2006;34:427-433

[99] Wagener G, Gubitasa G, Renz J, Kinkhabwaia M, Brentjens T, et al. Liver Transplantation. 2008;14:1664-1670

[100] Baik SK, Jeong PH, Ji SW, Yoo BS, Kim HS, et al. Acute hemodynamic effects of octreotide and terlipressin in patients with cirrhosis: A randomized comparison. American Journal of Gastroenterology. 2005;100:631-635

[101] Kam PC, Williams S, Yoong FF. Vasopressin and terlipressin: Pharmacology and its clinical relevance. Anaesthesia. 2004;59:993-1001

[102] Mandell MS, Katz JJ, Wachs M, Gill E, Kam I. Circulatory pathophysiology and options in hemodynamic management during adult liver transplantation. Liver Transplantation and Surgery. 1997;3:379-387

[103] Vitin AA, Martay K, Vater Y, Dembo G, Maziarz M. Effects of vasoactive agents on blood loss and transfusion requirements during pre-reperfusion stages of the Orthotopic Liver Transplantation. Journal of Anesthesia and Clinical Research. 2010;1:104

[104] Swygert TH, Roberts LC, Valek TR, Brajtbord D, Brown MR, Gunning TC, Paulsen AW, Ramsay MA. Effect of intraoperative low-dose dopamine on renal function in liver transplant recipients. Anesthesiology. 1991 Oct;75(4):571-576

[105] Manaker S. Use of Vasopressors and Inotropes. https://www.uptodate.com/contents/use-of-vasopressors-and-inotropes

[106] Ho-Geol R, Chul-Woo J, Hyung-Chul L, Youn-Joung C. Epinephrine and phenylephrine pretreatments for preventing postreperfusion syndrome during adult liver transplantation. Liver Transplantation. 2012;18:1430-1439

[107] Takashi M, Hilmi IA,. Planinsic RM, Humar A, Sakai A. Cardiac arrest during adult liver transplantation: A single institution's experience with 1238 deceased donor transplants. Liver Transplantation. 2012;18:1430-1439

[108] Fischer, W, Bengtsson Y, Scarola S, Cohen E. Methylene Blue for vasopressor-resistant vasoplegia syndrome during liver transplantation. Journal of Cardiothoracic & Vascular Anesthesia. 2010 June;24(3):463-466

[109] Kimmoun A, Novy E, Auchet T, Ducrocq N, Levy B. Hemodynamic consequences of severe lactic acidosis in shock states: From bench to bedside. Critical Care. 2015;19:175

[110] Levy B, Collin S, Sennoun N, Ducrocq N, Kimmoun A, Asfar P, et al. Vascular hyporesponsiveness to vasopressors in septic shock: From bench to bedside. Intensive Care Medicine. 2010;36:2019-2029

[111] Nahas GG, Sutin KM, Fermon C, Streat S, Wiklund L, Wahlander S, Yellin P, Brasch H, Kanchuger M, Capan L, Manne J, Helwig H, Gaab M, Pfenninger E, Wetterberg T, Holmdahl M, Turndorf H. Guidelines for the treatment of acidaemia with THAM. Drugs. 1998 Feb;55(2):191-224

[112] Pearl RG, Rosenthal MH, Schroeder JS, Ashton JP. Acute hemodynamic effects of nitroglycerin in pulmonary hypertension. Annals of Internal Medicine. 1983 Jul;99(1):9-13

8

Pharmacological Therapy of Ascites

Aziza Ajlan, Waleed K. Al-hamoudi and
Hussein Elsiesy

Abstract

Ascites refer to accumulation of fluids in the peritoneal cavity. Ascites is caused by multiple causes, among which liver cirrhosis is the commonest. Confirming the etiology is the first and most important step toward proper management. Assuming that ascites is always caused by cirrhosis can lead to unnecessarily sending patients with different etiologies for liver transplantation, particularly patients with non-cirrhotic portal hypertension. Calculating serum albumin ascitic gradient is important in differentiating ascites due to portal hypertension from other etiologies. The first-line therapy for ascites in cirrhosis is low salt diet and diuretics. It is important to avoid nonsteroidal anti-inflammatory drugs (NSAIDs) and nephrotoxic medications in these patients.

Keywords: ascites, treatment, pharmacological therapy, liver cirrhosis

1. Introduction

Even though liver disease remains the main cause of ascites, there are several other causes including renal diseases, infections (tuberculosis), malignancies, and heart disease (**Table 1**).

It is important to diagnose the etiology of ascites in order to properly treat it.

Detailed history, physical examination, laboratory blood test, abdominal ultrasound, and serum albumin ascitic gradient are important in narrowing the differential diagnosis of ascites.

Cirrhosis is the eighth leading cause of death in the United States [1]. Ascites is one of the most common complications of cirrhosis that leads to hospital admissions [2]. It occurs due

High SAAG ascites (>1.1)	Low SAAG ascites (<1.1)
Liver cirrhosis	Tuberculosis
Budd-Chiari syndrome	Malignancy
Sinusoidal obstructive syndrome	Pancreatic
Heart failure (high protein)	Renal
Alcoholic hepatitis	Serositis
Acute liver failure	

Table 1. Causes of ascites.

to portal hypertension and is primarily related to an inability to excrete an adequate amount of sodium into urine, leading to positive sodium balance leading to fluid retention [3]. Many patients are referred for liver transplantation after development of ascites. Evidence suggests that arterial splanchnic vasodilation leads to renal sodium and water retention in patients with cirrhosis. This permits dropping in effective arterial blood capacity with stimulation of arterial as well as cardiopulmonary volume receptors, in addition to homeostatic stimulation of vasoconstrictor and sodium-retaining systems (i.e., the RAAS (renin-angiotensin-aldosterone system) as well as the sympathetic nervous system). Renal sodium preservation causes extension of the extracellular fluid volume and accumulation of ascites and edema [4, 5]. The occurrence of ascites is directly linked to worse prognosis and compromised life quality; therefore, patients should be turned over to liver transplant center for evaluation [6]. Nearly 75% of the patients with ascites in Western Europe or the United States have cirrhosis as the primary cause. The remaining 25% of the ascites is caused by malignancy, heart failure, tuberculosis, pancreatic disease, or other miscellaneous causes [7].

Determining the cause of ascites is very important for appropriate management. The serum-ascites albumin gradient (SAAG) can be helpful for both diagnostic and therapeutic purposes. Patients with a high SAAG (≥1.1 g/dL) have portal hypertension and usually are responsive to diuretic therapy measures [8].

1.1. First-line treatment

One of the most important steps in treating ascites in this setting is to treat the underlying liver disease. In patients with alcoholic liver disease, abstinence from alcohol intake can result in dramatic improvement in the reversible component of alcoholic liver disease. This measure alone can lead to an around 75% 3-year survival. If the patient does not succeed in refraining from alcohol intake, they may die within 3 years [9]. Abstinence from alcohol intake alone may lead to either complete resolution of ascites or at least a better response to medical therapy.

Ascites in decompensated hepatitis B virus infection-related cirrhosis and autoimmune hepatitis can also have a great response to specific drug therapy, although liver disease is unlikely to be revisable by the time ascites is manifested (**Table 2**) [10].

Treatment of ascites due to liver cirrhosis
1. Treatment of the underlying cause: stop alcohol, treat AIH, and HBV
2. Low-salt diet and diuretics
3. Water restriction if sodium <120 mmol
4. Vaptans (not effective)
5. Albumin and colloid replacement
6. Avoid nephrotoxic medications

Table 2. Treatment of ascites due to liver cirrhosis.

2. Diet and diuretics

The first-line treatment of patients with cirrhosis and ascites includes (1) dietary sodium restriction (2000 mg/day [88 mmol/day]) and (2) oral diuretics [11]. Evidence suggests that renal sodium retention in these patients is mainly caused by increased proximal as well as distal tubular sodium reabsorption instead of reduction of filtered sodium load [12, 13]. Although the mechanism by which enhanced proximal tubular reabsorption of sodium occurs has not been fully established, the increased reabsorption of sodium along the distal tubule is mainly due to hyperaldosteronism [14]. Therefore, aldosterone antagonists are considered the treatment of choice and are more effective than loop diuretics. Amiloride (with doses of 10–40 mg/day), a diuretic acting in the collecting duct, is less effective than the active metabolite spironolactone and much more expensive and should be used as an alternative only in those patients who develop side effects with aldosterone antagonists (e.g., tender gynecomastia) [15]. There has been a long argument, whether aldosterone should be administered alone or coupled with loop diuretics. Two studies have assessed both approaches. The first used aldosterone antagonists in a stepwise increase every 7 days (up to 400 mg/day) in combination with furosemide (40–160 mg/day, in 40 mg/day steps) considered only in patients not exhibiting proper response to maximum doses of aldosterone antagonists versus joint treatment of aldosterone antagonists and furosemide from the commencement of treatment (100 in addition to 40 mg/day with the option to build the dose in a stepwise manner every 7 days in view of lack of response up to 400 and 160 mg/day) [16, 17]. The results of the two studies were inconsistent with each other probably due to differences in patient populations, in particular, with regard to the percentage of patients with the first episode of ascites [17]. Initiation of both drugs appears to be the favored approach in attaining quick natriuresis and preserving normokalemia. Single morning dosing enhances adherence. Dosing more than once daily decreases adherence and may lead to nocturia.

The maximum doses are 400 mg/day of spironolactone and 160 mg/day of furosemide [8, 11]. Furosemide can be suspended for a short period of time in patients with hypokalemia, which is very common in the setting of alcoholic hepatitis.

Other diuretics including triamterene, metolazone, and hydrochlorothiazide have also been used to treat ascites [11].

Eplerenone is a newer aldosterone antagonist that has been used in heart failure [18]. There is only one study evaluating the use of eplerenone in ascites with comparable results to alda-ctone [19]. It could also serve as substitute of spironolactone in patients who develop tender gynecomastia [20].

Other loop diuretics, such as torasemide and bumetanide, are currently not being used as they did not seem to demonstrate superiority to the current agents, let alone their cost.

It's important to mention though, in all patients, diuretic therapy should aim to achieve weight loss of no more than 0.5 kg/day if peripheral edema is absent and 1 kg/day in those with peripheral edema to avoid diuretic-related renal failure and/or hyponatremia which is mainly due to intravascular volume depletion [7]. Other complications of diuretic therapy include hepatic encephalopathy, electrolyte disorders, gynaecomastia, and muscle cramps [13, 21–37]. If cramps are severe, diuretic dose should be decreased or stopped, and albumin infusion [37], baclofen, and l-carnitine may relieve symptoms [23–27, 37].

3. Fluid restriction

Fluid restriction is not necessary in treating most patients with cirrhosis and ascites unless sodium is less than 120. The chronic hyponatremia commonly observed in cirrhotic ascites patients is occasionally fatal if not corrected. One study with 997 cirrhotic patients with ascites showed that the serum sodium is ≤120 mmol/L in 1.2% of the patients and ≤ 125 mmol/L in only 5.7%. Rapidly correcting serum sodium with hypertonic saline in this setting makes the patients prone to more complications rather than the hyponatremia itself.

4. Vaptans

Vaptans are "vasopressin receptor antagonists" and have been studied, mainly in heart failure and in the setting of cirrhosis [38, 39]. Their value in treating hyponatremia and in reduc-ing fluid overload has been investigated. They appear to be useful in treating mild hypona-tremia. However, correction of hyponatremia solely may not associate with more important clinical outcomes. The intravenous agent conivaptan has been approved for use for treat-ment of euvolemic and hypervolemic hyponatremia in hospitalized patients [38]. The manu-facturer advises clinician to exercise extra precaution as rapid correction of hyponatremia can have serious/irreversible clinical outcomes, i.e., central pontine myelinolysis. An oral formulation—tolvaptan—increases serum sodium in patients who have baseline values of <130 mmol/L [40]. Of note, correction of sodium is not permanent, and hyponatremia may return when medication is stopped [41].

Recently, satavaptan was particularly investigated to define its effectiveness in managing ascites rather than hyponatremia, was found to be "not clinically beneficial" in the controlling of ascites in cirrhosis, and was linked with higher mortality compared to placebo [42]. It is also more expensive than first-line therapy.

5. Intravenous albumin

An open-label, randomized controlled trial in patients with new onset ascites demonstrates that weekly 25 g infusions of albumin for 1 year followed by infusions every 2 weeks improved survival and decreased the risk of ascite recurrence compared to diuretics alone [43].

In patients who undergo large-volume paracentesis (LVP) > 5 L secondary to refractory ascites, the administration of albumin prevents post-paracentesis circulatory dysfunction (PPCD) [44]. Circulatory homeostasis has detrimental effects in cirrhotic patients as it leads to rapid rebuildup of ascites [45]. Around 20% of these patients develop dilutional hyponatremia secondary to hepatorenal syndrome and/or water retention. The portal pressure usually rises in patients developing circulatory dysfunction after LVP, probably due to a raised intrahepatic resistance due to the action of vasoconstrictor systems on the hepatic vascular bed [46–54]. Finally and most importantly, circulatory dysfunction is usually linked to decreased survival [44, 53].

LVP coupled with albumin infusion is more effective than diuretics and significantly cuts the length of hospital stay. It also has lower frequency of hyponatremia, renal impairment, and hepatic encephalopathy when compared with diuretics. However, there were no differences between the two approaches with respect to hospital readmission or survival [45, 55].

Albumin has shown to be more effective than dextran-70 and polygeline (other plasma expanders) for the stoppage of PPCD [44]. If <5 L of ascites are eliminated, dextran-70 (8 g/L of ascites removed) and polygeline (150 mL/L of ascites removed) show effectiveness comparable to that of albumin. Nevertheless, albumin has higher efficacy than these other plasma expanders if in the case of removal of more than 5 L of ascetic fluid [44]. In spite of that, randomized trials did not show survival advantage in patients treated with albumin versus those treated with other plasma expanders [44, 53, 56]. To demonstrate survival benefit of albumin, larger trials are warranted. Of note, a published meta-analysis included 17 trials involving 1225 patients, demonstrating a lessening in mortality with an odds ratio of death of 0.64 (95% CI, 0.41–0.98) in the albumin group [57, 58]. Albumin was superior to other plasma expanders in which a mean volume of ascetic fluid removed was 5.5–15.9 L [58]. Studies have administered between 5 and 10 g of albumin per liter of fluid removed; 6–8 g/L have been the most frequently used doses [58]. Another study compared albumin doses in 70 patients; the 4 g/L group had comparable PPCD and renal impairment to the 8 g/L group [46, 59].

Albumin is usually infused throughout and/or shortly after the paracentesis. In Europe, only a 20% intravenous solution is available. While in the United States, 5% and 25% intravenous solutions are available, all are isotonic. Using the 5% solution increases the sodium load five times.

6. Drugs to be avoided or used with caution

Angiotensin-converting enzyme inhibitors and angiotensin receptor blockers should be avoided in patients with cirrhosis and ascites even in low doses as they can induce arterial hypotension and renal failure [60, 61]. If used, blood pressure and renal function must be monitored carefully [7].

The administration of nonsteroidal anti-inflammatory drugs (NSAIDs), such as indomethacin, ibuprofen, and aspirin, in patients with cirrhosis and ascites is associated with a high risk of development of acute renal failure and hyponatremia and lowers the effect of diuretics [7]. This occurs primarily due to inhibition of renal prostaglandin synthesis leading to deficiency in glomerular filtration rate, which is due to a reduced renal perfusion [62]. Cyclooxygenase-2 (COX-2) inhibitors may provide an alternative for short term as preliminary data show that short-term administration of celecoxib does not impair renal function and does not alter response to diuretics [62].

Beta-blockers have been shown to reduce survival in patients with refractory ascites [63, 64]. This has been linked to their undesirable effect on blood pressure and the increase in the rate of paracentesis-induced circulatory dysfunction [63, 64].

Both blood pressure and renal function should be monitored closely in patients who have refractory ascites with consideration not to initiate or discontinue beta-blockers in such setting.

7. Colloid replacement

Colloid replacement therapy remains as a contentious issue in therapeutic paracentesis. One study compared the use of albumin (10 g/L of fluid removed) versus no albumin in 105 patients with tense ascites, following therapeutic paracentesis [65]. The no-albumin group had statistically significantly more changes in electrolytes, plasma renin, and serum creatinine, but no more clinical morbidity or mortality compared to the albumin group [65]. There are no studies that demonstrate decreased survival in patients without plasma expander compared to patients given with albumin after paracentesis [44].

Polygeline (plasma expander) is no longer used in many countries because of the possible risk of transmission of prions. Some evidence suggest that the use of saline is not linked to a high risk to develop PPCD after small-volume paracentesis [53]; there are no randomized controlled studies comparing saline versus albumin in patients who require paracentesis of less than 5 L. The use of starch as a plasma expander has been addressed in few studies in patients with cirrhosis and grade 3 ascites treated with LVP, revealing some concerning issues regarding the likelihood for starch to induce renal failure and hepatic accumulation of starch [66, 67].

On the other hand, a health economic analysis model suggested that it is more cost-effective to use albumin after LVP compared with alternative cheaper plasma volume expanders. This finding was mainly attributed to the fact that the administration of albumin post-paracentesis is associated with a smaller number of liver-related complications within the first 30 days which leads to increased total health cost [56].

8. Other treatment options

Activation of neurohumoral systems with sodium and water retention plays a major role in the pathogenesis of refractory ascites; thus, drugs that may improve circulatory and renal function, principally vasoconstrictors, have been investigated. Vasoconstrictors such as the α1-adrenergic agonist midodrine or terlipressin improve circulatory and renal function in patients with and without refractory ascites. Terlipressin is given in intravenous boluses (1 mg at onset of paracentesis, 1 mg at 8 h and 1 mg at 16 h) in addition to oral midodrine (for 72 h post-paracentesis), which appear to be as good as albumin in suppressing plasma renin elevation in randomized trials; terlipressin is not commercially offered in the United States [51, 68, 69].

9. Spontaneous bacterial peritonitis (SBP)

Ascitic fluid infection is common (12% in older series) and is associated with mortality rate that surpassed 90% [70–72]. This mortality rate can be reduced to 20% with early diagnosis and treatment [6, 73]. The diagnosis of spontaneous bacterial peritonitis (SBP) is made in the presence of raised ascitic fluid absolute polymorphonuclear leukocyte (PMN) count (i.e., $\geq$250 cells/mm^3 [0.25 × 10^9/L]). Treatment of SBP is a separate topic; we will discuss the importance of albumin and other therapies in addition to antibiotic use.

10. Empiric treatment

Empiric antibiotic therapy should be initiated in patients with ascitic fluid PMN counts greater than or equal to 250 cells/mm^3 (0.25 × 10^9/L). About 60% of the patients present with culture-negative ascites. If cultures are positive, however, the most common pathogens include Gram-negative bacteria (GNB), usually *Escherichia coli* and Gram-positive cocci (mainly streptococcus species and enterococci) [71, 74]. The epidemiology of bacterial infections differs between community-acquired (in which GNB infections predominate) and nosocomial infections (in which Gram-positive infections predominate).

Moderately broad-spectrum therapy is necessary in patients with suspected ascitic fluid infection unless otherwise indicated by culture and sensitivity when available. In a controlled trial, cefotaxime, a cephalosporin from the third generation, is shown to be superior to ampicillin plus tobramycin [75]. Cefotaxime or a similar third-generation cephalosporin seems to be the best therapeutic option for anticipated SBP; it is used to cover 95% of the flora including the three most common isolates: *E. coli*, *Klebsiella pneumoniae*, and *Streptococcus pneumoniae* [75]; usually, a 5-day treatment is as effective as 10 days in the treatment [76]. To achieve ascetic fluid levels that are 20-fold above the killing power after 1 dose of cefotaxime, 2 g intravenously every 8 h is required [77]. In neutrocytic ascites, a 5-day course of ceftriaxone 1 g intravenously twice per day was sufficient in treating culture-negative ascites [78].

Amoxicillin/clavulanic acid, intravenously and then orally, has comparable outcomes with respect to SBP resolution and mortality, compared with cefotaxime [79] and at reduced cost.

Another antibiotic that produces a similar SBP resolution rate and hospital survival compared with cefotaxime is ciprofloxacin. Ciprofloxacin is administered as either for 7 days intravenously or for 2 days intravenously followed by 5 days orally. Nevertheless, the cost is higher compared with cephalosporin-based options [80]. However, the use of intravenous antibiotic at the start, followed by oral step-down administration with ciprofloxacin, is more cost-effective than intravenous cefotaxime [81]. Ofloxacin also has produced similar results to intravenous cefotaxime when given orally in uncomplicated SBP, without renal failure, hepatic encephalopathy, gastrointestinal bleeding, ileus, or shock [82].

It is important to mention that, if ascitic fluid neutrophil count does not decrease to less than 25% of the pretreatment value after 48 h of antibiotic treatment, there is a high likelihood of failure to respond to therapy [83, 84]. In such scenarios antibiotic therapy should be broaden to cover more resistant pathogens.

11. Secondary prophylaxis of spontaneous bacterial peritonitis

The ideal prophylactic agent should be safe, affordable, and effective at decreasing the episodes of SBP while preserving the protective anaerobic flora (selective intestinal decontamination) [73]. Given the high cost and the risk of developing resistant organisms, the use of prophylactic antibiotics must be strictly restricted to patients with the following risk factors: (1) patients with acute gastrointestinal hemorrhage, (2) patients with low total protein content in ascitic fluid and no prior history of SBP (primary prophylaxis), and (3) patients with a previous history of SBP (secondary prophylaxis).

The cumulative recurrence rate at 1 year is approximately 70% in patients who survive an episode of SBP with survival rate of up to 30–50% and falls to 25–30% at 2 years [73]. Several antimicrobial regimens have been proposed as secondary prophylaxis. Norfloxacin was studied in a randomized, double-blind, placebo-controlled trial of (400 mg/day orally) in patients who had a previous episode of SBP [85, 86]. Norfloxacin was found to reduce the likelihood of SBP recurrence from 68 to 20% and the likelihood of SBP due to Gram-negative bacteria from 60 to 3%. Other studies evaluated the impact of ciprofloxacin, trimethoprim-sulfamethoxazole, and norfloxacin on SBP recurrence, but they included patients with and without previous episodes of SBP. All studies showed a reduced incidence of SBP with antibiotic prophylaxis [87–89].

The emergence of resistant, extended-spectrum B-lactamase-producing *Enterobacteriaceae* has occurred as a result of the extensive use of quinolones to prevent SBP [90–92].

Alternatively, ofloxacin, dosed at 400 mg bid for about 8 days, was found to be as good as parenteral cefotaxime in the treatment of SBP in patients without vomiting, shock, grade II (or higher) hepatic encephalopathy, or serum creatinine greater than 3 mg/dL [82]. A more cost-effective choice when compared to intravenous ceftazidime in a randomized trial would be the administration of intravenous ciprofloxacin followed by oral administration in patients who had not received quinolone prophylaxis [93]. Patients' flora may become resistant to quinolone prophylaxis, and hence treatment with alternative agents is warranted.

Reduction in mortality was reported in one trial when patients with SBP were randomized to receive cefotaxime alone versus cefotaxime plus 1.5 g albumin per kg body weight within 6 h of enrollment and 1.0 g/kg on day 3. A reduction in mortality from 29 to 10% was described [93]. Another study has revealed that albumin must be administered when the serum creatinine is >1 mg/dL, total bilirubin >4 mg/dL, or blood urea nitrogen >30 mg/dL. If the patient does not meet these prerequisite criteria, then albumin is not indicated [94–97]. Albumin is superior to hydroxyethyl starch in spontaneous bacterial peritonitis [98].

Author details

Aziza Ajlan[1], Waleed K. Al-hamoudi[2,3] and Hussein Elsiesy[2,4]*

*Address all correspondence to: helsiesy@gmail.com

1 Department of Pharmacy, King Faisal Specialist Hospital & Research Center, Riyadh, Saudi Arabia

2 Department of Liver Transplantation, King Faisal Specialist Hospital & Research Center, Riyadh, Saudi Arabia

3 Division of Gastroenterology, King Saud University, Riyadh, Saudi Arabia

4 Department of Medicine, Alfaisal University, Riyadh, Saudi Arabia

References

[1] Asrani SK, Larson JJ, Yawn B, Therneau TM, Kim WR. Underestimation of liver-related mortality in the United States. Gastroenterology. 2013;**145**(2):375-82 e1-2.

[2] Lucena MI, Andrade RJ, Tognoni G, Hidalgo R, De La Cuesta FS, Spanish Collaborative Study Group on Therapeutic Management in Liver D. Multicenter hospital study on pre-scribing patterns for prophylaxis and treatment of complications of cirrhosis. European Journal of Clinical Pharmacology. 2002;**58**(6):435-40.

[3] Ripoll C, Groszmann R, Garcia-Tsao G, Grace N, Burroughs A, Planas R, et al. Hepatic venous pressure gradient predicts clinical decompensation in patients with compen-sated cirrhosis. Gastroenterology. 2007;**133**(2):481-88.

[4] Schrier RW, Arroyo V, Bernardi M, Epstein M, Henriksen JH, Rodes J. Peripheral arterial vasodilation hypothesis: A proposal for the initiation of renal sodium and water reten-tion in cirrhosis. Hepatology. 1988;**8**(5):1151-7.

[5] Schomerus H, Heinrich R. Systemic manifestations of liver cirrhosis. Heart, circulation, lung. Zeitschrift für Gastroenterologie. Verhandlungsband. 1986;**21**:21-6.

[6] Tandon P, Garcia-Tsao G. Bacterial infections, sepsis, and multiorgan failure in cirrhosis. Seminars in Liver Disease. 2008;**28**(1):26-42.

[7] European Association for the Study of the L. EASL clinical practice guidelines on the management of ascites, spontaneous bacterial peritonitis, and hepatorenal syndrome in cirrhosis. Journal of Hepatology. 2010;**53**(3):397-417.

[8]   BA R. Sleisenger and Fordtran's Gastrointestinal and Liver Disease. Philadelphia: Saunders Elsevier; 2010. pp. 1517-41.

[9]   Veldt BJ, Laine F, Guillygomarc'h A, Lauvin L, Boudjema K, Messner M, et al. Indication of liver transplantation in severe alcoholic liver cirrhosis: Quantitative evaluation and optimal timing. Journal of Hepatology. 2002;36(1):93-98.

[10] Garg H, Sarin SK, Kumar M, Garg V, Sharma BC, Kumar A. Tenofovir improves the outcome in patients with spontaneous reactivation of hepatitis B presenting as acute-on-chronic liver failure. Hepatology. 2011;53(3):774-80.

[11] Montero E, Miguel J, Lopez-Alvarez J. Care of patients with ascites. The New England Journal of Medicine. 1994;330(25):1828.

[12] Angeli P, Gatta A, Caregaro L, Menon F, Sacerdoti D, Merkel C, et al. Tubular site of renal sodium retention in ascitic liver cirrhosis evaluated by lithium clearance. European Journal of Clinical Investigation. 1990;20(1):111-7.

[13] Angeli P, De Bei E, Dalla Pria M, Caregaro L, Ceolotto G, Albino G, et al. Effects of amiloride on renal lithium handling in nonazotemic ascitic cirrhotic patients with avid sodium retention. Hepatology. 1992;15(4):651-4.

[14] Bernardi M, Servadei D, Trevisani F, Rusticali AG, Gasbarrini G. Importance of plasma aldosterone concentration on the natriuretic effect of spironolactone in patients with liver cirrhosis and ascites. Digestion. 1985;31(4):189-93.

[15] Angeli P, Dalla Pria M, De Bei E, Albino G, Caregaro L, Merkel C, et al. Randomized clinical study of the efficacy of amiloride and potassium canrenoate in nonazotemic cirrhotic patients with ascites. Hepatology. 1994;19(1):72-9.

[16] Angeli P, Fasolato S, Mazza E, Okolicsanyi L, Maresio G, Velo E, et al. Combined versus sequential diuretic treatment of ascites in non-azotaemic patients with cirrhosis: Results of an open randomised clinical trial. Gut. 2010;59(1):98-104.

[17] Santos J, Planas R, Pardo A, Durandez R, Cabre E, Morillas RM, et al. Spironolactone alone or in combination with furosemide in the treatment of moderate ascites in nonazotemic cirrhosis. A randomized comparative study of efficacy and safety. Journal of Hepatology. 2003;39(2):187-92.

[18] Pitt B, Remme W, Zannad F, Neaton J, Martinez F, Roniker B, et al. Eplerenone, a selective aldosterone blocker, in patients with left ventricular dysfunction after myocardial infarction. The New England Journal of Medicine. 2003;348(14):1309-21.

[19] Singh HJ, Singh S, Chander R, Charan S. Comparative study of spironolactone and eplerenone in management of ascites in cirrhosis liver. The Journal of the Association of Physicians of India. 2016;64(1):48.

[20] Mimidis K, Papadopoulos V, Kartalis G. Eplerenone relieves spironolactone-induced painful gynaecomastia in patients with decompensated hepatitis B-related cirrhosis. Scandinavian Journal of Gastroenterology. 2007;42(12):1516-7.

[21] Elfert AA, Abo Ali L, Soliman S, Zakaria S, Shehab El-Din I, Elkhalawany W, et al. Randomized placebo-controlled study of baclofen in the treatment of muscle cramps in patients with liver cirrhosis. European Journal of Gastroenterology & Hepatology. 2016;28(11):1280-4.

[22] Chatrath H, Liangpunsakul S, Ghabril M, Otte J, Chalasani N, Vuppalanchi R. Prevalence and morbidity associated with muscle cramps in patients with cirrhosis. The American Journal of Medicine. 2012;125(10):1019-25.

[23] Atluri DK, Veluru C, Mullen K. An alternative treatment for muscle cramps in patients with liver cirrhosis. Liver International: Official Journal of the International Association for the Study of the Liver. 2013;33(3):496-7.

[24] Henry ZH, Northup PG. Baclofen for the treatment of muscle cramps in patients with cirrhosis: A new alternative. Hepatology. 2016;64(2):695-6.

[25] Angeli P, Albino G, Carraro P, Dalla Pria M, Merkel C, Caregaro L, et al. Cirrhosis and muscle cramps: Evidence of a causal relationship. Hepatology. 1996;23(2):264-73.

[26] Nakanishi H, Kurosaki M, Tsuchiya K, Nakakuki N, Takada H, Matsuda S, et al. L-carnitine reduces muscle cramps in patients with cirrhosis. Clinical Gastroenterology and Hepatology. 2015;13(8):1540-3.

[27] Mehta SS, Fallon MB. Muscle cramps in cirrhosis: A moving target. Clinical Gastroenterology and Hepatology. 2015;13(8):1544-6.

[28] Corbani A, Manousou P, Calvaruso V, Xirouchakis I, Burroughs AK. Muscle cramps in cirrhosis: The therapeutic value of quinine. Is it underused? Digestive and Liver Disease: Official Journal of the Italian Society of Gastroenterology and the Italian Association for the Study of the Liver. 2008;40(9):794-9.

[29] Abrams GA, Concato J, Fallon MB. Muscle cramps in patients with cirrhosis. The American Journal of Gastroenterology. 1996;91(7):1363-6.

[30] Marotta PJ, Graziadei IW, Ghent CN. Muscle cramps: A 'complication' of cirrhosis. Canadian Journal of Gastroenterology. 2000;14(Suppl D):21D-5D.

[31] Marchesini G, Bianchi G, Amodio P, Salerno F, Merli M, Panella C, et al. Factors associated with poor health-related quality of life of patients with cirrhosis. Gastroenterology. 2001;120(1):170-8.

[32] Qavi AI I, Kamal R, Schrier RW. Clinical use of diuretics in heart failure, cirrhosis, and nephrotic syndrome. International Journal of Nephrology. 2015;2015:975934.

[33] Knauf H, Mutschler E. Liver cirrhosis with ascites: Pathogenesis of resistance to diuretics and long-term efficacy and safety of torasemide. Cardiology. 1994;84(Suppl 2):87-98.

[34] Porayko MK, Wiesner RH. Management of ascites in patients with cirrhosis. What to do when diuretics fail. Postgraduate Medicine. 1992;92(8):155-158 61-6.

[35] Bernardi M. Optimum use of diuretics in managing ascites in patients with cirrhosis. Gut. 2010;59(1):10-1.

[36] Planas R, Pardo A, Durandez R, Cabre E, Morillas RM, Granada ML, et al. Spironolactone alone or in combination with furosemide in the treatment of moderate ascites in non-azotemic cirrhosis. A randomized comparative study of efficacy and safety. Journal of Hepatology. 2003;**39**(2):187-92.

[37] Vidot H, Carey S, Allman-Farinelli M, Shackel N. Systematic review: The treatment of muscle cramps in patients with cirrhosis. Alimentary Pharmacology & Therapeutics. 2014;**40**(3): 221-32.

[38] Wong F, Blei AT, Blendis LM, Thuluvath PJ. A vasopressin receptor antagonist (VPA-985) improves serum sodium concentration in patients with hyponatremia: A multi-center, randomized, placebo-controlled trial. Hepatology. 2003;**37**(1):182-191.

[39] Schrier RW, Gross P, Gheorghiade M, Berl T, Verbalis JG, Czerwiec FS, et al. Tolvaptan, a selective oral vasopressin V2-receptor antagonist, for hyponatremia. The New England Journal of Medicine. 2006;**355**(20):2099-2112.

[40] Yamada T, Ohki T, Hayata Y, Karasawa Y, Kawamura S, Ito D, et al. Potential effectiveness of tolvaptan to improve ascites unresponsive to standard diuretics and overall survival in patients with decompensated liver cirrhosis. Clinical Drug Investigation. 2016;**36**(10):829-35.

[41] Cardenas A, Gines P, Marotta P, Czerwiec F, Oyuang J, Guevara M, et al. Tolvaptan, an oral vasopressin antagonist, in the treatment of hyponatremia in cirrhosis. Journal of Hepatology. 2012;**56**(3):571-8.

[42] Wong F, Watson H, Gerbes A, Vilstrup H, Badalamenti S, Bernardi M, et al. Satavaptan for the management of ascites in cirrhosis: Efficacy and safety across the spectrum of ascites severity. Gut. 2012;**61**(1):108-16.

[43] Romanelli RG, La Villa G, Barletta G, Vizzutti F, Lanini F, Arena U, et al. Long-term albumin infusion improves survival in patients with cirrhosis and ascites: An unblinded randomized trial. World Journal of Gastroenterology. 2006;**12**(9):1403-7.

[44] Gines A, Fernandez-Esparrach G, Monescillo A, Vila C, Domenech E, Abecasis R, et al. Randomized trial comparing albumin, dextran 70, and polygeline in cirrhotic patients with ascites treated by paracentesis. Gastroenterology. 1996;**111**(4):1002-10.

[45] Sola R, Vila MC, Andreu M, Oliver MI, Coll S, Gana J, et al. Total paracentesis with dextran 40 vs diuretics in the treatment of ascites in cirrhosis: A randomized controlled study. Journal of Hepatology. 1994;**20**(2):282-8.

[46] Hoefs JC. Prevention of the paracentesis-induced circulatory dysfunction (PICD) in cirrhosis: Is the SPA treatment worthwhile? Digestive Diseases and Sciences. 2016;**61**(10):2773-5.

[47] Tan HK, James PD, Wong F. Albumin may prevent the morbidity of Paracentesis-induced circulatory dysfunction in cirrhosis and refractory ascites: A pilot study. Digestive Diseases and Sciences. 2016;**61**(10):3084-92.

[48] Kim JH. What we know about paracentesis induced circulatory dysfunction? Clinical and Molecular Hepatology. 2015;**21**(4):349-51.

[49] Bai M, Han G. Midodrine for paracentesis-induced circulatory dysfunction. Journal of Clinical Gastroenterology. 2014;**48**(3):300.

[50] Hamdy H, ElBaz AA, Hassan A, Hassanin O. Comparison of midodrine and albumin in the prevention of paracentesis-induced circulatory dysfunction in cirrhotic patients: A randomized pilot study. Journal of Clinical Gastroenterology. 2014;**48**(2):184-8.

[51] Singh V, Dheerendra PC, Singh B, Nain CK, Chawla D, Sharma N, et al. Midodrine versus albumin in the prevention of paracentesis-induced circulatory dysfunction in cirrhotics: A randomized pilot study. The American Journal of Gastroenterology. 2008;**103**(6):1399-405.

[52] Appenrodt B, Wolf A, Grunhage F, Trebicka J, Schepke M, Rabe C, et al. Prevention of paracentesis-induced circulatory dysfunction: Midodrine vs albumin. A randomized pilot study. Liver International: Official Journal of the International Association for the Study of the Liver. 2008;**28**(7):1019-25.

[53] Sola-Vera J, Minana J, Ricart E, Planella M, Gonzalez B, Torras X, et al. Randomized trial comparing albumin and saline in the prevention of paracentesis-induced circulatory dysfunction in cirrhotic patients with ascites. Hepatology. 2003;**37**(5):1147-53.

[54] Ruiz-del-Arbol L, Monescillo A, Jimenez W, Garcia-Plaza A, Arroyo V, Rodes J. Paracentesis-induced circulatory dysfunction: Mechanism and effect on hepatic hemodynamics in cirrhosis. Gastroenterology. 1997;**113**(2):579-86.

[55] Acharya SK, Balwinder S, Padhee AK, Nijhawan S, Tandon BN. Large volume paracentesis and intravenous dextran to treat tense ascites. Journal of Clinical Gastroenterology. 1992;**14**(1):31-5.

[56] Moreau R, Valla DC, Durand-Zaleski I, Bronowicki JP, Durand F, Chaput JC, et al. Comparison of outcome in patients with cirrhosis and ascites following treatment with albumin or a synthetic colloid: A randomised controlled pilot trail. Liver International: Official Journal of the International Association for the Study of the Liver. 2006;**26**(1):46-54.

[57] Bernardi M, Caraceni P, Navickis RJ. Does the evidence support a survival benefit of albumin infusion in patients with cirrhosis undergoing large-volume paracentesis? Expert Review of Gastroenterology & Hepatology. 2017;**11**(3):191-192.

[58] Bernardi M, Caraceni P, Navickis RJ, Wilkes MM. Albumin infusion in patients undergoing large-volume paracentesis: A meta-analysis of randomized trials. Hepatology. 2012;**55**(4):1172-81.

[59] Alessandria C, Elia C, Mezzabotta L, Risso A, Andrealli A, Spandre M, et al. Prevention of paracentesis-induced circulatory dysfunction in cirrhosis: Standard vs half albumin doses. A prospective, randomized, unblinded pilot study. Digestive and Liver Disease: Official Journal of the Italian Society of Gastroenterology and the Italian Association for the Study of the Liver. 2011;**43**(11):881-6.

[60] Pariente EA, Bataille C, Bercoff E, Lebrec D. Acute effects of captopril on systemic and renal hemodynamics and on renal function in cirrhotic patients with ascites. Gastroenterology. 1985;**88**(5 Pt 1):1255-9.

[61] Gentilini P, Romanelli RG, La Villa G, Maggiore Q, Pesciullesi E, Cappelli G, et al. Effects of low-dose captopril on renal hemodynamics and function in patients with cirrhosis of the liver. Gastroenterology. 1993;**104**(2):588-94.

[62] Claria J, Kent JD, Lopez-Parra M, Escolar G, Ruiz-Del-Arbol L, Gines P, et al. Effects of celecoxib and naproxen on renal function in nonazotemic patients with cirrhosis and ascites. Hepatology. 2005;**41**(3):579-87.

[63] Kurt M. Deleterious effects of beta-blockers on survival in patients with cirrhosis and refractory ascites. Hepatology. 2011;**53**(4):1411-2.

[64] Serste T, Melot C, Francoz C, Durand F, Rautou PE, Valla D, et al. Deleterious effects of beta-blockers on survival in patients with cirrhosis and refractory ascites. Hepatology. 2010;**52**(3): 1017-22.

[65] Gines P, Tito L, Arroyo V, Planas R, Panes J, Viver J, et al. Randomized comparative study of therapeutic paracentesis with and without intravenous albumin in cirrhosis. Gastroenterology. 1988;**94**(6):1493-502.

[66] Brunkhorst FM, Engel C, Bloos F, Meier-Hellmann A, Ragaller M, Weiler N, et al. Intensive insulin therapy and pentastarch resuscitation in severe sepsis. The New England Journal of Medicine. 2008;**358**(2):125-39.

[67] Christidis C, Mal F, Ramos J, Senejoux A, Callard P, Navarro R, et al. Worsening of hepatic dysfunction as a consequence of repeated hydroxyethylstarch infusions. Journal of Hepatology. 2001;**35**(6):726-32.

[68] Angeli P, Volpin R, Piovan D, Bortoluzzi A, Craighero R, Bottaro S, et al. Acute effects of the oral administration of midodrine, an alpha-adrenergic agonist, on renal hemodynamics and renal function in cirrhotic patients with ascites. Hepatology. 1998;**28**(4):937-43.

[69] Krag A, Moller S, Henriksen JH, Holstein-Rathlou NH, Larsen FS, Bendtsen F. Terlipressin improves renal function in patients with cirrhosis and ascites without hepatorenal syndrome. Hepatology. 2007;**46**(6):1863-71.

[70] Zhang JM, Weng XH. Diagnosis, treatment and prophylaxis of spontaneous bacterial peritonitis. Zhonghua Gan Zang Bing Za Zhi. 2005;**13**(6):459-60.

[71] Rimola A, Garcia-Tsao G, Navasa M, Piddock LJ, Planas R, Bernard B, et al. Diagnosis, treatment and prophylaxis of spontaneous bacterial peritonitis: A consensus document. International ascites Club. Journal of Hepatology. 2000;**32**(1):142-53.

[72] Navasa M, Casafont F, Clemente G, Guarner C, de la Mata M, Planas R, et al. Consensus on spontaneous bacterial peritonitis in liver cirrhosis: Diagnosis, treatment, and prophylaxis. Gastroenterología y Hepatología. 2001;**24**(1):37-46.

[73] Garcia-Tsao G. Current Management of the Complications of cirrhosis and portal hypertension: Variceal hemorrhage, ascites, and spontaneous bacterial peritonitis. Digestive Diseases. 2016;**34**(4):382-6.

[74] Fernandez J, Navasa M, Gomez J, Colmenero J, Vila J, Arroyo V, et al. Bacterial infections in cirrhosis: Epidemiological changes with invasive procedures and norfloxacin prophylaxis. Hepatology. 2002;**35**(1):140-8.

[75] Felisart J, Rimola A, Arroyo V, Perez-Ayuso RM, Quintero E, Gines P, et al. Cefotaxime is more effective than is ampicillin-tobramycin in cirrhotics with severe infections. Hepatology. 1985;**5**(3):457-62.

[76] Runyon BA, McHutchison JG, Antillon MR, Akriviadis EA, Montano AA. Short-course versus long-course antibiotic treatment of spontaneous bacterial peritonitis. A randomized controlled study of 100 patients. Gastroenterology. 1991;**100**(6):1737-42.

[77] Runyon BA, Akriviadis EA, Sattler FR, Cohen J. Ascitic fluid and serum cefotaxime and desacetyl cefotaxime levels in patients treated for bacterial peritonitis. Digestive Diseases and Sciences. 1991;**36**(12):1782-6.

[78] Baskol M, Gursoy S, Baskol G, Ozbakir O, Guven K, Yucesoy M. Five days of ceftriaxone to treat culture negative neutrocytic ascites in cirrhotic patients. Journal of Clinical Gastroenterology. 2003;**37**(5):403-5.

[79] Ricart E, Soriano G, Novella MT, Ortiz J, Sabat M, Kolle L, et al. Amoxicillin-clavulanic acid versus cefotaxime in the therapy of bacterial infections in cirrhotic patients. Journal of Hepatology. 2000;**32**(4):596-602.

[80] Terg R, Cobas S, Fassio E, Landeira G, Rios B, Vasen W, et al. Oral ciprofloxacin after a short course of intravenous ciprofloxacin in the treatment of spontaneous bacterial peritonitis: Results of a multicenter, randomized study. Journal of Hepatology. 2000;**33**(4):564-9.

[81] Angeli P, Guarda S, Fasolato S, Miola E, Craighero R, Piccolo F, et al. Switch therapy with ciprofloxacin vs. intravenous ceftazidime in the treatment of spontaneous bacterial peritonitis in patients with cirrhosis: Similar efficacy at lower cost. Alimentary Pharmacology & Therapeutics. 2006;**23**(1):75-84.

[82] Navasa M, Follo A, Llovet JM, Clemente G, Vargas V, Rimola A, et al. Randomized, comparative study of oral ofloxacin versus intravenous cefotaxime in spontaneous bacterial peritonitis. Gastroenterology. 1996;**111**(4):1011-7.

[83] Guarner C, Soriano G. Spontaneous bacterial peritonitis. Seminars in Liver Disease. 1997; **17**(3):203-17.

[84] Brahmbhatt R, Tapper EB. Optimizing the outcomes associated with spontaneous bacterial peritonitis. Journal of Clinical Gastroenterology. 2017;**51**(3):191-4.

[85] Gines P, Rimola A, Planas R, Vargas V, Marco F, Almela M, et al. Norfloxacin prevents spontaneous bacterial peritonitis recurrence in cirrhosis: Results of a double-blind, placebo-controlled trial. Hepatology. 1990;**12**(4 Pt 1):716-24.

[86]   Bauer TM, Follo A, Navasa M, Vila J, Planas R, Clemente G, et al. Daily norfloxacin is more effective than weekly rufloxacin in prevention of spontaneous bacterial peritonitis recurrence. Digestive Diseases and Sciences. 2002;**47**(6):1356-61.

[87]   Soriano G, Guarner C, Teixido M, Such J, Barrios J, Enriquez J, et al. Selective intestinal decontamination prevents spontaneous bacterial peritonitis. Gastroenterology. 1991;**100**(2): 477-81.

[88]   Rolachon A, Cordier L, Bacq Y, Nousbaum JB, Franza A, Paris JC, et al. Ciprofloxacin and long-term prevention of spontaneous bacterial peritonitis: Results of a prospective controlled trial. Hepatology. 1995;**22**(4 Pt 1):1171-4.

[89]   Singh N, Gayowski T, Yu VL, Wagener MM. Trimethoprim-sulfamethoxazole for the prevention of spontaneous bacterial peritonitis in cirrhosis: A randomized trial. Annals of Internal Medicine. 1995;**122**(8):595-8.

[90]   Fernandez J, Acevedo J, Castro M, Garcia O, de Lope CR, Roca D, et al. Prevalence and risk factors of infections by multiresistant bacteria in cirrhosis: A prospective study. Hepatology. 2012;**55**(5):1551-61.

[91]   Ariza X, Castellote J, Lora-Tamayo J, Girbau A, Salord S, Rota R, et al. Risk factors for resistance to ceftriaxone and its impact on mortality in community, healthcare and nosocomial spontaneous bacterial peritonitis. Journal of Hepatology. 2012;**56**(4):825-32.

[92]   Runyon BA. Changing Flora of bacterial infections in patients with cirrhosis. Liver International : Official Journal of the International Association for the Study of the Liver. 2010;**30**(9):1245-6.

[93]   Sort P, Navasa M, Arroyo V, Aldeguer X, Planas R, Ruiz-del-Arbol L, et al. Effect of intravenous albumin on renal impairment and mortality in patients with cirrhosis and spontaneous bacterial peritonitis. The New England Journal of Medicine. 1999;**341**(6):403-9.

[94]   Verma A, Lalchandani A, Giri R, Agarwal S, Priyadarshi BP. Evaluation of relation between spontaneous bacterial peritonitis and serum ascites albumin gradient as a prognostic risk factor in chronic liver disease. The Journal of the Association of Physicians of India. 2016;**64**(1):48.

[95]   Jamtgaard L, Manning SL, Cohn B. Does albumin infusion reduce renal impairment and mortality in patients with spontaneous bacterial peritonitis? Annals of Emergency Medicine. 2016;**67**(4):458-9.

[96]   Salerno F, Navickis RJ, Wilkes MM. Albumin infusion improves outcomes of patients with spontaneous bacterial peritonitis: A meta-analysis of randomized trials. Clinical Gastroenterology and Hepatology. 2013;**11**(2):123-30 e1.

[97]   Sigal SH, Stanca CM, Fernandez J, Arroyo V, Navasa M. Restricted use of albumin for spontaneous bacterial peritonitis. Gut. 2007;**56**(4):597-9.

[98]   Grange JD, Amiot X. Effect of intravenous albumin on renal impairment and mortality in patients with cirrhosis and spontaneous bacterial peritonitis. Gastroentérologie Clinique et Biologique. 2000;**24**(3):378-9.

9

Nutritional Status in Liver Cirrhosis

Kazuyuki Suzuki, Ryujin Endo and Akinobu Kato

Abstract

The metabolism of many nutritional elements (carbohydrate, protein, fat, vitamins, and minerals) is gradually disturbed with progressive chronic liver diseases. In particular, protein-energy malnutrition (PEM) is known as the most characteristic manifestation of liver cirrhosis (LC) and is closely related to its prognosis. Recently, while sarcopenia (loss of muscle mass and strength or physical performance) has been discussed as an independent factor associated with prognosis in patients with LC, obesity and insulin resistance in patients with LC also contribute to carcinogenesis in LC. Deficiencies of zinc and carnitine are involved in the malnutrition in LC and are associated with hyperammonemia, which is related to the pathogenesis of hepatic encephalopathy. Because the nutritional and metabolic disturbances in LC are fundamentally influenced by many factors, such as the severity of liver damage, the existence of portal-systemic shunting, and inflammation, proper nutritional assessment is necessary for the nutritional management of patients with LC.

Keywords: liver cirrhosis, malnutrition, protein-energy malnutrition, sarcopenia, glucose intolerance

1. Introduction

The liver plays a central role in the metabolism of many nutritional elements (carbohydrate, protein, fat, vitamins, and minerals). The metabolism of these nutritional elements is gradually disturbed with progressive chronic liver disease. Protein-energy malnutrition (PEM) is the most characteristic manifestation and is closely related to the prognosis and the quality of life in liver cirrhosis (LC) [1–7]. PEM can lead to muscle atrophy and reduced strength [8–12], which is defined as sarcopenia and has recently been considered an independent prognostic factor in LC with PEM [13–16], while overweight or obesity has been seen as one of the important factors related to carcinogenesis in LC [17]. The relationships among PEM, sarcopenia, and prognosis in LC are shown in **Figure 1**. Furthermore, glucose intolerance or diabetes mellitus (DM) is also an independent factor related to carcinogenesis in LC [18–23]. Serum zinc (Zn) and carnitine (CA) status are involved in the malnutrition in LC and are associated with hyperammonemia, which is related to the pathogenesis of hepatic encephalopathy (HE) [24–31].

Malnutrition in LC is affected by many factors, such as the severity of liver damage, the existence of portal-systemic shunting, and inflammation [10, 32]. Therefore, for the proper nutritional management of patients with LC, precise nutritional assessment is needed.

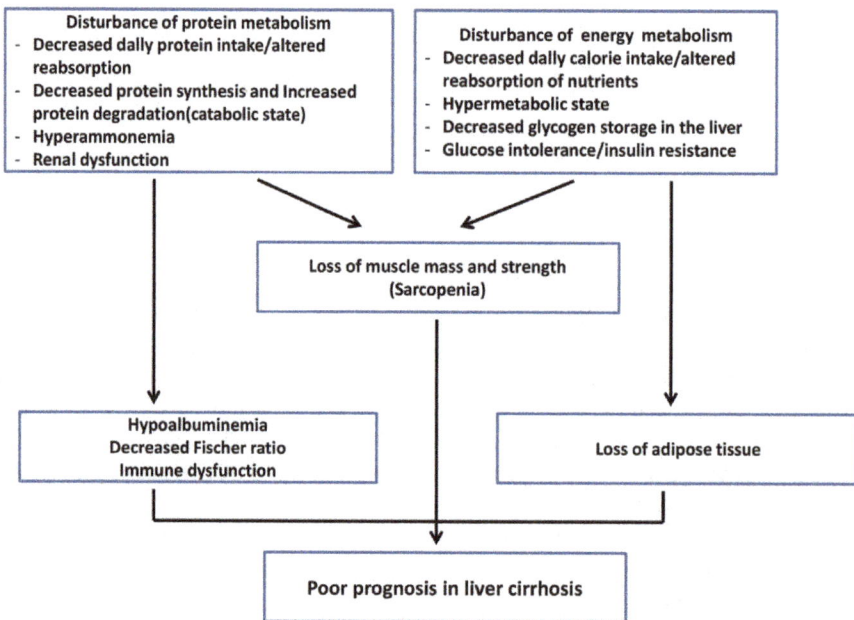

Figure 1. Relationships among protein-energy malnutrition, sarcopenia, and prognosis in liver cirrhosis patients.

This chapter focuses on the association between nutritional assessment and malnutrition in patients with LC.

2. Nutritional assessments

Recommended nutritional assessments in patients with LC are shown in **Table 1**. Static and dynamic status of nutrition should be necessary. Dietary assessment by a skilled dietitian is the first step in assessing nutritional status. Simple and easy applied methods, such as the subjective global assessment (SGA), mini nutritional assessment (MNA), and anthropometric parameters, are recommended in the assessment of nutritional status [32]. Biomarkers representing serum albumin (Alb) are important to assess nutritional status. However, because many biomarkers

1. **Static status of nutrition**

    a. Daily food intake

    b. Body composition analysis

        Height, body weight, body mass index, anthropometric parameters,

        bioelectrical impedance analysis (BIA)

    c. Biomarkers

        Red blood cell count, hemoglobin, routine liver function tests, cholesterol, cholinesterase, albumin, rapid
        turnover proteins, adipocytokines (adiponectin, leptin, resistin, etc.), tumor necrosis factor-α, ghrelin,
        vitamins, minerals, creatinine height index in urine

    d. Immune reaction

        Total lymphocyte count, delated cutaneous hypersensitivity, purified protein derivate of tuberculin

    e. Imaging

        Computer tomography (abdomen)

2. **Dynamic status of nutrition**

    a. Energy metabolism using indirect calorimetry

    b. Nitrogen balance

    c. Biomarkers: plasma free amino acids pattern (Fischer ratio and BTR*)

    d. Urinary 3-methylhistidine excretion

*Fischer ratio, branched chain amino acids (BCAA)/phenylalanine + tyrosine; BTR, BCAA/tyrosine ratio.

Table 1. Recommended nutritional assessment in patients with liver cirrhosis.

are often affected by complications such as infection and renal dysfunction, the data must be
carefully interpreted. Energy metabolism assessment (e.g., resting energy expenditure (REE),
nonprotein respiratory quotient (npQR), and substrate oxidation rates for glucose, protein, and
fat) using indirect calorimetry is the most useful method to assess whether patients with LC
have PEM [32–35]. However, this method cannot be used routinely and easily to examine outpatients, because the indirect calorimeter has a high cost, and it takes time to perform the test.

2.1. Changes of body composition

Analysis of body composition includes height, body weight, body mass index (BMI), and
anthropometric parameters. Anthropometric parameters include percent ideal body weight
(IBM), triceps skin fold thickness (TSF), arm circumference (AC), and arm muscle circumference (AMC). Among these parameters, TSF and AMC are significantly correlated with muscle
volume or the volume of total body fat mass [34, 35]. However, these parameters cannot
be accurately estimated in patients with LC who have edema and/or ascites. Recently, new
methods of body mass composition analysis using computer tomography and bioelectrical
impedance analysis have been developed in daily clinical practice, but this method also cannot provide accurate results in patients with LC who have edema and/or ascites [12–14].

In various chronic liver diseases including LC, several previous reports have shown skeletal
muscle loss using anthropometric parameters [1–4, 11]. This status has recently been defined

as sarcopenia, which shows loss of muscle mass and muscle strength or physical performance [8–12]. Although multiple factors, including differences in the etiology of LC, duration of disease, and the severity of liver damage, are related to the prevalence of sarcopenia in LC, sarcopenia is seen in approximately 30–70% of patients with LC [11–14, 35]. Additionally, a recent study showed that sarcopenia is a risk factor for recurrence in LC patients with hepatocellular carcinoma who undergo curative treatment [14].

Muscle mass is the result of a dynamic balance between protein synthesis and degradation [36–39]. This balance is regulated by two major branches of AKT (also known as protein kinase B) signaling pathways: the AKT/mammalian target of rapamycin (mTOR) pathway that controls protein synthesis and the AKT/forkhead box O (FOXO) pathway that controls protein degradation. Recent reports have shown that myostatin, a member of the transforming growth factor-β superfamily, has emerged as a key regulator of skeletal muscle mass [39]. Myostatin is also a key mediator between energy metabolism and endurance capacity of skeletal muscle [37–39].

On the other hand, the prevalence of LC patients with obesity has increased in the last decade [17]. The definition of obesity is different between Japan and European countries (body mass index (BMI) ≥ 25 kg/m^2 in Japan and ≥ 30 kg/m^2 in European countries). Obesity in patients with LC is associated with insulin resistance, which has been discussed as an important factor in carcinogenesis in LC [17–22].

2.2. Changes of biomarkers

Serum Alb is a main secretion protein synthesized by the liver and has multiple functions, such as the maintenance of colloid osmotic pressure, ligand binding and transport, and enzymatic and antioxidative activities [40, 41]. The synthesis and degradation rates of Alb in patients with LC are decreased compared with those in healthy individuals whose liver function is normal. In particular, the half-life of serum Alb is extended in patients with LC [42]. The serum Alb concentration is affected by the volume of daily food intake, digestion and absorption from the intestine, the degree of severity of liver damage, the imbalances of various hormone dynamics, and nutritional and catabolic status, such as that conferred by infections and burns [43]. However, serum Alb concentration is still frequently used as a biomarker of malnutrition and as an item of both the Child-Pugh classification score and the modified end-stage liver disease (MELD) score [44, 45]. Serum Alb is microheterogeneous with oxidized and reduced forms. Serum Alb concentration decreases, while the ratio of oxidized Alb increases, with LC progression [46, 47]. A recent report has shown that this ratio improved in patients with LC after supplemental treatment with a branched-chain amino acid (BCAA; valine, leucine, and isoleucine)-enriched formula [48]. These findings suggest that the oxidative status of serum Alb could provide a better assessment of malnutrition, though the measurement of serum levels of oxidized and reduced forms of Alb is time-consuming and inconvenient in the clinical setting.

Rapid turnover proteins such as transthyretin (prealbumin), retinol-binding protein, and transferrin are useful biomarkers of short-term nutritional status in patients with LC. The half-life time is 2 days for transthyretin, 0.4–0.7 days for retinol-binding protein, and 7–10 days for transferrin [49, 50]. These proteins are also influenced by baseline conditions such as surgery, infection, and anemia [50]. Recent reports have suggested that serum retinol-binding protein 4 (RBP-4) is a biomarker for assessing malnutrition in patients with LC. Serum RBP-4 levels are decreased in patients with LC and directly related to the severity of liver damage according to the Child-Pugh classification, while these levels are not correlated with insulin resistance [51, 52].

The profiles of plasma amino acids show characteristic changes in patients with LC. In particular, the plasma concentration of BCAAs is decreased, while that of aromatic amino acids (AAA; phenylalanine (Phe) and tyrosine (Tyr)) is increased, resulting in a decreased BCAA/ AAA molar ratio (namely, the Fischer ratio) or the BCAA/Tyr ratio (BTR) [53–55]. BCAA is mainly metabolized and used to detoxify ammonia and for energy production in the skeletal muscle. AAA is metabolized in the liver and is a representative precursor of a neurotransmitter (dopamine) and a pseudo-neurotransmitter (octopamine), which are closely associated with the pathogenesis of HE [53]. The plasma Fischer ratio and serum BTR are significantly correlated with the serum Alb concentration and the severity of liver damage according to the Child-Pugh classification (**Figure 2**), but not with the degree of HE [32, 55]. Furthermore, serum BTR can help predict a decrease in serum Alb concentration associated with chronic liver diseases [56].

Adipocytokines are also biomarkers of nutritional status in patients with LC. Leptin, adiponectin, and resistin are representative peptide hormones that are produced by adipose tissue, and they are closely associated with insulin resistance and arteriosclerosis [32]. Serum leptin levels are higher in females than males among healthy individuals and patients with LC. These levels are correlated with AMC and TSF, but they are not correlated with the severity of liver

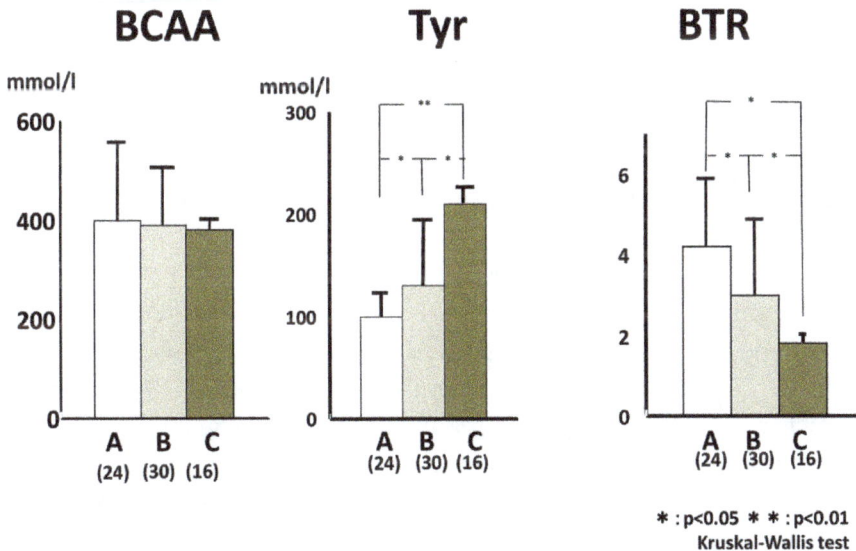

Figure 2. Plasma branched-chain amino acids, tyrosine, and the branched-chain amino acid to tyrosine ratio in patients with liver cirrhosis. Seventy cirrhotic patients with or without hepatocellular carcinoma who were admitted to Iwate Medical University Hospital were investigated. Serum amino acid concentrations were measured by an enzymatic method. The severity of liver damage was classified into grades A, B, and C based on the Child-Pugh classification. BCAA, branched-chain amino acid (valine + leucine + isoleucine); BTR, BCAA/tyrosine ratio. Each value is shown as the mean ± standard deviation. *P < 0.05, **P < 0.01 (Kruskal-Wallis test). (), number of patients with LC.

damage [57–59]. Plasma adiponectin assumes three forms: low molecular weight, medium molecular weight, and high molecular weight [60–62]. In patients with LC, the high molecular weight form of plasma adiponectin is significantly increased compared with healthy individuals and is correlated with the severity of liver damage [32, 62]. Plasma resistin levels associated with insulin resistance are also correlated with the severity of liver damage in patients with LC [63, 64].

Ghrelin, an orexigenic hormone and stimulator of growth hormone, is mainly found in the gastric wall [65, 66]. Ghrelin plays a role in the hypothalamic centers to regulate feeding and caloric intake [65–67]. Furthermore, ghrelin controls feeding behavior and the long-term regulation of body weight in association with leptin in the hypothalamic centers [66, 67]. The plasma ghrelin level has been considered a marker of pathological conditions such as obesity, insulin resistance, type 2 DM, and hypertension. However, the plasma ghrelin level in patients with LC was controversial in previous reports [68–70]. Our study has shown that the plasma ghrelin level (desacyl form) is higher in LC patients than in healthy controls, while it is not correlated with the severity of liver damage. Rather, the plasma ghrelin level is significantly correlated with BMI, AMC, TSF, and non-protein respiratory quotient (npRQ) [70].

Vitamins (fat-soluble: A, D, E, and K, and water-soluble: thiamine, riboflavin, niacin, B_6, B_{12}, C, and folate), carnitine (CA), minerals, trace elements (copper, zinc, iron, manganese, and selenium), and hormones (insulin-like growth factor 1, insulin-like growth factor-binding protein 3, reverse triiodothyronine, etc.) need to be examined when assessing the nutritional status of LC patients. In particular, evaluations of serum zinc and CA (total CA, free CA, and acyl-CA) are necessary in LC patients with sarcopenia and hyperammonemia [23–32].

2.3. Disturbances of energy metabolism

PEM is a characteristic state of malnutrition in advanced LC and is closely associated with the survival rate, the carcinogenic risk, and the outcome of liver transplantation in patients with LC. The serum Alb concentration is generally a marker of protein malnutrition. The npRQ using indirect calorimetry is a marker of energy malnutrition [71]. Therefore, indirect calorimetry would be the best method to assess PEM. The results of REE, npRQ, and the oxidation rates of three nutrients (carbohydrate, protein, and fat) are obtained by indirect calorimetry. Many previous reports indicated that the npRQ decreases, the oxidation rate of fat increases, and the oxidation rate of carbohydrate decreases according to the Child-Pugh classification [5, 72, 73]. It has been considered that a decreased npRQ (<0.85) after an overnight fast predicts a catabolic state and is related to a lower survival rate in LC patients [5]. Decreased carbohydrate oxidation is explained by both the lower production rate of glucose from glycogen in the liver and decreases in peripheral glucose use due to insulin resistance [74]. In fact, patients with LC cannot store sufficient glycogen due to liver atrophy, and their energy generation pattern after an overnight fast is equivalent to that observed in healthy individuals after 2–3 days of starvation [74, 75]. Increased fat oxidation is caused by an increased rate of lipolysis in fat tissue [76]. Our earlier results are generally similar to previous reports (**Figures 3** and **4**). However, because measurement by indirect calorimetry is not easy, it cannot be routinely performed in outpatients with LC. The serum free fatty acid (FAA)

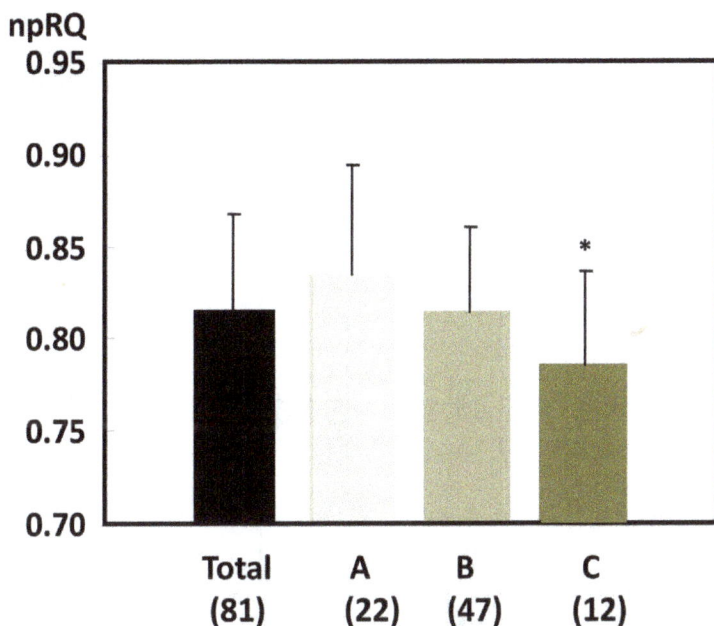

Figure 3. Nonprotein respiratory quotients in patients with liver cirrhosis. Eighty-one cirrhotic patients with or without hepatocellular carcinoma who were admitted to Iwate Medical University Hospital were investigated. Energy metabolism was measured by indirect calorimetry (Deltatrac-II Metabolic Monitor, Datax Division Inst. Corp., Helsinki, Finland) in the morning after overnight fasting. npRQ, nonprotein respiratory quotient. Each value is shown as the mean ± standard deviation. *$P < 0.05$ (compared to grade A). ( ), number of patients with LC.

concentration has recently been reported as an alternative marker to represent npRQ measured by indirect calorimetry to evaluate energy malnutrition in LC [77]. The serum FFA concentration is also a predictor of minimal hepatic encephalopathy diagnosed by computerized neuropsychological testing [78]. Furthermore, our previous study showed that the serum FAA concentration is correlated with the serum acyl-CA to total CA ratio, which would indirectly reflect intracellular mitochondrial function [30]. These findings suggest that the serum FAA concentration in the fasting state may be useful in the assessment of nutritional status in patients with LC.

2.4. Glucose intolerance and diabetes mellitus

Glucose intolerance and/or diabetes mellitus is seen in about 30% of patients with LC, though 80% of LC patients have a normal fasting blood glucose level [79]. These manifestations are mainly caused by obesity and increased insulin resistance and hepatitis C virus (HCV) infection. HCV is a major cause of LC and is induced by increased insulin resistance, excess secretion of pancreatic β cells, and portal-systemic shunting [80, 81]. However, insulin resistance improves after eradication of HCV [82]. Age, sex, smoking, excessive alcohol intake, and chronic viral infection (hepatitis B virus and HCV) are established risk factors for HCC [20]. Furthermore, many recent studies have reported that obesity and DM are risk factors for HCC [17–22]. These findings suggest that not only PEM, but also obesity and glucose intolerance or DM might be important factors in the nutritional status that affect the prognosis of LC.

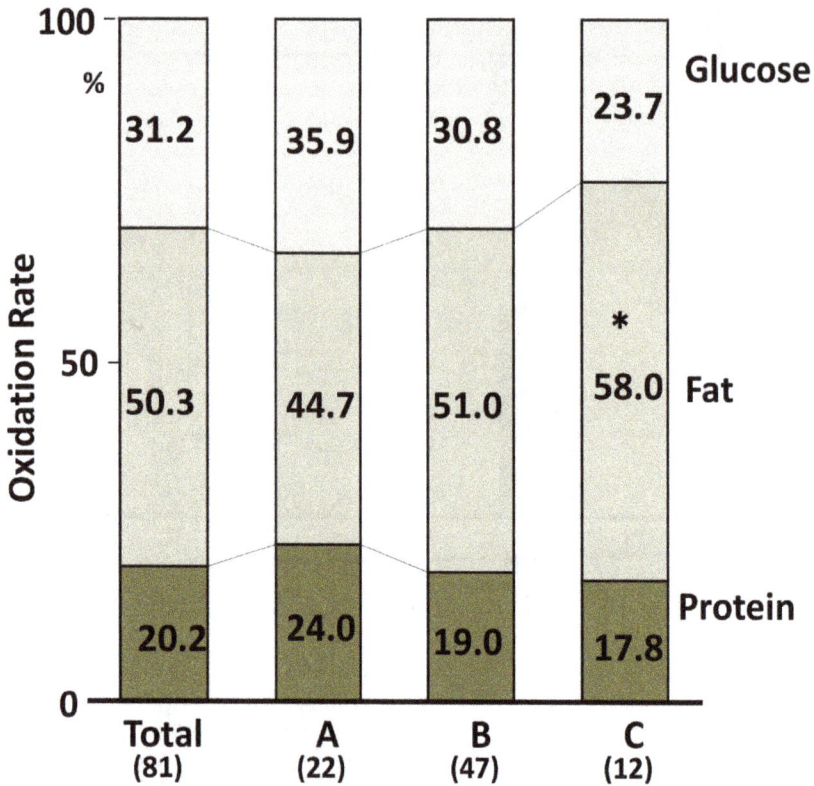

Figure 4. Substrate oxidation rates of glucose, fat, and protein using indirect calorimetry in patients with liver cirrhosis. Eighty-one cirrhotic patients with or without hepatocellular carcinoma who were admitted to Iwate Medical University Hospital were investigated. Energy metabolism was measured using indirect calorimetry (Deltatrac-II Metabolic Monitor, Datax Division Inst. Corp., Helsinki, Finland) in the morning after overnight fasting. Each value is shown as the mean. *$P < 0.05$ (compared to grade A). ( ), number of patients with LC.

3. Nutritional management

Based on previous many studies associated with malnutrition including obesity and glucose impairment (DM) in patients with LC, several guidelines on enteral nutrition have been proposed [83–85]. Here, flow chart on nutritional managements for patients with LC shows in **Figure 5**. The recommended dietary managements include energy, protein, fat, sodium chloride, iron, and other nutrient requirement. However, recommended energy intake and protein intake are different between Japan and European Society for parenteral and enteral Nutrition (ESPEN) guidelines (energy intake: 25–35 kcal/kg/day in Japan guideline and 35–40 kcal/kg/day in ESPEN guidelines, and protein intake: 1.0–1.5 g/kg/day in Japan guideline and 1.2–1.5 g/kg/day in ESPEN guidelines). Energy intake should be reduced (25 kcal/kg/day) in patients complicated with DM [85]. Moreover, protein intake involves the protein content of BCAA formulas (BCAA granules or BCAA-enriched nutrient mixture), and it should be reduced to 0.5–0.7 g/kg/day in patients with protein intolerance [85]. Late evening snack (LES) reduces overnight catabolic state in patients with LC

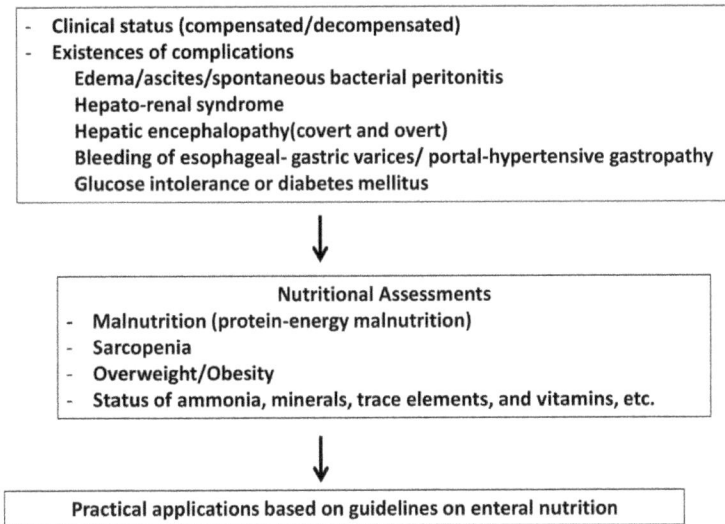

Figure 5. Flow chart on nutritional managements for patients with liver cirrhosis.

[86–89]. LES is particularly recommended to the patients with PEM and also useful for managing the blood glucose level in patients with glucose intolerance or DM [90]. As LES, snacks (approximately amounts of 200 kcal) and BCAA-enriched nutrient mixture are usually used. As excess deposition of iron in the liver causes oxidative stress and also promotes hepatocarcinogenesis, so unless severe anemia is observed, an iron-restricted diet 6 mg/kg/day) should be the standard [85, 91]. Zinc supplementation improves the status of hyperammonemia [24–26].

4. Conclusion

Nutritional assessment in patients with LC is necessary for the appropriate management of LC patients. PEM, sarcopenia, and obesity are closely associated with adverse outcomes such as liver failure and HCC, as well as graft survival after liver transplantation in patients with LC. However, traditional and newly developed methods of measuring nutritional status are confounded by the changes in metabolism, body composition, and immune function that occur in LC independent of nutritional status. Further studies of precise assessments of malnutrition are needed to improve the prognosis of patients with LC.

Acknowledgements

The authors would like to thank Dr Yasuhiro Takikawa, Professor at the Division of Hepatology, Department of Internal Medicine, Iwate Medical University, for his assistance in creating this article.

Author details

Kazuyuki Suzuki[1]*, Ryujin Endo[2] and Akinobu Kato[3]

*Address all correspondence to: kasuzuki@morioka-u.ac.jp

1 Department of Nutritional Science, Morioka University, Takizawa, Japan

2 Division of Hepatology, Department of Internal Medicine, Iwate Medical University, Morioka, Japan

3 Department of Gastroenterology, Morioka Municipal Hospital, Morioka, Japan

References

[1] Caregaro L, Alberino F, Amodio P, et al. Malnutrition in alcoholic and virus-related cirrhosis. The American Journal of Clinical Nutrition. 1996;**63**:602-609

[2] Campillo B, Richardet JP, Scherman E, Bories PN. Evaluation of nutritional practice in hospitalized cirrhotic patients: results of a prospective study. Nutrition. 2003;**19**:515-521

[3] Riggio O, Angeloni S, Ciuffa L, et al. Malnutrition is not related to alterations in energy balance in patients with stable liver cirrhosis. Clinical Nutrition. 2003;**22**:553-559

[4] Cabré E, Gassull MA. Nutrition in liver disease. Current Opinion in Clinical Nutrition & Metabolic Care. 2005;**8**:545-551

[5] Tajika M, Kato M, Mohri H, et al. Prognostic value of energy metabolism in patients with viral liver cirrhosis. Nutrition 2002;**18**:229-234

[6] Rojas-Loureiro G, Servín-Caamaño A, Pérez-Reyes E, et al. Malnutrition negatively impacts the quality of life of patients with cirrhosis: An observational study. World Journal of Hepatology. 2017;**18**:263-269

[7] Tsiaousi ET, Hatzitolios AI, Trygonis SK, Savopoulos CG. Malnutrition in end stage liver disease: recommendations and nutritional support. Journal of Gastroenterology and Hepatology. 2008;**23**:527-533

[8] Rosenberg I. Sarcopenia: Origins and clinical relevance. Journal of Nutrition. 1997;**127**: 990S-991S

[9] Cruz-Jentoft AJ, Baeyens JP, Bauer JM, et al. European working group on sarcopenia in older people. sarcopenia: Report of the European working group on sarcopenia in older people. Age Aging. 2010;**39**:412-423

[10] Periyalwar P, Dasarathy S. Malnutrition in cirrhosis: Contribution and consequences of sarcopenia on metabolic and clinical responses. Clinical Liver Disease. 2012;**16**:95-131

[11] Kalafateli M, Konstantakis C, Thomopoulos K, Triantos C. Impact of muscle wasting on survival in patients with liver cirrhosis. World Journal of Gastroenterology. 2015;**21**:7357-7360

[12] Nishikawa H, Shiraki M, Hiramatsu A, et al. Japan Society of Hepatology guidelines for sarcopenia in liver disease (1st edition): Recommendation from the working group for creation of sarcopenia assessment criteria. Hepatology Research. 2016;**46**:951-963

[13] Hanai T, Shiraki M, Nishimura K, et al. Sarcopenia impairs prognosis of patients with liver cirrhosis. Nutrition. 2015;**31**:193-199

[14] Hanai T, Shiraki M, Ohnishi S, et al. Rapid skeletal wasting predicts worse survival in patients with liver cirrhosis. Hepatology Research. 2016;**46**:743-751

[15] Sinlair M, Gow PJ, Grossmann M, Angus PW. Review article: sarcopenia in cirrhosis– Aetiology, implications and potential therapeutic interventions. Alimentary Pharmacology & Therapeutics. 2016;**43**:765-777

[16] Kamachi S, Mizuta T, Otsuka T, et al. Sarcopenia is a risk factor for the recurrence of hepatocellular carcinoma after curative treatment. Hepatology Research. 2016;**46**:201-208

[17] Muto Y, Sato S, Watanabe A, et al. Overweight and obesity increases the risk for liver cancer in patients with liver cirrhosis and long-term oral supplementation with branched-chain amino acid granules inhibits liver carcinogenesis in heavier patients with liver cirrhosis. Hepatology Research.. 2006;35:204-214

[18] White DL, Ratziu V, El-Serag HB. Hepatitis C infection and risk of diabetes: A systemic review and meta- analysis. Journal of Hepatology. 2008;**49**:831-844

[19] El-Serag HB, Hampel H, Javadi F. The association between diabetes and hepatocellular carcinoma: a systemic review of epidemiologic evidence. Clinical Gastroenterology and Hepatology. 2006;**4**:369-380

[20] Kawaguchi T, Kohjima M, Ichikawa T, et al. The morbidity and associated risk factors of cancer in chronic liver disease patients with diabetes mellitus: A multicenter field survey. Journal of Gastroenterology. 2015;**50**:33-41

[21] Garcia-Compeán D, González-González JA, Lavalle-González JL, et al. Current concept in diabetes mellitus and chronic liver disease: Clinical outcomes, hepatitis C virus association, and therapy. Digestive Diseases and Sciences. 2016;**61**:371-380

[22] Dyal HK, Aguilar M, Bartos G, et al. Diabetes mellitus increases risk of hepatocellular carcinoma in chronic hepatitis C viral patients: A systemic review. Digestive Diseases and Sciences. 2016;**61**:636-645

[23] Knobler H, Malnick S. Hepatitis C and insulin action: An intimate relationship. World Journal of Hepatology. 2016;**18**:131-138

[24] Marchesini G, Fabbri A, Bianchi G, et al. Zinc supplementation and amino acid-nitrogen metabolism in patients with advanced cirrhosis. Hepatology. 1996;**23**:1084-1092

[25] Stamoulis I, Kouraklis G, Theocharis S. Zinc and the liver: An active interaction. Digestive Diseases and Sciences. 2007;**52**:1595-1612

[26] Katayama K, Saito M, Kawaguchi T, et al. Effect of zinc on liver cirrhosis with hyperammonemia: A preliminary randomized, placebo-controlled double-blind trial. Nutrition. 2014;**30**:1409-1414

[27] Gatti R, Palo CB, Spinella P, De Paul EF. Free carnitine and acetyl carnitine plasma levels and their relationship with body muscular mass in athletes. Amino Acid. 1998;**14**:361-369

[28] Rudman D, Sewell CW, Ansley JD. Deficiency of carnitine in cachectic cirrhotic patients. Journal of Clinical Investigation. 1997;**60**:716-723

[29] Amodio P, Angeli P, Merkel C, et al. Plasma carnitine levels in liver cirrhosis: relationship with nutritional status and liver damage. Journal of Clinical Chemistry and Clinical Biochemistry. 1990;**28**:619-626

[30] Krahenbuhl S, Reichen J. Carnitine metabolism in patients with chronic liver disease. Hepatology 1997;**25**:148-153

[31] Suzuki K, Onodera M, Kuroda H, et al. Reevaluation of serum carnitine status in patients with liver cirrhosis. Journal of Liver Research, Disorders & Therapy. 2016;**2**:25-32

[32] Suzuki K, Takikawa Y. Biomarkers of malnutrition in liver cirrhosis. In: Preedy VR, Lakshman R, Srirajaskanthan R and Watson RR, editors. Nutrition, Diet Therapy, and the Liver. London: CRC Press; 2009. Pp203-215. ISBN: 978-1-4200-8549-5

[33] Madden AM, Morgan YM. Resting energy expenditure should be measured in patients with cirrhosis, not predict. Hepatology. 1999;**30**:655-664

[34] Peng SLD, Plank LD, McCall JL, et al. Body composition, muscle function, and energy expenditure in patients with liver cirrhosis: A comprehensive study. The American Journal of Clinical Nutrition. 2007;**85**:1257-1266

[35] Guglielmi FW, Panella C, Buda A, et al. Nutritional state and energy balance in cirrhotic patients with or without hypermetabolism. Multicenter prospective study by the 'Nutritional Problems in Gastroenterology' Section of the Italian Society of Gastroenterology (SIGE). Digestive and Liver Disease. 2005;**37**:681-688

[36] Ruegg MA, Glass DJ. Molecular mechanism and treatment options for muscle wasting diseases. Annual Review of Pharmacology and Toxicology. 2011;**51**:373-395

[37] Glass DJ. Skeletal muscle hypertrophy and atrophy signaling pathways. The International Journal of Biochemistry & Cell Biology. 2005;**37**:1974-1984

[38] Sandri M. Signaling in muscle atrophy and hypertrophy. Physiology. 2008;**23**:160-170

[39] Rodriguez J, Vernus B, Chelh L, et al. Myostatin and the skeletal muscle atrophy and hypertrophy signaling pathways. Cellular and Molecular Life Sciences. 2014;**71**:4361-4371

[40] Quinlan GJ, Martin GS, Evans TW. Albumin: Biochemical properties and therapeutic potential. Hepatology. 2005;**41**:1211-1219

[41] Moriwaki H, Miwa Y, Tajika M, et al. Branched-chain amino acids as a protein- and energy-source in liver cirrhosis. Biochemical and Biophysical Research Communications. 2004;**313**:405-409

[42] Johnson AM. Low levels of plasma proteins malnutrition or inflammation? Clinical Chemistry and Laboratory Medicine. 1999;**37**:91-96

[43] Pugh RNH, Murry-Lyon IM, Dawson L, et al. Transection of the oesophagus for bleeding oesophageal varices. British Journal of Surgery. 1973;**60**:646-649

[44] Kamath PS, Kim WR, Advanced liver study group. The model for end-stage liver disease (MELD). Hepatology. 2007;**45**:797-805

[45] Kawakami A, Kubota K, Yamada N, et al. Identification and characterization of oxidized human serum albumin. A slight structural change impairs its ligand-binding and antioxidant functions. FEBS. 2006;3346-57

[46] Watanabe A, Mastuzaki H, Moriwaki H, et al. Problem in serum albumin measurement and clinical significance of albumin microheterogeneity in cirrhosis. Nutrition. 2004;**20**:351-357

[47] Fukushima H, Miwa Y, Shiraki M, et al. Oral branched-chain amino acid supplementation improves the oxidized/reduced albumin ratio in patients with liver cirrhosis. Hepatology Research. 2007;**37**:765-770

[48] Brose L. Prealbumin as a marker of nutritional status. Journal of Burn Care & Research. 1990;**11**:372-375

[49] Gabay C, Kushner I. Acute-phase proteins and other systemic responses to inflammation. The New England Journal of Medicine. 1999;**340**:448-454

[50] Calamita A, Dichi I, Papini-Berto SJ, et al. Plasma levels of transthyretin and retinol-binding protein in Child-A cirrhotic patient in relation to protein-calorie status and plasma amino acids, zinc, vitamin A and plasma thyroid hormones. Arq Gastroenterol. 1997;**34**:139-147

[51] Bahr M, Boeker KH, Manns MP, et al. Decrease hepatic RBP4 secretion is correlated with reduced hepatic glucose production but not associated with insulin resistance in patients with liver cirrhosis. Clinical Endocrinology. 2008;**68**:1-22

[52] Yagmur E, Weiskirchen R, Gressner AM, et al. Insulin resistance in liver cirrhosis is not associated with circulating retinol-binding protein 4. Diabetes Care. 2007;**30**:1168-1172

[53] Fischer JE, Rosen HM, Ebeid AM, et al. The effect of normalization of plasma amino acids on hepatic encephalopathy. Surgery. 1976;**80**:77-91

[54] Azuma Y, Maekawa Y, Kuwabara Y, et al. Determination of branched-chain amino acid and tyrosine in serum of patients with various hepatic diseases and its clinical usefulness. Clinical Chemistry. 1989;**35**:1399-1403

[55] Suzuki K, Kato A, Iwai M. Branched-chain amino acid treatment in patients with liver cirrhosis. Hepatology Research. 2004;**30S**:S25-29

[56]   Suzuki T, Suzuki K, Koizumi K, et al. Measurement of serum branched-chain amino acid to tyrosine ratio is useful in a prediction of a change of serum albumin level in chronic liver disease. Hepatology Research. 2008;**38**:267-272

[57]   McCullough AJ, Bugianesi E, Marchesini G, et al. Gender-dependent alterations in serum leptin in alcoholic cirrhosis. Gastroenterology. 1998;**115**:947-953

[58]   Campillo B, Sherman E, Richardet JP, et al. Serum leptin levels in alcoholic liver cirrhosis: Relationship with gender, nutritional status, liver function and energy metabolism. European Journal of Clinical Nutrition. 2001;**55**:980-988

[59]   Onodera MK, Kato A, Suzuki K. Serum leptin concentrations in liver cirrhosis: Relationship to the severity of liver dysfunction and their characteristic diurnal profiles. Hepatology Research. 2001;**21**:205-212

[60]   Schere PE, Williams S, Fogliano M, et al. Novel serum protein similar to Clq produced exclusively in adipocytes. The Journal of Biological Chemistry. 1995;**270**:26746-26749

[61]   Sohara N, Takagi H, Kakizaki S, et al. Elevated plasma adiponectin concentration in patients with liver cirrhosis correlate with plasma insulin levels. Liver International. 2004;**25**:28-32

[62]   Hara K, Horikoshi M, Yamauchi T, et al. Measurement of the high-molecular weight form adiponectin in plasma is useful for the prediction of insulin resistance and metabolic syndrome. Diabetes Care. 2006;**29**:1357-1362

[63]   Bahr MJ, Ockenga J, Böker KHW, et al. Elevated resistin levels in cirrhosis are associated but not with insulin resistance. American Physiological Society. 2006;**11**:372-375

[64]   Kakizaki S, Sohara N, Yamazaki Y, et al. Elevated plasma resistin concentrations in patients with liver cirrhosis. Journal of Gastroenterology and Hepatology. 2008;**23**:73-77

[65]   Kojima M, Hosoda H, Date Y, et al. Ghrelin is a growth-hormone-releasing acylated peptide form stomach. Nature 1999;**402**:656-660

[66]   Cummings DE, Weigle DS, Frayo S, et al. Plasma ghrelin levels after diet-induced weight loss or gastric bypass surgery. The New England Journal of Medicine. 2003;**346**:1623-1630

[67]   Nakazato M, Murakami N, Date Y, et al. A role of ghrelin in the central regulation of feeding. Nature. 2001;**409**:194-198

[68]   Tacke FG, Brabant E, Kruck E, et al. Ghrelin in chronic liver disease. Journal of Hepatology. 2003;**38**:447-454

[69]   Marchesini G, Villanova N, Bianchi G, et al. Plasma ghrelin concentrations, food intake, and anorexia in liver disease. The Journal of Clinical Endocrinology & Metabolism. 2004;**89**:2136-2141

[70]   Takahashi T, Kato A, Onodera K, et al. Fasting plasma ghrelin levels reflect malnutrition state in patients with liver cirrhosis. Hepatology Research. 2006;**24**:117-123

[71]   Ziegler TR. Parenteral nutrition in the critically ill patients. The New England Journal of Medicine. 2009;**361**:1088-1097

[72] Terakura Y, Shiraki M, Nishimura K, et al. Indirect calorimetry and anthropometry to estimate energy metabolism in patients with liver cirrhosis. Journal of Nutritional Science and Vitaminology. 2010;**56**:372-379

[73] Nishikawa H, Enomoto H, Iwata Y, et al. Prognostic significance of nonprotein respiratory quotient in patients with cirrhosis. Medicine. 2017;**96:3** e5800

[74] Proietto J, Alford FP, Dudley FJ. The mechanism of the carbohydrate intolerance of cirrhosis. The Journal of Clinical Endocrinology & Metabolism. 1980;**51**:1030-1036

[75] Riggio O, Merli M, Cantafora A, et al. Total and individual free fatty acid concentrations in liver cirrhosis. Metabolism 1984;**33**:646-651

[76] Owen OE, Trapp VE, Reichard GA, et al. Nature and quantity of fuels consumed in patients with alcoholic cirrhosis. Journal of Clinical Investigation. 1983;**72**:1821-1832

[77] Hanai T, Shiraki M, Nishimura K, et al. Free fatty acid as a marker of energy malnutrition in liver cirrhosis. Hepatology Research. 2014;**44**:218-228

[78] Taniguchi E, Kawaguchi T, Sakata M, et al. Lipid profile is associated with the incidence of cognitive dysfunction in viral cirrhotic patients: A data-mining analysis. Hepatology Research. 2013;**43**:418-424

[79] Garcia-Compean D, Jaquez-Quintana JO, Lavalle-Gonzalez FJ, et al. The prevalence and clinical characteristics of glucose metabolism disorders in patients with liver cirrhosis: A prospective study. Annals of Hepatology. 2012;**11**:240-248

[80] Sakata M, Kawahara A, Kawaguchi T, et al. Decreased expression of insulin and increased expression of pancreatic transcription factor PDX-1 in islets in patients with liver cirrhosis: A comparative investigation using human autopsy specimens. Journal of Gastroenterology. 2013;**48**:277-285

[81] Kawaguchi T, Yoshida T, Harada M, et al. Hepatitis C virus down-regulates insulin receptor substrates 1 and 2 through up-regulation of suppressor of cytokine signaling 3. American Journal of Pathology. 2004;**165**:1499-1508

[82] Milner KL, Jenkins AB, Trenell M, et al. Eradicating hepatitis C virus ameliorates insulin resistance without change in adipose depots. Journal of Viral Hepatitis. 2014;**21**:325-352

[83] Plauth M, Cabre E, Riggio O, et al. ESPEN guidelines on enteral nutrition: Liver disease. Clinical Nutrition. 2006;**25**:285-294

[84] Plauth M, Cabre E, Campillo O, et al. ESPEN guidelines on parenteral nutrition: hepatology. Clinical Nutrition. 2009;**28**:436-444

[85] Suzuki K, Endo R, Kohgo Y, et al. Guidelines on nutritional management in Japanese patients with liver cirrhosis from the perspective of preventing hepatocellular carcinoma. Hepatology Research. 2012;**42**:621-626

[86] Chang WK, Chao YC, Tang HS, et al. Effects of exra-carbohydrate supplementation in the late evening on energy expenditure and substrate oxidation in patients with liver cirrhosis. Journal of Parenteral and Enteral Nutrition. 1997;**21**:96-99

[87] Yamanaka-Okumura H, Nakamura T, Takeuchi H, et al. Effects of late evening snack with rice ball on energy metabolism in liver cirrhosis. European Journal of Clinical Nutrition. 2006;**60**:1067-1072

[88] Miwa Y, Shiraki M, Kato M, et al. Improvement of fuel metabolism by nocturnal energy supplementation in patients with liver cirrhosis. Hepatology Research. 2000;**18**:184-189

[89] Nakaya Y, Okita K, Suzuki K, et al. Hepatic nutritional Therapy (HNT) Study Group. BCAA-enriched snack improves nutritional state of cirrhosis. Nutrition. 2007;**23**:113-120

[90] Korenaga K, Korenaga M, Uchida K, et al. Effects of a late evening snack combined with alpha-glucosidase inhibitor on liver cirrhosis. Hepatology Research. 2008;**38**:1087-1097

[91] Kohgo Y, Ikuta K, Ohtake T, et al. Body iron metabolism and pathophysiology of iron overload. International Journal of Hematology. 2008;**88**:7-15

10

The Promising Role of Anti-Fibrotic Agent Halofuginone in Liver Fibrosis/Cirrhosis

Berna Karakoyun

Abstract

Liver fibrosis is a complex inflammatory and fibrogenic process that results from chronic liver injury and represents an early step in the progression of cirrhosis. Several cell types [hepatic stellate cells (HSCs), hepatocytes, liver sinusoidal endothelial cells (LSECs), and Kupffer cells (KCs)], cytokines [platelet-derived growth factor (PDGF), transforming growth factor (TGF)-β, tumor necrosis factor (TNF)-α, interferons (IFNs), interleukins (ILs)], oxidative stress, and microRNAs (miRNAs) are involved in the initiation and progression of liver fibrosis/cirrhosis. Generally, liver fibrosis begins with the stimulation of inflammatory immune cells to secrete cytokines, growth factors, and other activator molecules. These chemical mediators direct HSCs to activate and synthesize large amounts of extracellular matrix (ECM) components. Therefore, HSC activation is a pivotal event in the development of fibrosis and a major contributor to collagen (specifically type I) accumulation. The inhibitory effect of halofuginone on collagen type α1(I) synthesis and ECM deposition has been shown in several experimental models of fibrotic diseases. Halofuginone inhibits TGF-β–induced phosphorylation of Smad3, which is a key phenomenon in the fibrogenesis. It also regulates cell growth and differentiation, apoptosis, cell migration, and immune cell function in liver fibrosis/cirrhosis. This review discusses the etiology and mechanisms of liver fibrosis/cirrhosis and the promising role of anti-fibrotic agent halofuginone.

Keywords: liver fibrosis, liver cirrhosis, hepatic stellate cells, pathogenesis, anti-fibrotic, halofuginone

1. Introduction

Liver cirrhosis is the end-stage condition of several chronic liver diseases, and fibrosis is the critical pre-stage of cirrhosis. On a worldwide perspective, liver cirrhosis can be induced by a number of well-defined etiological causes/factors or conditions such as chronic infection by hepatitis B, C viruses, chronic alcoholism and/or chronic exposure to toxins or drugs, infections, chronic exposure to altered metabolic conditions, inherited metabolic diseases such as hematochromatosis and Wilson's disease, auto-immune diseases such as primary biliary cirrhosis, and auto-immune hepatitis [1–3]. These etiologies may work separately or in combination with each other to produce cumulative effects. While the causes of liver cirrhosis are multifactorial, there are some pathological characteristics that are common to all cases of cirrhosis, including degeneration and necrosis of hepatocytes, replacement of healthy liver parenchyma by fibrotic scar tissues and regenerative nodules, and loss of liver function [4–7].

Fibrosis is characterized by high levels of extracellular matrix (ECM, non-functional connective tissue) components extremely rich in collagen type I. The matrix metalloproteinases (MMPs, matrix degradation enzymes), and the tissue inhibitor of metalloproteinases (TIMPs) play a crucial role in the fine regulation of ECM turnover, which is altered in most pathological states associated with liver fibrosis [8]. The key cellular mediator of fibrosis comprises the activated hepatic stellate cells (HSCs), which serve as the primary ECM-producing cells. HSCs, which play a key role in the development of liver fibrosis [9, 10], are activated by several inflammatory cytokines and growth factors in a paracrine and autocrine manner [11, 12].

Liver fibrosis and cirrhosis are dynamic and highly integrated molecular, tissue and cellular processes that can progress and regress over time [13] and that require cellular cross-talk between various liver cell types [14]. At early stages of fibrosis, initiating signals [such as DNA, reactive oxygen species (ROS)], responding cells [Kupffer cells (KCs), platelets, liver sinusoidal endothelial cells (LSECs)], and soluble mediators [such as platelet-derived growth factor (PDGF), transforming growth factor (TGF)-β] induce accompanying wound-healing responses to liver injury. With time, cells, cytokine responses, and ECM components become more specialized but continue to have strong interactions with each other [15].

Halofuginone is a non-toxic plant alkaloid [7-bromo-6-chloro-3-(3-hydroxy-2-piperidine)-2-oxopropyl-4(3H)-quinazoline] isolated from the roots of *Dichroa febrifuga*, and is used worldwide as an anti-parasitic drug [16]. Independent of this effect, halofuginone was found to be a potent inhibitor of collagen type $\alpha 1$ (I) gene expression [17], which was demonstrated in a broad range of cell types both *in vitro* and *in vivo* [16–20]. Due to its inhibitory effects on collagen synthesis (collagen type $\alpha 1$) and ECM deposition, halofuginone treatment was used in several experimental disease models characterized by excessive collagen accumulation, such as pulmonary, pancreatic and renal fibrosis [21–23], scleroderma and chronic graft-versus-host disease [24], post-operative peritendinous and abdominal adhesions [25, 26], urethral and esophageal strictures [27, 28], wound repair [29], burn injury [30], renal injury [31, 32], injury-induced arterial intimal hyperplasia [33], colitis [34], and liver fibrosis and cirrhosis [35–39]. Although the exact anti-fibrotic mechanism of halofuginone is not well understood, it was found that halofuginone affects collagen synthesis probably by inhibiting TGF-β-mediated Smad3 (intracellular protein) activation [40]. Halofuginone also regulates cell growth and differentiation, apoptosis, cell migration, and immune cell function [41]. It prevents concanavalin A-induced liver fibrosis by affecting T helper 17 (Th17) cell differentiation, which suggests a direct connection between the myofibroblasts/fibrosis pathway and the Th17 pro-inflammatory pathway [38]. In addition, halofuginone treatment effectively inhibits the delayed-type hypersensitivity response, indicating suppression of T cell–mediated inflammation *in vivo* [42]. Moreover, it is a potent inhibitor of nuclear factor (NF)-κB, pro-inflammatory cytokines and p38 mitogen-activated protein kinase (p38 MAPK) phosphorylation in activated T cells *in vitro* [42]. Also, it inhibits HSC proliferation and migration and up-regulates their expressions of fibrolytic MMP-3 and -13 via activation of p38 MAPK and NF-κB [43].

Although there are no highly effective anti-fibrogenic agents currently available, the potential candidates that can specifically inhibit ECM components in general and specifically inhibit collagen type I in particular, are considered to be promising for the prevention and treatment of liver fibrosis/cirrhosis. The present review aims to clarify the etiology and mechanisms of liver fibrosis/cirrhosis and focus on the anti-fibrotic potential of a novel and promising agent, halofuginone.

2. Role of different cell types in liver fibrosis/cirrhosis

The liver is composed of parenchymal cells (hepatocytes) and non-parenchymal cells (HSCs, LSECs, and KCs). Both parenchymal and non-parenchymal cells are involved in the initiation and progression of liver fibrosis/cirrhosis (**Table 1**).

Cell types	Role in liver fibrosis/cirrhosis	References
Hepatic stellate cells (HSCs)	Main function is storage of vitamin A and other retinoids	[7, 44]
	Undergo a phenotypic switch from a quiescent type into an activated type (myofibroblast-like cells) by several inflammatory cytokines	[46]
	Activated HSCs are major contributors to collagen accumulation	[47, 48]
Hepatocytes	Hepatocyte-derived apoptotic bodies stimulate secretion of fibrogenic cytokines from KCs and promote HSC activation	[50–53]
	Hypoxic hepatocytes become a primary source of TGF-β in cirrhotic stage	[55]
Liver sinusoidal endothelial cells (LSECs)	Defenestration and capillarization of LSECs lead to impaired substrate exchange and HSC activation	[57, 61, 62]
	Secrete IL-33 to activate HSCs	[63]
Kupffer cells (KCs)	Activated KCs secrete inflammatory cytokines, promote HSC activation, and stimulate cell proliferation	[65–69]
	KC-derived TGF-β1 stimulates proliferation and collagen formation of HSCs	[66]
	Activated KCs kill HSCs by a caspase 9-dependent mechanism via TRAIL	[72, 73]

Abbreviations: TGF-β, transforming growth factor-β; IL, interleukin; TRAIL, tumor necrosis factor-related apoptosis-inducing ligand.

Table 1. Role of different cell types in liver fibrosis/cirrhosis.

2.1. Hepatic stellate cells (HSCs)

HSCs are one of the non-parenchymal cells of the liver located in the perisinusoidal space (space of Disse) between hepatocytes and sinusoidal endothelial cells. HSCs are also known as fat-storing cells, perisinusoidal cells, lipocytes, or vitamin A-rich cells, and their main function is storage of vitamin A and other retinoids [7, 44]. HSCs show two different phenotypes: quiescent type in the healthy liver and activated type in the diseased one. Quiescent HSCs mostly function as vitamin A reserves [45]. However, in response to liver injury, inflammatory cytokines such as tumor necrosis factor (TNF)-α, TGF-β, interleukin (IL)-1, and PDGF promote HSCs to undergo a phenotypic switch from a quiescent, vitamin A storing cell into proliferative, α-smooth muscle actin (α-SMA)-positive, myofibroblast-like cells which contribute to fibrosis by producing the abnormal ECM components [46]. Therefore, HSC activation is a pivotal phenomenon in initiation and progression of liver fibrosis and a major contributor to collagen accumulation [47, 48].

2.2. Hepatocytes

Hepatocytes are the primary parenchymal component of the liver and play an important role in fibrosis/cirrhosis. They are the main targets of several hepatotoxic agents including hepatitis viruses, alcohol metabolites, and bile acids [11]. Liver injury either promotes apoptosis or triggers compensatory regeneration of hepatocytes [49]. Hepatocyte-derived apoptotic bodies stimulate secretion of fibrogenic cytokines from KCs and promote HSC activation via interaction of toll-like receptor (TLR)-9 with DNA, which is released from apoptotic hepatocytes [50–53]. On the other hand, activated HSCs also act as phagocytes and phagocytize hepatocyte apoptotic bodies, which promote myofibroblasts survival and fibrogenesis [54]. Therefore, apoptosis of hepatocytes is a crucial event in liver injury and contributes to tissue inflammation, fibrogenesis, and development of cirrhosis. Also, in the cirrhotic stage, hypoxic hepatocytes become a primary source of TGF-β, which may augment liver fibrosis [55].

2.3. Liver sinusoidal endothelial cells (LSECs)

LSECs constitute the sinusoidal wall, also known as endothelium, or endothelial lining. The main characteristic of LSECs is having the fenestrae on the surface of the endothelium [56, 57]. The endothelial fenestrae control exchange of fluids, solutes, and particles between sinusoidal blood and hepatocytes [58]. In the healthy liver, the fenestrated endothelial cells prevent HSC activation through vascular endothelial growth factor-stimulated nitric oxide production [59]. However, LSECs have high endocytotic capacity [56, 60]. Upon liver injury, defenestration and capillarization of LSECs lead to impaired substrate exchange which is the major cause of hepatic dysfunction [57, 58] and HSC activation [61, 62]. It has been also revealed that LSECs can secrete the cytokine IL-33 to activate HSCs and promote liver fibrosis [63].

2.4. Kupffer cells (KCs)

KCs, also called stellate macrophages, are interspersed throughout the liver, situated within the sinusoids. KCs are responsible for the removal of circulating microorganisms, immune complexes, and debris from the blood stream. They are usually activated by many injurious factors such as viral infection and alcohol [64]. Activation of KCs is a key phenomenon in initiation and preservation of liver fibrosis. Activated KCs express chemokine receptors, secret inflammatory cytokines (such as TNF-α, IL-1, IL-6) and serve as antigen-presenting cells, which lead to progression of fibrosis [65–68]. KCs are also involved in the activation of HSCs and formation of liver fibrosis. For example, KC-conditioned medium promotes activation of cultured rat HSCs with enhanced ECM production and stimulates cell proliferation via induction of PDGF receptors on the membrane of HSCs [69]. KC-derived TGF-β1 stimulates proliferation and collagen formation of HSCs in a rat model of alcoholic liver fibrogenesis [66]. Moreover, macrophage ablation has been shown to attenuate liver fibrosis. For example, gadolinium chloride-mediated depletion of KCs has been shown to result in attenuation of carbon tetrachloride (CCl_4)-induced fibrosis in rats with prevention of the increased TGF-β expression [70]. Conversely, KCs produce interstitial collagenase MMP-13 when treated with gadolinium chloride, which reduces ECM deposition during experimental liver fibrosis [71]. In addition, activated KCs can effectively kill HSCs by a caspase 9-dependent mechanism via possible involvement of TNF-related apoptosis-inducing ligand (TRAIL) [72, 73].

3. Role of cytokines in liver fibrosis/cirrhosis

Cytokines, which mediate several immune and inflammatory reactions, are small signaling proteins that facilitate intercellular communication between various cells. They function through cell-surface receptors, and down-stream signaling induces an alteration of cell functions. Liver fibrosis/cirrhosis is a result of interaction of a complex network of cytokines, which modify activities of circulating immune cells, HSCs, KCs, LSECs, and hepatocytes. The role of cytokines in liver fibrosis/cirrhosis is summarized in **Table 2**.

3.1. Platelet-derived growth factor (PDGF)

PDGF is one of the most potent mitogen for HSCs isolated from mouse, rat, or human liver [74]. PDGF and its receptors are significantly overexpressed in fibrotic tissues, and its activity increases with the degree of liver fibrosis [75, 76]. Hepatocyte damage resulting from factors, such as viruses, chemicals, or hepatotoxins, can induce KCs to synthesize and release PDGF [77]. When PDGF binds to its specific receptor on the membrane of HSCs, it activates corresponding signal molecules and transcription factors, leading to the activation of its downstream target genes and activation of HSCs [74]. PDGF has been shown to up-regulate the expression of MMP-2, MMP-9, and TIMP-1, and inhibit collagenase activity, thereby decreasing ECM degradation [78].

3.2. Transforming growth factor (TGF)-β

Among fibrotic mediators, TGF-β is one of the most important pro-fibrotic cytokine. The direct targets in TGF-β pathway, Smads (especially Smad3) are critical mediators in fibrogenesis [79, 80]. The intracellular effectors of TGF-β signaling, the Smad proteins, are activated by receptors and

Mediators	Mechanism of action	References
Platelet-derived growth factor (PDGF)	Activates HSCs	[74]
	Up-regulates expression of MMP-2, MMP-9, and TIMP-1 and inhibits collagenase activity	[78]
Transforming growth factor (TGF)-β	Stimulates HSC activation	[81, 82]
	Induces expression of matrix-producing genes, inhibits ECM degradation, and promotes TIMPs	[84, 85]
	Inhibits DNA synthesis and induces apoptosis of hepatocytes	[86–88]
Tumor necrosis factor (TNF)-α	Induces hepatocyte death by apoptosis	[90]
	Activates HSCs and stimulates ECM synthesis	[91, 92]
	Induces/reduces apoptosis of activated HSCs	[73, 93]
	Reduces glutathione and inhibits pro-collagen α1 mRNA expression	[94]
Interferons (IFNs)		
IFN-α	Triggers apoptosis of HSCs	[96]
	Elicits an anti-apoptotic effect on activated HSCs	[100]
IFN-β	Decreases α-SMA and collagen expression and inhibits HSC activation through inhibition of TGF-β and PDGF	[97]
IFN-γ	Reduces ECM deposition by inhibiting HSC activation	[98]
	Exerts a pro-apoptotic effect on activated HSCs	[100]
Interleukins (ILs)		
IL-1	Activates HSCs and stimulates them to produce MMP-9, MMP-13 and TIMP-1	[102]
	Increases MCP-1 in hepatocytes and augments TLR-4-dependent up-regulation of inflammatory signaling in macrophages	[105]
IL-17	Regulates production of TGF-β1 by KCs, induces activation of HSCs and induces production of collagen and α-SMA in HSCs via STAT3 pathway	[108]
IL-6	Attenuates hepatocyte apoptosis and induces regeneration of hepatocytes through NF-κB pathway	[112]
IL-10	Inhibits expression of TGF-β1, MMP-2 and TIMP-1	[115]
	Inhibits HSC activity	[117]
	Reduces TGF-β1, TNF-α, collagen α1, and TIMP mRNA up-regulation	[120]
IL-22	Inhibits hepatocyte apoptosis via STAT3	[121, 122]
	Induces HSC senescence	[123]

Abbreviations: HSC, hepatic stellate cell; MMP, matrix metalloproteinase; TIMP, tissue inhibitor of metalloproteinase; ECM, extracellular matrix; SMA, smooth muscle actin; MCP, monocyte chemoattractant protein; TLR, toll-like receptor; KC, Kupffer cell; STAT, signal transducer and activator of transcription; NF-κB, nuclear factor-κB.

Table 2. Role of cytokines in liver fibrosis/cirrhosis.

translocate into the nucleus, where they regulate transcription [79]. The main effect of TGF-β is to stimulate HSC activation, and the TGF-β autocrine cycle in activated HSCs is an important positive feedback to the progression of liver fibrosis [81, 82]. Though the main source of TGF-β in fibrotic liver is activated HSCs, LSECs, KCs, and hepatocytes also contribute to synthesis of this growth factor [83]. The level of TGF-β1 expression is increased during liver fibrosis and reaches a maximum at cirrhosis [55]. TGF-β1 induces expression of the matrix-producing genes, inhibits ECM degradation, and promotes TIMPs, leading to excessive collagen accumulation and promoting the development of liver fibrosis [84, 85]. Furthermore, TGF-β1 has been shown to inhibit DNA synthesis and induces apoptosis of hepatocytes. In particular, TGF-β1-induced apoptosis is thought to be responsible for tissue loss and decrease in liver size seen in cirrhosis [86–88].

3.3. Tumor necrosis factor (TNF)-α

TNF-α is a pro-inflammatory cytokine produced by different cell types. However, it is mainly produced by activated KCs in the liver. TNF-α is an important mediator in several processes such as cell proliferation, inflammation, and apoptosis [89]. TNF-α can induce cell death by apoptosis, and KCs can be stimulated by apoptotic hepatocytes to produce more TNF-α [90]. Furthermore, TNF-α plays an essential role in the HSC activation and ECM synthesis in liver fibrosis [91, 92]. TNF-α may act as surviving factor for activated rat HSCs by up-regulating the anti-apoptotic factors (NF-κB, bcl-xL, and p21WAF1) and by down-regulating the pro-apoptotic factor (p53) [93]. On the other hand, TNF-α can induce apoptosis in HSCs [73]. It has been also demonstrated that TNF-α shows anti-fibrogenic effect in rat HSCs by reducing glutathione and inhibiting pro-collagen α1 mRNA expression [94].

3.4. Interferons (IFNs)

IFNs are potent pleiotropic cytokines that broadly alter cellular functions in response to viral and other infections. Leukocytes synthesize IFN-α and IFN-β in response to viruses, and T cells secrete IFN-γ upon stimulation with various antigens and mitogens. Although the primary action of IFN-α is to eradicate viruses, patients with hepatitis C treated with IFN-α exhibit a regression of liver fibrosis even if viral eradication is not achieved [95], indicating that IFN-α itself has anti-fibrotic activity via triggering the apoptosis of HSCs [96]. IFN-β treatment decreases α-SMA and collagen expression and inhibits HSC activation through inhibition of TGF-β and PDGF pathways [97]. Similarly, IFN-γ reduces ECM deposition *in vivo* by inhibiting HSC activation [98] via TGFβ1/Smad3 signaling pathways [99]. Interestingly, IFN-α and IFN-γ may exert opposite effects on apoptosis in HSCs. IFN-α was shown to elicit an anti-apoptotic effect on activated HSCs, whereas IFN-γ was found to exert pro-apoptotic effect on HSCs by down-regulating heat-shock protein 70 [100].

3.5. Interleukins (ILs)

ILs are immunomodulatory cytokines that are critically involved in the regulation of immune responses. They are produced by a variety of cell types such as CD4+ T lymphocytes, monocytes, macrophages, and endothelial cells. KCs and LSECs can rapidly produce ILs in response to liver injury. ILs can have pro- and anti-inflammatory functions in chronic liver diseases, dependent on the inflammatory stimulus and, the producing and the responding cell type.

The main function of pro-inflammatory ILs is to stimulate immune responses that result in the elimination of invading pathogens or damaged cells. On the other hand, anti-inflammatory ILs are produced to protect the host's body from exaggerated immune responses and to limit organ damage. As soon as the pathogenic stimuli are removed, ILs production is no longer needed, and inflammation diminishes. If the stimulus continues, inflammation can become chronic and induce a variety of inflammatory diseases [101].

IL-1 is a pro-inflammatory and pro-fibrotic cytokine that directly activates HSCs and stimulates them to produce MMP-9, MMP-13, and TIMP-1, resulting in liver fibrogenesis [102]. IL-1 receptor-deficient mice exhibits ameliorated liver damage and reduced fibrogenesis [102]. Similarly, IL-1 receptor antagonist protects rats from developing fibrosis in dimethylnitrosamine-induced liver fibrosis [103]. Lack of IL-1α or IL-1β also makes the mice less susceptible to develop liver fibrosis in experimental model of steatohepatitis [104]. It has been also shown that IL-1β at physiological doses increases the inflammatory and prosteatotic chemokine monocyte chemoattractant protein (MCP)-1 in hepatocytes, and augments TLR-4-dependent up-regulation of inflammatory signaling in macrophages [105]. Thus, IL-1 is an important participant, along with other cytokines, and controls the progression from liver injury to fibrogenesis.

Another pro-inflammatory and pro-fibrotic cytokine IL-17 has been reported to be involved in many immune processes, most notably in inducing and mediating pro-inflammatory responses. Its expression increases with increasing degree of liver fibrosis [106, 107], suggesting that IL-17 may not only induce inflammation but also contribute to disease progression and chronicity [106]. IL-17 regulates production of TGF-β1 by KCs, which in turn, induces activation of HSCs into myofibroblasts, and further facilitates differentiation of IL-17 expressing cells [108]. Also, IL-17 directly induces production of collagen and α-SMA in HSCs via the signal transducer and activator of transcription (STAT)3 signaling pathway [108]. Furthermore, abrogation of IL-17 signaling by deletion of IL-17RA protects mice from fibrogenesis [108]. Similarly, blockade of endogenous IL-17 with neutralizing IL-17-specific antibody reduces liver fibrosis, whereas treatment with recombinant IL-17 increases fibrosis development [109].

IL-6 is a pleiotropic cytokine, which may affect differentiation of fibroblast to myofibroblast, and it plays an important role in fibrotic diseases [110, 111]. On the other hand, IL-6 has beneficial effects for the liver. For example, IL-6 reduces CCl_4-induced acute and chronic liver injury and fibrosis [112]. Also, it attenuates hepatocyte apoptosis and induces regeneration of hepatocytes through NF-κB signaling pathway [112]. In an experimental model of concavaline A-induced hepatitis, IL-6 pretreatment protects mice from liver injury. This protection requires gp130 signaling in hepatocytes and is mediated via the gp130/STAT3 signaling cascade [113]. Furthermore, systemic injection of IL-6 followed by intrahepatic transplantation of mesenchymal stem cells is also able to reduce hepatocyte apoptosis and liver fibrogenesis after CCl_4 treatment [114].

IL-10 is one of the major anti-inflammatory cytokines, with tissue protective functions during fibrogenesis. It down-regulates the pro-inflammatory response and has a modulatory effect on liver fibrogenesis [115, 116]. IL-10 has been shown to exert anti-fibrotic effects through inhibiting HSC activity [117]. IL-10-deficient mice show higher liver fibrosis with larger inflammatory infiltrates in CCl_4-induced liver fibrosis compared to wild-type mice [118, 119]. IL-10 gene therapy reverses CCl_4-induced murine liver fibrosis by inhibiting the expression of TGF-β1, MMP-2, and TIMP-1 [115]. Additionally, IL-10 gene therapy reverses liver fibrosis and prevents cell apoptosis in a thioacetamide-treated murine liver, and reduces TGF-β1, TNF-α, collagen α1, and TIMP mRNA up-regulation, suggesting a therapeutic potential for treatment with IL-10 [120].

IL-22 is known to play important roles in the modulation of tissue immune responses to inflammation. It reduces inflammation-induced damage of hepatocytes both *in vitro* and *in vivo* by promoting their survival and inhibiting apoptosis [121]. This protective function is dependent on STAT3 signaling, as STAT3-deficient mice were not protected when treated with IL-22 [122]. Similarly, in CCl_4-induced liver fibrogenesis, IL-22 is protective through induction of senescence in HSCs via STAT3 signaling pathway [123]. Moreover, IL-22 is also involved in the restoration of functional liver mass after organ damage. Liver progenitor cells have been shown to express IL-22R, and IL-22 derived from inflammatory cells induces proliferation of liver progenitor cells [124].

4. Role of oxidative stress in liver fibrogenesis

Oxidative stress is caused by an imbalance between production of ROS and their elimination by anti-oxidant defenses [125]. As liver is an essential organ for detoxification and nutrients metabolism, it is more vulnerable to oxidative stress [125]. Oxidative stress-related molecules and pathways modulate tissue and cellular events involved in the liver fibrogenesis [126]. The generation of ROS plays a crucial role in producing liver damage and initiating liver fibrogenesis [126]. Oxidative stress disrupts lipids, proteins and DNA, induces necrosis and apoptosis of hepatocytes, resulting in the initiation of fibrosis [127]. ROS stimulate the production of pro-fibrogenic mediators from KCs and circulating inflammatory cells. Remarkably, ROS directly activate HSCs. The elevated oxidative stress contributes to fibrogenesis via stimulating collagen production from activated HSCs and release of other pro-fibrogenic cytokines and growth factors [126, 128].

5. Role of microRNAs (miRNAs) in liver pathophysiology

miRNAs are a family of small non-coding RNAs (20–25 nucleotides in length) that control gene expression by binding to mRNAs to repress translation or induce mRNA cleavage [129]. Many researchers have reported that the unusual expression of miRNAs in liver tissue was related to the pathogenesis of liver disease of any etiology [130, 131]. Recently, miRNAs have been found to play fundamental roles in liver fibrosis, including those in HSC activation and ECM production [132]. For example, miRNA-21 exhibits an important role in the pathogenesis and progression of liver fibrosis. A natural product 3,3'-Diindolylmethane (DIM) inhibits TGF-β signaling pathway by down-regulating the miRNA-21 expression in thioacetamide-induced experimental liver fibrosis. Furthermore, DIM can suppress HSC activation via down-regulating miRNA-21 levels in HSCs by inhibiting activity of the transcription factor AP-1 [133]. Inhibition of miRNA-21 also reduces liver fibrosis through concomitant reduction of CD24+ liver progenitor cells [134]. In mouse and human studies, the expression levels of miRNA-199a, antisense miRNA-199a*, miRNA-200a, and miRNA-200b are found to be positively and significantly correlated with progression of liver fibrosis. Overexpression of these miRNAs dramatically increases the expression of fibrosis-related genes in HSCs [135]. Also, miRNA-221 and miRNA-222 are up-regulated in human liver in a fibrosis progression-dependent manner [136]. Similarly, in isolated primary human liver cells, miRNA-571 is up-regulated in hepatocytes and HSCs in response to the pro-fibrogenic cytokine TGF-β [137]. miRNA-214 appears to participate in the development of liver fibrosis by modulating the epidermal growth factor (EGF) receptor and TGF-β signaling pathways. Also, inhibition of miRNA-214 by locked nucleic acid-antimiRNA-214 ameliorates liver fibrosis in PDGF c transgenic mice [138]. In addition, miRNA-214-5p may play crucial roles in HSC activation and progression of liver fibrosis. The overexpression of miRNA-214-5p in human stellate cells increases the expression of fibrosis-related genes such as MMP-2, MMP-9, α-SMA, and TGF-β1 [139].

miRNAs may also play anti-fibrogenic roles. It has been demonstrated that both miRNA-150 and miRNA-194 inhibit HSC activation and ECM production in rats with liver fibrosis by decreasing the expression of c-myb (target for miRNA-150) and rac 1 (target for miRNA-194) [140]. Interestingly, miRNAs such as miRNA-19b, miRNA-29, miRNA-133a, and miRNA-146a are significantly down-regulated in HSCs isolated from experimental animals with liver fibrosis, and restoration of these miRNAs alleviates fibrogenesis [47, 141, 142]. Moreover, miRNA-133a overexpression inhibits both human and murine primary HSCs proliferation and prevents the progression of liver fibrosis [142].

Multiple studies have proposed that miRNAs may serve as biomarkers for HSC activation and liver fibrosis progression, and can be possible candidates for future therapies targeting liver fibrosis/cirrhosis.

6. Pathogenesis of liver fibrosis/cirrhosis

Liver fibrosis and its end-stage consequence, cirrhosis, represent the final common pathway of almost all chronic liver diseases. Fibrosis and cirrhosis of the liver remain major medical problems with significant morbidity and mortality worldwide. Liver fibrosis is in fact a wound-healing response to liver injury and is characterized by accumulation of fibrotic scar tissue. Although the scar tissue formation is beneficial at first because it encapsulates the injury, the chronic activation of this healing process eventually progresses to advanced fibrosis/cirrhosis. This leads to altered vascular architecture and microcirculation, ischemia, and widespread hepatocyte cell death [143]. Also, in cirrhosis, collagen strands become so prevalent and divide the liver parenchyma into distinct structurally abnormal regenerative nodules, resulting in organ dysfunction [143].

In fact, liver damage leading to cirrhosis is the result of a complex mechanism involving, from direct toxic effects to a sustained inflammatory process, driving to the death of hepatocytes via apoptosis and liver fibrosis, mediated by secretion of several cytokines [144]. The inflammatory reaction is the coordinated process by which the liver responds to local insults, trying to restore the hepatic architecture and function after acute liver injury [128]. However, if the liver is faced to a sustained local damage, the chronic inflammatory response gives rise to a progressive replacement of healthy liver tissue by non-functional fibrotic scar tissue. The imbalance between tissue regeneration and fibrosis determines the outcome toward health recovery or liver cirrhosis [144].

6.1. Imbalance between extracellular matrix synthesis and degradation

Liver fibrosis can be defined as a dynamic and highly integrated molecular, tissue and cellular process regarded as the result of an imbalance between ECM synthesis and degradation. In the healthy liver, ECM is composed of several components such as collagens (mainly the interstitial types I, III, V, VI, and the basement membrane types IV, XV, XVIII, and XIX), glycoproteins (such as laminin isoforms and fibronectin), proteoglycans and elastin [145–147]. Normally, ECM components comprise less than 3% of the relative area of a liver tissue section and approximately 0.5% of the wet weight. During the development of liver fibrosis, there is a 5- to 10-fold increase in the content of collagenous and non-collagenous components, particularly of fibrillar collagen type I and III [146], and an increase of elastin, laminins, and proteoglycans [148]. The total amount of ECM is not only dependent on the rate of synthesis but also largely on the balance between the matrix MMPs, and the TIMPs, especially TIMP-1 [15].

The MMPs are a family of zinc-dependent endopeptidases that can degrade both collagenous and non-collagenous components of ECM in the extracellular space [149]. MMP activity is regulated by TIMPs, which bind to MMPs, blocking their proteolytic activity. The MMPs and TIMPs play a crucial role in the fine regulation of the ECM turnover and the resulting increase in the TIMPs/MMPs ratio in liver promotes fibrosis by protecting accumulated matrix from degradation by MMPs (**Figure 1**) [8].

6.2. Mechanisms and mediators of liver fibrogenesis

Liver fibrosis, which is characterized by the excessive deposition of ECM (non-functional connective tissue) components [150], involves both parenchymal and non-parenchymal cells, as well as infiltrating immune cells [151, 152]. Furthermore, several critical signaling pathways have important roles in liver fibrosis. The complex interactions between these signaling pathways and different cells contribute to the progression of liver fibrosis [153].

HSCs are central effectors of fibrogenesis although other cells and processes can make significant contributions. In the healthy liver, HSCs are in a quiescent state with low proliferation rates, store dietary vitamin A, control the ECM synthesis, regulate the local vascular contractility, and serve as the pericytes for the sinusoidal endothelial cells. Damage to hepatocytes activates HSCs transformation into myofibroblast-like cells that play a fundamental role in the development of fibrotic liver response [14]. Myofibroblast-like cells with high proliferative capacity, without vitamin A, exhibit increased expression of α-SMA fibers [3]. These cells contribute to fibrosis by producing large amounts of ECM components and collagens (specifically type I) to encapsulate

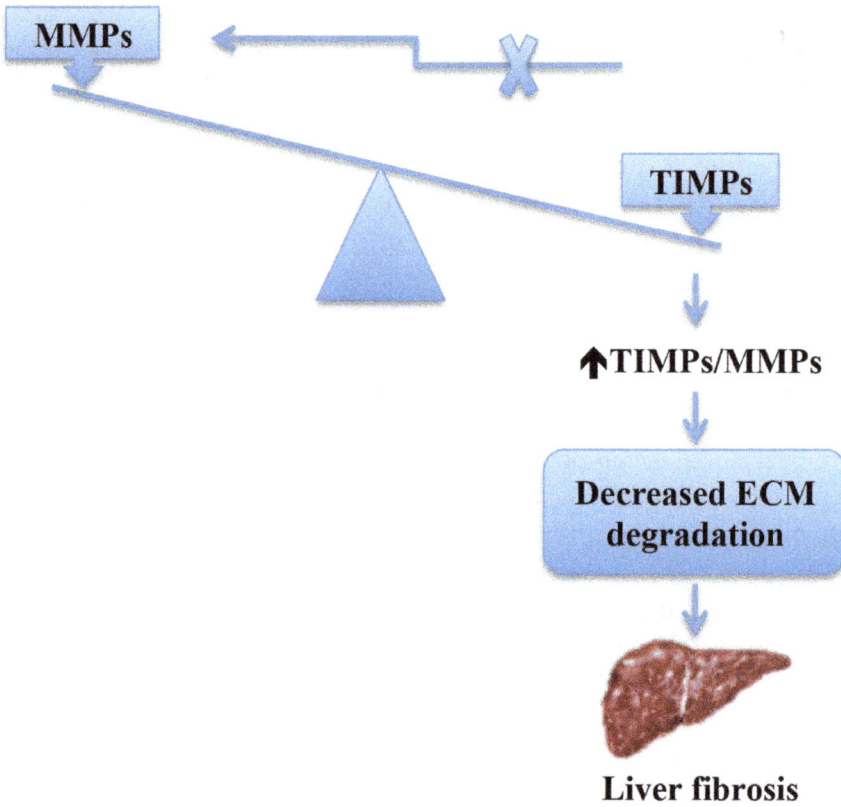

Figure 1. Imbalances in ECM synthesis and degradation result in liver fibrosis. Regulation of degradation is determined by the balance between the activity of MMPs and TIMPs. The MMPs degrade both collagenous and non-collagenous components of ECM in the extracellular space. MMP activity is regulated by TIMPs, which bind to MMPs, blocking their proteolytic activity. Increase in the TIMPs/MMPs ratio in liver promotes fibrosis by protecting accumulated matrix from degradation by MMPs. ECM, extracellular matrix; MMPs, matrix metalloproteinases; TIMPs, tissue inhibitor of metalloproteinases.

the injury [152]. Although HSCs are classically considered to be a major source of myofibroblasts [154, 155], other cell types like portal myofibroblasts and cells recruited from the bone marrow also contribute to the expansion of the myofibroblast population observed during the liver injury [154]. Activated HSCs also secrete an increased amount of MMPs and their inhibitors, TIMPs, which are necessary for the ECM remodeling [154, 156]. HSC activation leads to the up-regulation of TIMPs and TGF-β1 with the inhibition of MMP activity. The TIMP activation thus stimulates collagen type I synthesis and ECM deposition in the extracellular space [157]. Besides injured hepatocytes, hepatic macrophages (KCs), endothelial cells, and lymphocytes also drive HSC activation [158].

HSC activation is still the primary pathway leading to the liver fibrosis and it consists of two main stages: initiation and perpetuation (**Figure 2**) [126]. The initiation stage is related with the early changes in gene expression and phenotype that render the cells responsive to several cytokines and stimuli. Initiation of HSC activation is stimulated by several soluble factors such as oxidant stress signals (ROS), apoptotic bodies, and paracrine stimuli from neighboring cell types including hepatocytes, KCs, sinusoidal endothelium, and platelets [8, 72]. Hepatocytes

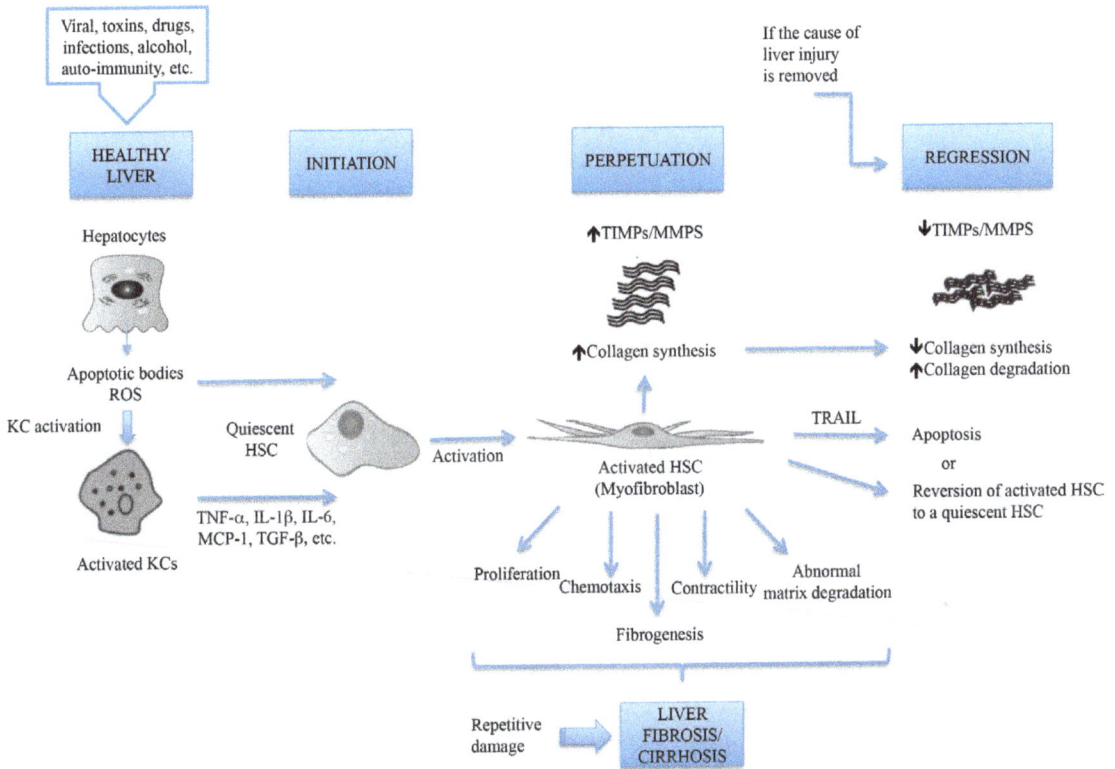

Figure 2. Initiation, perpetuation, and regression of liver fibrogenesis involving HSCs. The pathways of HSC activation consist of initiation and perpetuation. Initiation is stimulated by soluble factors such as apoptotic bodies, oxidant stress signals (ROS), and paracrine stimuli from neighboring cell types. Perpetuation includes HSC activation (phenotypic switch from a quiescent type into an activated type) and related cellular changes such as proliferation, chemotaxis, fibrogenesis, contractility, and abnormal matrix degradation. Repetitive damage to liver causes perpetuation of activated HSCs in the liver. Activated HSCs produce excessive collagen, down-regulate release of MMPs and enhance expression of the physiological inhibitors of the MMPs (TIMPs). Imbalances in collagen synthesis and degradation result in liver fibrosis/cirrhosis. During regression, activated HSCs undergo apoptosis or inactivation if the cause of liver injury is removed. ROS, reactive oxygen species; KC, Kupffer cell; HSC, hepatic stellate cell; TNF-α, tumor necrosis factor-α; IL, interleukin; MCP-1, monocyte chemoattractant protein-1; TGF-β, transforming growth factor-β; TIMPs, tissue inhibitor of metalloproteinases; MMPs, matrix metalloproteinases; TRAIL, TNF-related apoptosis-inducing ligand.

are believed to represent a major source of ROS as well as of other oxidative stress-related reactive mediators or intermediates [1]. Hepatocyte apoptosis leads to the release of cellular contents such as DNA and ROS that activate KCs to release pro-inflammatory (such as TNF-α, IL-1β, IL-6, MCP-1) and pro-fibrogenic (especially TGF-β) factors [158]. Hepatocyte apoptosis following injury also promotes initiation of HSC activation through a process mediated by Fas, and this process may involve the TRAIL [159]. After stimulation by cytokines or engulfment of apoptotic bodies, KCs stimulate matrix synthesis and cell proliferation through the actions of cytokines including TGF-β1 and ROS/lipid peroxides [64]. Endothelial cells are also likely to participate by conversion of TGF-β from the latent to the active, pro-fibrogenic form [126]. Platelets are another important source of paracrine stimuli, including PDGF, TGF-β1, and EGF [126]. On the other hand, perpetuation stage results from the effects of these stimuli on maintaining the activated phenotype and generating liver fibrosis. This stage involves autocrine as well as paracrine cycles. It includes HSC activation and related cellular changes such as proliferation, chemotaxis, fibrogenesis, contractility, and matrix degradation [126]. Activated HSCs proliferate in response to various kinds of cytokines, chemokines, and growth factors such as TGF-β, EGF, and PDGF [2, 8]. TGF-β, which has been identified as the most pro-fibrotic cytokine, promotes expression of collagen type I by activated HSCs and inhibits ECM degradation through the expression of TIMPs [160]. In parallel, PDGF has emerged as the most potent proliferative cytokine for HSCs [8]. Also, activated HSCs show chemotactic response, migrate toward damaged area and start to accumulate [3]. They express the cytoskeleton protein (α-SMA), equipping the cells with a contractile apparatus and collagens (especially type I) [12, 161, 162]. Thus, HSCs are able to constrict individual sinusoids as well as the entire fibrotic liver [3]. The net effect of these changes is to increase ECM deposition. In addition, cytokine release by HSCs can expand the inflammatory and fibrogenic tissue responses, and matrix proteases may hasten the replacement of normal matrix with fibrotic scar [126]. Briefly, activated HSCs are major effectors of liver fibrogenesis by integrating all incoming paracrine or autocrine signals released from both parenchymal and non-parenchymal cells (pro-inflammatory cytokines, growth factors, chemokines, ROS, and others).

Chronic inflammation and fibrosis are inseparably linked and the interactions between immune cells, local fibroblasts and especially subsets of macrophages determine the outcome of liver injury [8]. Macrophage phenotype and function are critical determinants of fibrotic scarring or resolution of injury. Macrophages, which are typically categorized into classically activated (M1) or alternatively activated (M2) phenotypes, play dual roles in the progression and resolution of liver fibrosis [163]. Typically, M1 macrophages play a pro-inflammatory role in liver injury and produce inflammatory cytokines, while M2 macrophages exert an anti-inflammatory role during tissue repair and fibrosis. The imbalance of M1 and M2 macrophages mediates the progression and resolution of liver fibrosis [164]. During the early stages of liver injury, bone marrow-derived monocytes are extensively recruited to the liver and then differentiate into inflammatory macrophages (mostly M1 macrophages) to produce pro-inflammatory and pro-fibrotic cytokines, thereby promoting inflammatory responses and HSC activation. Afterwards, recruited macrophages switch their phenotypes (mostly M2 macrophages) to secrete MMPs for the successful resolution in hepatic scar [153, 165, 166]. Therefore, a complicated interplay between M1 and M2 types of macrophages plays a critical role in fibrogenesis [128].

6.3. Liver fibrosis is potentially reversible

Liver fibrosis is thought to be a potentially reversible condition if the cause of liver injury is removed (such as virus suppression or alcohol absence) (**Figure 2**). Regression of liver fibrosis is associated either with elimination of activated HSCs via apoptosis or senescence or with reversion of activated HSCs to a more quiescent phenotype. It has been shown that HSCs are sensitive to Fas and TRAIL-mediated apoptosis, and natural killer cells can induce apoptosis of HSCs by a TRAIL-mediated mechanism [167]. Similarly, TRAIL expressed by KCs is also thought to mediate HSC apoptosis [168]. In addition, apoptosis of activated HSCs is for sure followed by a decrease in collagen production as well as a reduction in TIMP synthesis with an increase in the hepatic MMP expression [1]. Therefore, activated HSCs, the primary source of ECM, are the most attractable target for reversing liver fibrosis [169].

7. Halofuginone

Halofuginone, a non-toxic and low molecular weight plant alkaloid [7-bromo-6-chloro-3-(3-hydroxy-2-piperidine)-2-oxopropyl-4(3H)-quinazoline] (**Figure 3**) isolated from the roots of *Dichroa febrifuga* (Chinese medicinal plant), is used worldwide as an anti-parasitic drug in commercial poultry production [16]. At first, halofuginone was identified as a potent inhibitor of collagen type α1 gene expression and ECM deposition. At present, it is being evaluated in clinical trial for Duchenne muscular dystrophy, in which fibrosis is the main complication.

7.1. Halofuginone and its effect on collagen synthesis

Halofuginone was found to be a potent inhibitor of collagen type α1 gene expression [17], which was demonstrated in a broad range of cell types including rat, mouse, chicken, and human, both *in vitro* and *in vivo* [16–20]. The discovery of the inhibitory effect of halofuginone on collagen synthesis and ECM deposition has led to intensive studies that were aimed to control many diseases associated with excessive collagen accumulation, such as pulmonary, pancreatic and renal fibrosis [21–23], scleroderma and chronic graft-versus-host disease [24], post-operative peritendinous and abdominal adhesions [25, 26], urethral and esophageal strictures [27, 28], wound repair [29], burn injury [30], renal injury [31, 32], injury-induced arterial intimal hyperplasia [33], colitis [34], and liver fibrosis and cirrhosis [35–39]. Inhibition is independent of the route of administration (intraperitoneally, administered locally, or given orally).

Halofuginone was found to inhibit collagen type I synthesis but not that of type II [17] or III [170] *in vitro*. The inhibitor effect of halofuginone on collagen α1 synthesis appears not to be a direct effect but rather dependent on new protein synthesis, because concurrent treatment of fibroblasts with protein synthesis inhibitors blocks the suppressive effect of halofuginone on collagen α1 mRNA gene expression [18].

Because of the significant impact of fibrosis on human health, there is an unmet need for safe and effective therapies that directly target fibrosis. In animal models of fibrosis, regardless of the tissue, halofuginone had a minimal effect on collagen levels in the control (non-fibrotic) animals; however, it displayed a strong inhibitory effect in the fibrotic organs. This suggests that the regulation of the low-level expression of collagen type I genes differs from that of the

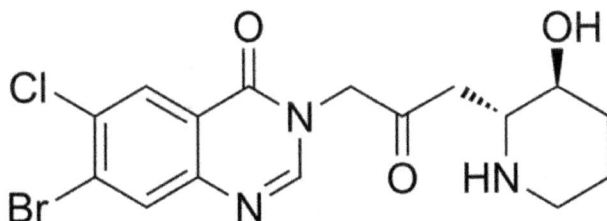

Figure 3. Chemical structure of halofuginone.

overexpression induced by the fibrogenic stimulus, which is usually an aggressive and rapid process [171]. Halofuginone mainly affects the stimulated collagen synthesis, therefore, when it is administered systemically, it is actually targeted to the desired fibrotic location without affecting collagen synthesis in other regions.

7.2. Halofuginone and TGF-β pathway

TGF-β is a "master switch" in chronic liver disease, being involved in all stages of the disease progression, from initial liver injury, inflammation, fibrosis, to cirrhosis and hepatocellular carcinoma at the end [172]. TGF-β signals through transmembrane receptor serine/threonine kinases to activate novel signaling intermediates called Smad proteins, which then modulate transcription of target genes [173]. TGF-β, signaling via Smad3, is the most pro-fibrogenic cytokine present in the liver and the major promoter of ECM synthesis [173, 174]. It induces pro-fibrotic cellular and transcriptional responses such as induction of the synthesis of ECM components, especially collagen, as well as fibronectin and laminin, and it inhibits the matrix degradation enzymes [175]. In various experimental fibrotic models, no effect of halofuginone was observed on the expression of the TGF-β receptors gene or on TGF-β levels [176–178]. This finding supports the hypothesis that the halofuginone target is down-stream in the TGF-β pathway. Halofuginone is an inhibitor of Smad3 phosphorylation down-stream of the TGF-β signaling pathway [177, 179, 180]. In chemically induced liver fibrosis, halofuginone affects TGF-β regulated genes through inhibition of Smad3 phosphorylation of activated HSCs [181]. It inhibits TGF-β-induced phosphorylation of Smad3 and also increases the expression of the inhibitory Smad7 in several cell types (such as fibroblasts, hepatic and pancreatic stellate cells, tumor cells and myoblasts) [178, 181–183]. The inhibition of Smad3 phosphorylation is associated with the halofuginone-dependent activation of Akt MAPK/ERK and p38 MAPK phosphorylation [182]. Thus, drugs that selectively target individual signaling pathways down-stream of the TGF-β receptor are likely to be more successful.

7.3. Halofuginone affects pre-existing fibrosis

Halofuginone affects fibrosis as a preventive agent when it was administered before or together with the fibrotic stimulus [21, 26, 27, 35, 184]. It can elicit resolution of established fibrosis, a capability that sets it apart from all other preventive anti-fibrotic agents. For example, in rats with established thioacetamide-induced liver fibrosis, addition of halofuginone to the diet results in almost complete resolution of the fibrotic condition as measured by hydroxyproline levels in the liver [36]. This is probably due to up-regulation of the collagen degradation pathway by inhibition of the TIMP-1, and activation of MMPs [43]. In addition, halofuginone given orally before fibrosis induction prevents the activation of most of the stellate cells and the remaining cells expressed low levels of collagen α1 gene, resulting in low levels of collagen [36]. Furthermore, halofuginone administration in low concentrations prior to and following partial hepatectomy in cirrhotic rats does not inhibit normal liver regeneration, despite the reduced levels of collagen type I mRNA [37]. When given to rats with established fibrosis, halofuginone causes significant reductions in α-SMA, TIMP-2, collagen type I gene expression, and collagen accumulation [37]. These animals demonstrate improved capacity for regeneration, suggesting the possible beneficial use of halofuginone before and during fibrotic/cirrhotic liver regeneration.

7.4. Halofuginone as an anti-fibrotic agent

In recent years, much attention was focused on halofuginone against liver fibrosis (**Table 3**). Although the exact anti-fibrotic mechanism of halofuginone is not well understood, it is found to be associated with inhibition of TGF-β signaling [179], which is known to inhibit mesengial

Models	Effects	Mechanisms	References
DMN-induced liver fibrosis/cirrhosis in rats	Prevents liver cirrhosis	Prevents increase in collagen type I gene expression	[35]
TAA-induced liver fibrosis in rats	Causes almost complete resolution of fibrosis	Reduces collagen levels, collagen α1(I) gene expression, TIMP-2 content, and SMA-positive cells	[36]
TAA-induced liver cirrhosis in rats	Improves liver regeneration	Reduces α-SMA, TIMP-2, collagen type I gene expression, and collagen accumulation	[37]
ConA-induced liver fibrosis in rats	Prevents liver fibrosis	Decreases Th17 cell differentiation and its related cytokines production	[38]
ConA-induced liver fibrosis in rats	Attenuates liver fibrosis	Suppresses synthesis of collagen 1, α-SMA and TIMP-2; down-regulates TGF-β1/Smad3 signaling pathway; decreases pro-inflammatory cytokines	[39]
TAA-induced liver fibrosis in rats	Up-regulates MMP-3 and -13 and down-regulates TIMP-1 (*in vivo*); inhibits HSC proliferation and migration (*in vitro*)	Activates p38 MAPK and NF-κB	[43]
TAA-induced liver fibrosis in rats	Inhibits HSC activation and collagen synthesis; prevents activation of TGF-β-dependent genes	Inhibits Smad3 phosphorylation	[181]
TAA-induced liver fibrosis in rats	Affects cross-talk between hepatocytes and HSCs	Up-regulates synthesis and secretion of IGFBP-1	[192]
TAA-induced liver fibrosis in rats	Prevents liver fibrosis and improves cirrhotic liver regeneration	Increases expression of early genes of regeneration (PRL-1 and IGFBP-1)	[193]
Human hepatoma cell injected mice	Suppresses tumor growth	Increases IFN-γ and IL-2	[196]
Diethylnitrosamine and N-nitrosomorpholine-induced HCC in rats	Suppresses lung metastasis	Inhibits MMP	[197]

Abbreviations: DMN, dimethylnitrosamine; TAA, thioacetamide; TIMP, tissue inhibitor of metalloproteinase; SMA, smooth muscle actin; ConA, Concanavalin A; Th17, T helper 17; TGF-β, transforming growth factor-β; MMP, matrix metalloproteinase; HSC, hepatic stellate cell; p38 MAPK, p38 mitogen-activated protein kinase; NF-κB, nuclear factor-κB; IGFBP-1, insulin-like growth factor binding protein-1; PRL-1, tyrosine phosphatase; IFN-γ, interferon-γ; IL-2, interleukin-2; HCC, hepatocellular carcinoma.

Table 3. Effects of halofuginone in various experimental liver diseases.

cell proliferation and ECM deposition [185]. In several animal models of fibrosis, in which excess collagen is the characteristic of the disease, halofuginone prevents transition of the fibroblasts to myofibroblasts by inhibition of Smad3 phosphorylation down-stream of the TGF-β signaling pathway [186, 187], thereby inhibits collagen synthesis [186]. Halofuginone also regulates cell growth and differentiation, apoptosis, cell migration, and immune cell function [41]. It prevents concanavalin A-induced liver fibrosis by affecting Th17 cell differentiation, which suggests a direct link between the myofibroblasts/fibrosis pathway and the Th17 pro-inflammatory pathway [38]. Th17 cells, a distinct subset of CD4+ T cells with IL-17 as their major cytokine, orchestrate the pathogenesis of inflammation [171]. It has been suggested that halofuginone-dependent inhibition of fibrosis includes selective inhibition of the Th17 cell development by activating the amino acid starvation response [188, 189]. Halofuginone activates the amino acid starvation response by directly inhibiting the prolyl-tRNA synthetase activity of glutamyl-prolyl-tRNA synthetase [190]. Furthermore, addition of exogenous proline reverses a broad range of halofuginone-induced cellular effects, indicating that glutamyl-prolyl-tRNA synthetase-inhibition underlies the therapeutic activities of halofuginone [190]. TGF-β is required for facilitation of differentiation of the inflammatory Th17 cell subset [191], which suggests the presence of a connection between the TGF-β signaling inhibition and the amino acid starvation response [187]. Treatment with halofuginone also effectively inhibits the delayed-type hypersensitivity response, indicating suppression of T cell–mediated inflammation *in vivo* [42]. Moreover, it was shown that halofuginone is a potent inhibitor of NF-κB, pro-inflammatory cytokines, and p38 MAPK phosphorylation in activated T cells *in vitro* [42]. Also, submicromolar concentrations of halofuginone inhibit HSC proliferation and migration and up-regulate their expression of fibrolytic MMP-3 and -13 via activation of p38 MAPK and NF-κB. The remarkable induction of MMP-3 and -13 makes halofuginone a promising agent for anti-fibrotic combination therapies [43]. Halofuginone also affects the cross-talk between the hepatocytes and the HSCs by up-regulating the synthesis and secretion of insulin-like growth factor binding protein-1 (IGFBP-1), which inhibits HSC migration [192]. It also affects the expression of early genes of liver regeneration, IGFBP-1 whose synthesis and secretion is regulated in part by TGF-β [192] and tyrosine phosphatase (PRL-1) whose synthesis is regulated by transcription factor early growth response-1 (Egr-1) probably via TGF-β [193].

7.5. Anti-tumoral role of halofuginone

In many types of tumor, there is a strong relationship between tissue fibrosis and increased risk of tumor development. For example, the leading risk factor for hepatocellular carcinoma is liver cirrhosis, and its associated inflammation, regeneration, and fibrosis [194, 195]. Tumor cells develop and metastasize more effectively in fibrotic tissues; therefore, any reduction in tissue fibrosis reduces the risk of cancer [171]. Halofuginone reduces tumor growth and mortality in xenograph mice implanted with human hepatoma cells [196]. In diethylnitrosamine and N-nitrosomorpholine-induced, spontaneously metastasizing hepatocellular carcinoma, halofuginone suppresses lung metastasis in rats through MMP inhibition [197]. Moreover, halofuginone treatment results in effective inhibitory effects on the cascade of events leading to angiogenesis (formation of new blood vessels), such as abrogation of endothelial cell MMP-2 expression, basement membrane invasion, capillary tube formation, vascular sprouting, and deposition of sub-endothelial ECM *in vitro* [171]. Inhibition of angiogenesis is mostly accompanied by inhibition of the fibroblasts to myofibroblasts transition, reduction in tumor stroma ECM, and inhibition of tumor growth [171]. The high effectiveness of halofuginone in reducing fibrosis, which affects tumor growth and tissue regeneration in the liver, arises from its dual role in inhibiting the TGF-β signaling and Th17 cell development [187].

8. Conclusion

Fibrosis is a pathological process associated with excessive ECM deposition that leads to destruction of organ architecture and function. Fibrosis contributes enormously to deaths worldwide; thus, effective therapies are of a great need. Halofuginone has great potential as an anti-fibrotic therapeutic. Systemic administration of halofuginone in animal models and humans is well tolerated [24]. Additionally, in most animal models of fibrosis, halofuginone has a minimal effect on collagen levels in non-fibrotic animals, while exerting strong inhibitory effects in fibrotic organs. It mainly affects stimulated collagen synthesis without altering the usual low physiological level of collagen expression. Because halofuginone inhibits collagen type I synthesis on the transcriptional level and reduces ECM deposition, it is a promising candidate for treatment of diseases associated with excessive ECM, such as liver fibrosis/cirrhosis. Thus, halofuginone meets the criteria as a promising anti-fibrotic drug for further evaluation in the treatment of liver fibrosis/cirrhosis.

Conflicts of Interest

The author reports no conflicts of interest.

Author details

Berna Karakoyun

Address all correspondence to: bernakarakoyun@gmail.com; berna.lacin@marmara.edu.tr

Department of Basic Health Sciences, Faculty of Health Sciences, Marmara University, Istanbul, Turkey

References

[1] Novo E, Cannito S, Paternostro C, Bocca C, Miglietta A, Parola M. Cellular and molecular mechanisms in liver fibrogenesis. Archives of Biochemistry and Biophysics. 2014;**548**:20-37. DOI: 10.1016/j.abb.2014.02.015

[2] Zhou WC, Zhang QB, Qiao L. Pathogenesis of liver cirrhosis. World Journal of Gastroenterology. 2014;**20**(23):7312-7324. DOI: 10.3748/wjg.v20.i23.7312

[3]   Ahmad A, Ahmad R. Understanding the mechanism of hepatic fibrosis and potential therapeutic approaches. Saudi Journal of Gastroenterology. 2012;**18**(3):155-167. DOI: 10.4103/1319-3767.96445

[4]   Anthony PP, Ishak KG, Nayak NC, Poulsen HE, Scheuer PJ, Sobin LH. The morphology of cirrhosis. Recommendations on definition, nomenclature, and classification by a working group sponsored by the World Health Organization. Journal of Clinical Pathology. 1978;**31**(5):395-414. DOI: 10.1136/jcp.31.5.395

[5]   Wanless IR, Nakashima E, Sherman M. Regression of human cirrhosis. Morphologic features and the genesis of incomplete septal cirrhosis. Archives of Pathology & Laboratory Medicine. 2000;**124**(11):1599-1607. DOI: 10.1043/0003-9985(2000)124<1599:ROHC>2.0.CO;2

[6]   Ferrell L. Liver pathology: Cirrhosis, hepatitis, and primary liver tumors. Update and diagnostic problems. Modern Pathology. 2000;**13**(6):679-704. DOI: 10.1038/modpathol. 3880119

[7]   Elsharkawy AM, Oakley F, Mann DA. The role and regulation of hepatic stellate cell apoptosis in reversal of liver fibrosis. Apoptosis. 2005;**10**(5):927-939. DOI: 10.1007/s10495-005-1055-4

[8]   Xu R, Zhang Z, Wang F. Liver fibrosis: Mechanisms of immune-mediated liver injury. Cellular and Molecular Immunology. 2012;**9**(4):296-301. DOI: 10.1038/cmi.2011.53

[9]   Zhang D, Zhao Y, Wei D, Li Y, Zhang Y, Wu J, et al. HAb18G/CD147 promotes activation of hepatic stellate cells and is a target for antibody therapy of liver fibrosis. Journal of Hepatology. 2012;**57**(6):1283-1291. DOI: 10.1016/j.jhep.2012.07.042

[10] Kisseleva T, Brenner DA. Role of hepatic stellate cells in fibrogenesis and the reversal of fibrosis. Journal of Gastroenterology and Hepatology. 2007;**22**(s1):S73–S78. DOI: 10.1111/j.1440-1746.2006.04658.x

[11] Bataller R, Brenner DA. Liver fibrosis. The Journal of Clinical Investigation. 2005;**115**:209-218. DOI: 10.1172/JCI24282

[12] Lotersztajn S, Julien B, Teixeira-Clerc F, Grenard P, Mallat A. Hepatic fibrosis: Molecular mechanisms and drug targets. Annual Review of Pharmacology and Toxicology. 2005;**45**(1):605-628. DOI: 10.1146/annurev.pharmtox.45.120403.095906

[13] Iredale JP. Hepatic stellate cell behavior during resolution of liver injury. Seminars in Liver Disease. 2001;**21**(03):427-436. DOI: 10.1055/s-2001-17557

[14] Kmiec Z. Cooperation of liver cells in health and disease. Advances in Anatomy, Embryology and Cell Biology. 2001;**161**:III–XIII. PMID: 11729749

[15] Mehal WZ, Schuppan D. Antifibrotic therapies in the liver. Seminars in Liver Disease. 2015;**35**(02):184-198. DOI: 10.1055/s-0035-1550055

[16] Granot I, Bartov I, Plavnik I, Wax E, Hurwitz S, Pines M. Increased skin tearing in broilers and reduced collagen synthesis in skin in vivo and in vitro in response to the coccidiostat halofuginone. Poultry Science. 1991;**70**(7):1559-1563. DOI: 10.3382/ps.0701559

[17] Granot I, Halevy O, Hurwitz S, Pines M. Halofuginone: An inhibitor of collagen type I synthesis. Biochimica et Biophysica Acta (BBA)—General Subjects. 1993;**1156**(2):107-112. DOI: 10.1016/0304-4165(93)90123-p

[18] Halevy O, Nagler A, Levi-Schaffer F, Genina O, Pines M. Inhibition of collagen type I synthesis by skin fibroblasts of graft versus host disease and scleroderma patients: Effect of halofuginone. Biochemical Pharmacology. 1996;**52**(7):1057-1063. DOI: 10.1016/0006-2952(96)00427-3

[19] Nagler A, Miao HQ, Aingorn H, Pines M, Genina O, Vlodavsky I. Inhibition of collagen synthesis, smooth muscle cell proliferation, and injury-induced intimal hyperplasia by halofuginone. Arteriosclerosis, Thrombosis, and Vascular Biology. 1997;**17**(1):194-202. DOI: 10.1161/01.atv.17.1.194

[20] Pines M, Nagler A: Halofuginone: A novel antifibrotic therapy. General Pharmacology. 1998;**30**(4):445-450. DOI: 10.1016/s0306-3623(97)00307-8

[21] Nagler A, Firman N, Feferman R, Cotev S, Pines M, Shoshan S. Reduction in pulmonary fibrosis in vivo by halofuginone. American Journal of Respiratory and Critical Care Medicine. 1996;**154**(4):1082-1086. DOI: 10.1164/ajrccm.154.4.8887611

[22] Benchetrit S, Yarkoni S, Rathaus M, Pines M, Rashid G, Bernheim J, Bernheim J. Halofuginone reduces the occurrence of renal fibrosis in 5/6 nephrectomized rats. Israel Medical Association Journal. 2007;**9**(1):30-34. PMID: 17274353

[23] Karatas A, Paksoy M, Erzin Y, Carkman S, Gonenc M, Ayan F, et al. The effect of halofuginone, a specific inhibitor of collagen type 1 synthesis, in the prevention of pancreatic fibrosis in an experimental model of severe hyperstimulation and obstruction pancreatitis. Journal of Surgical Research. 2008;**148**(1):7-12. DOI: 10.1016/j.jss.2008.03.015

[24] Pines M, Snyder D, Yarkoni S, Nagler A. Halofuginone to treat fibrosis in chronic graft-versus-host disease and scleroderma. Biology of Blood and Marrow Transplantation. 2003;**9**(7):417-425. DOI: 10.1016/s1083-8791(03)00151-4

[25] Nyska M, Nyska A, Rivlin E, Porat S, Pines M, Shoshan S, et al. Topically applied halofuginone, an inhibitor of collagen type I transcription, reduces peritendinous fibrous adhesions following surgery. Connective Tissue Research. 1996;**34**(2):97-103. DOI: 10.3109/03008209609021495

[26] Nagler A, Rivkind AI, Raphael J, Levi-Schaffer F, Genina O, Lavelin I, et al. Halofuginone—an inhibitor of collagen type I synthesis—prevents postoperative formation of abdominal adhesions. Annals of Surgery. 1998;**227**(4):575-582. DOI: 10.1097/00000658-199804000-00021

[27] Nagler A, Gofrit O, Ohana M, Pode D, Genina O, Pines M. The effect of halofuginone, an inhibitor of collagen type 1 synthesis, on urethral stricture formation: In vivo and in vitro study in a rat model. The Journal of Urology. 2000;**164**(5):1776-1780. DOI: 10.1016/s0022-5347(05)67105-4

[28] Özçelik M, Pekmezci S, Sarıbeyoğlu K, Ünal E, Gümüştaş K, Doğusoy G. The effect of halofuginone, a specific inhibitor of collagen type 1 synthesis, in the prevention

of esophageal strictures related to caustic injury. The American Journal of Surgery. 2004;**187**(2):257-260. DOI: 10.1016/j.amjsurg.2003.11.008

[29] Abramovitch R, Dafni H, Neeman M, Nagler A, Pines M. Inhibition of neovascularization and tumor growth, and facilitation of wound repair, by halofuginone, an inhibitor of collagen type I synthesis. Neoplasia. 1999;**1**(4):321-329. DOI: 10.1038/sj.neo.7900043

[30] Cerit KK, Karakoyun B, Yüksel M, Ercan F, Tuğtepe H, Dagli TE, et al. Halofuginone alleviates burn-induced hepatic and renal damage in rats. Journal of Burn Care & Research. 2017;**38**(1):e384-e394. DOI: 10.1097/bcr.0000000000000400

[31] Karakoyun B, Yuksel M, Turan P, Arbak S, Alican I. Halofuginone has a beneficial effect on gentamicin-induced acute nephrotoxicity in rats. Drug and Chemical Toxicology. 2009;**32**(4):312-318. DOI: 10.1080/01480540902976911

[32] Karadeniz Cerit K, Karakoyun B, Yüksel M, Özkan N, Çetinel Ş, Tolga Dağli E, et al. The antifibrotic drug halofuginone reduces ischemia/reperfusion-induced oxidative renal damage in rats. Journal of Pediatric Urology. 2013;**9**(2):174-183. DOI: 10.1016/j. jpurol.2012.01.015

[33] Liu K, Sekine S, Goto Y, Iijima K, Yamagishi I, Kondon K, et al. Halofuginone inhibits neointimal formation of cultured rat aorta in a concentration-dependent fashion in vitro. Heart and Vessels. 1998;**13**(1):18-23. DOI: 10.1007/bf02750639

[34] Karakoyun B, Yüksel M, Ercan F, Salva E, Işık I, Yeğen BC. Halofuginone, a specific inhibitor of collagen type 1 synthesis, ameliorates oxidant colonic damage in rats with experimental colitis. Digestive Diseases and Sciences. 2010;**55**(3):607-616. DOI: 10.1007/ s10620-009-0798-0

[35] Pines M, Knopov V, Genina O, Lavelin I, Nagler A. Halofuginone, a specific inhibitor of collagen type I synthesis, prevents dimethylnitrosamine-induced liver cirrhosis. Journal of Hepatology. 1997;**27**(2):391-398. DOI: 10.1016/s0168-8278(97)80186-9

[36] Bruck R, Genina O, Aeed H, Alexiev R, Nagler A, Avni Y, et al. Halofuginone to prevent and treat thioacetamide-induced liver fibrosis in rats. Hepatology. 2001;**33**(2):379-386. DOI: 10.1053/jhep.2001.21408

[37] Spira G, Mawasi N, Paizi M, Anbinder N, Genina O, Alexiev R, et al. Halofuginone, a collagen type I inhibitor improves liver regeneration in cirrhotic rats. Journal of Hepatology. 2002;**37**(3):331-339. DOI: 10.1016/s0168-8278(02)00164-2

[38] Liang J, Zhang B, Shen RW, Liu JB, Gao MH, Geng X, et al. The effect of antifibrotic drug halofugine on Th17 cells in concanavalin A-induced liver fibrosis. Scandinavian Journal of Immunology. 2014;**79**(3):163-172. DOI: 10.1111/sji.12144

[39] Liang J, Zhang B, Shen RW, Liu JB, Gao MH, Li Y, et al. Preventive effect of halofuginone on concanavalin A-induced liver fibrosis. PLoS ONE. 2013;**8**(12):e82232. DOI: 10.1371/ journal.pone.0082232

[40] Nelson EF, Huang CW, Ewel JM, Chang AA, Yuan C. Halofuginone down-regulates Smad3 expression and inhibits the TGF beta-induced expression of fibrotic markers in human corneal fibroblasts. Molecular Vision. 2012;**18**:479-487. PMID: 22393274

[41] Flanders KC. Smad3 as a mediator of the fibrotic response. International Journal of Experimental Pathology. 2004;**85**(2):47-64. DOI: 10.1111/j.0959-9673.2004.00377.x

[42] Leiba M, Cahalon L, Shimoni A, Lider O, Zanin-Zhorov A, Hecht I, et al. Halofuginone inhibits NF-kappaB and p38 MAPK in activated T cells. Journal of Leukocyte Biology. 2006;**80**(2):399-406. DOI: 10.1189/jlb.0705409

[43] Popov Y, Patsenker E, Bauer M, Niedobitek E, Schulze-Krebs A, Schuppan D. Halofuginone induces matrix metalloproteinases in rat hepatic stellate cells via activation of p38 and NFkappaB. Journal of Biological Chemistry. 2006;**281**(22):15090-15098. DOI: 10.1074/jbc.m600030200

[44] Friedman SL. Seminars in medicine of the Beth Israel Hospital, Boston. The cellular basis of hepatic fibrosis. Mechanisms and treatment strategies. New England Journal of Medicine. 1993;**328**(25):1828-1835. DOI: 10.1056/NEJM199306243282508

[45] Lepreux S, Desmoulière A. Human liver myofibroblasts during development and diseases with a focus on portal (myo)fibroblasts. Frontiers in Physiology. 2015;**6**:173. DOI: 10.3389/fphys.2015.00173

[46] Alison MR, Vig P, Russo F, Bigger BW, Amofah E, ThemisM, et al. Hepatic stem cells: From inside and outside the liver? Cell Proliferation. 2004;**37**(1):1-21. DOI: 10.1111/j.1365-2184.2004.00297.x

[47] Lakner AM, Steuerwald NM, Walling TL, Ghosh S, Li T, McKillop IH, et al. Inhibitory effects of microRNA 19b in hepatic stellate cell-mediated fibrogenesis. Hepatology. 2012;**56**(1):300-310. DOI: 10.1002/hep.25613

[48] Oakley F, Meso M, Iredale JP, Green K, Marek CJ, Zhou X, et al. Inhibition of inhibitor of kappa B kinases stimulates hepatic stellate cell apoptosis and accelerated recovery from rat liver fibrosis. Gastroenterology. 2005;**128**(1):108-120. DOI: 10.1053/j.gastro.2004.10.003

[49] Schattenberg JM, Nagel M, Kim YO, Kohl T, Wörns MA, Zimmermann T, et al. Increased hepatic fibrosis and JNK2-dependent liver injury in mice exhibiting hepatocyte-specific deletion of cFLIP. AJP: Gastrointestinal and Liver Physiology. 2012;**303**(4):G498-G506. DOI: 10.1152/ajpgi.00525.2011

[50] Canbay A, Taimr P, Torok N, Higuchi H, Friedman S, Gores GJ. Apoptotic body engulfment by a human stellate cell line is profibrogenic. Laboratory Investigation. 2003;**83**(5):655-663. DOI: 10.1097/01.lab.0000069036.63405.5c

[51] Zhan SS, Jiang JX, Wu J, Halsted C, Friedman SL, Zern MA, et al. Phagocytosis of apoptotic bodies by hepatic stellate cells induces NADPH oxidase and is associated with liver fibrosis in vivo. Hepatology. 2006;**43**(3):435-443. DOI: 10.1002/hep.21093

[52] Watanabe A, Hashmi A, Gomes DA, Town T, Badou A, Flavell RA, et al. Apoptotic hepatocyte DNA inhibits hepatic stellate cell chemotaxis via toll-like receptor 9. Hepatology. 2007;**46**(5):1509-1518. DOI: 10.1002/hep.21867

[53] Guicciardi ME, Gores GJ. Apoptosis as a mechanism for liver disease progression. Seminars in Liver Disease. 2010;**30**(04):402-410. DOI: 10.1055/s-0030-1267540

[54] Jiang JX, Mikami K, Venugopal S, Li Y, Török NJ. Apoptotic body engulfment by hepatic stellate cells promotes their survival by the JAK/STAT and Akt/NF-kappaB-dependent pathways. Journal of Hepatology. 2009;**51**(1):139-148. DOI: 10.1016/j.jhep. 2009.03.024

[55] Jeong WI, Do SH, Yun HS, Song BJ, Kim SJ, Kwak WJ, et al. Hypoxia potentiates trans-forming growth factor-beta expression of hepatocyte during the cirrhotic condition in rat liver. Liver International. 2004;**24**(6):658-668. DOI: 10.1111/j.1478-3231.2004.0961.x

[56] Braet F, Wisse E. Structural and functional aspects of liver sinusoidal endothelial cell fenestrae: A review. Comparative Hepatology. 2002;**1**(1):1. DOI: 10.1186/1476-5926-1-1

[57] Mori T, Okanoue T, Sawa Y, Hori N, Ohta M, Kagawa K. Defenestration of the sinusoidal endothelial cell in a rat model of cirrhosis. Hepatology. 1993;**17**(5):891-897. DOI: 10.1002/hep.1840170520

[58] Yokomori H, Oda M, Yoshimura K, Hibi T. Recent advances in liver sinusoidal endothe-lial ultrastructure and fine structure immunocytochemistry. Micron. 2012;**43**(2-3):129-134. DOI: 10.1016/j.micron.2011.08.002

[59] Deleve LD, Wang X, Guo Y. Sinusoidal endothelial cells prevent rat stellate cell activa-tion and promote reversion to quiescence. Hepatology. 2008;**48**(3):920-930. DOI: 10.1002/hep.22351

[60] Wisse E. An electron microscopic study of the fenestrated endothelial lining of rat liver sinusoids. Journal of Ultrastructure Research. 1970;**31**(1-2):125-150. DOI: 10.1016/S0022-5320(70)90150-4

[61] DeLeve LD. Liver sinusoidal endothelial cells in hepatic fibrosis. Hepatology. 2015;**61**(5): 1740-1746. DOI: 10.1002/hep.27376

[62] Xie G, Wang X, Wang L, Atkinson RD, Kanel GC, Gaarde WA, et al. Role of differentia-tion of liver sinusoidal endothelial cells in progression and regression of hepatic fibrosis in rats. Gastroenterology. 2012;**142**(4):918-927.e6. DOI: 10.1053/j.gastro.2011.12.017

[63] Marvie P, Lisbonne M, L'helgoualc'h A, Rauch M, Turlin B, Preisser L, et al. Interleukin-33 overexpression is associated with liver fibrosis in mice and humans. Journal of Cellular and Molecular Medicine. 2009;**14**(6b):1726-1739. DOI: 10.1111/j.1582-4934.2009.00801.x

[64] Bilzer M, Roggel F, Gerbes AL. Role of kupffer cells in host defense and liver disease. Liver International. 2006;**26**(10):1175-1186. DOI: 10.1111/j.1478-3231.2006.01342.x

[65] Xidakis C, Ljumovic D, Manousou P, Notas G, Valatas V, Kolios G, et al. Production of pro- and anti-fibrotic agents by rat Kupffer cells; the effect of octreotide. Digestive Diseases and Sciences. 2005;**50**(5):935-941. DOI: 10.1007/s10620-005-2668-8

[66] Matsuoka M, Tsukamoto H. Stimulation of hepatic lipocyte collagen production by kupffer cell-derived transforming growth factor beta: Implication for a pathogenetic role in alcoholic liver fibrogenesis. Hepatology. 1990;**11**(4):599-605. DOI: 10.1002/hep. 1840110412

[67] Luckey SW, Petersen DR. Activation of Kupffer cells during the course of carbon tetrachloride-induced liver injury and fibrosis in rats. Experimental and Molecular Pathology. 2001;**71**(3):226-240. DOI:10.1006/exmp.2001.2399

[68] Kolios G, Valatas V, Kouroumalis E. Role of Kupffer cells in the pathogenesis of liver disease. World Journal of Gastroenterology. 2006;**12**(46):7413-7420. DOI: 10.3748/wjg.v12.i46.7413

[69] Friedman SL, Arthur MJ. Activation of cultured rat hepatic lipocytes by Kupffer cell conditioned medium. Direct enhancement of matrix synthesis and stimulation of cell proliferation via induction of platelet-derived growth factor receptors. Journal of Clinical Investigation. 1989;**84**(6):1780-1785. DOI: 10.1172/JCI114362

[70] Rivera CA, Bradford BU, Hunt KJ, Adachi Y, Schrum LW, Koop DR, et al. Attenuation of CCl4-induced hepatic fibrosis by GdCl3 treatment or dietary glycine. AJP: Gastrointestinal and Liver Physiology. 2001;**281**(1):G200–G207. PMID: 11408273

[71] Hironaka K, Sakaida I, Matsumura Y, Kaino S, Miyamoto K, Okita K. Enhanced interstitial collagenase (matrix metalloproteinase-13) production of Kupffer cell by gadolinium chloride prevents pig serum-induced rat liver fibrosis. Biochemical and Biophysical Research Communications. 2000;**267**(1):290-295. DOI: 10.1006/bbrc.1999.1910

[72] Fischer R, Cariers A, Reinehr R, Haussinger D. Caspase 9-dependent killing of hepatic stellate cells by activated Kupffer cells. Gastroenterology. 2002;**123**(3):845-861. DOI: 10.1053/gast.2002.35384

[73] Taimr P, Higuchi H, Kocova E, Rippe RA, Friedman S, Gores GJ. Activated stellate cells express the TRAIL receptor-2/death receptor-5 and undergo TRAIL-mediated apoptosis. Hepatology. 2003;**37**(1):87-95. DOI: 10.1053/jhep.2003.50002

[74] Pinzani M. PDGF and signal transduction in hepatic stellate cells. Frontiers in Bioscience. 2002;**7**(1-3):d1720-d1726. DOI: 10.2741/pinzani

[75] Thieringer F, Maass T, Czochra P, Klopcic B, Conrad I, Friebe D, et al. Spontaneous hepatic fibrosis in transgenic mice overexpressing PDGF-A. Gene. 2008;**423**(1):23-28. DOI: 10.1016/j.gene.2008.05.022

[76] Cao S, Yaqoob U, Das A, Shergill U, Jagavelu K, Huebert RC, et al. Neuropilin-1 promotes cirrhosis of the rodent and human liver by enhancing PDGF/TGF-beta signaling in hepatic stellate cells. Journal of Clinical Investigation. 2010;**120**(7):2379-2394. DOI: 10.1172/JCI41203

[77] Borkham-Kamphorst E, Herrmann J, Stoll D, Treptau J, Gressner AM, Weiskirchen R. Dominant-negative soluble PDGF-beta receptor inhibits hepatic stellate cell activation and attenuates liver fibrosis. Laboratory Investigation. 2004;**84**(6):766-777. DOI: 10.1038/labinvest.3700094

[78] Czochra P, Klopcic B, Meyer E, Herkel J, Garcia-Lazaro JF, Thieringer F, et al. Liver fibrosis induced by hepatic overexpression of PDGF-B in transgenic mice. Journal of Hepatology. 2006;**45**(3):419-428. DOI: 10.1016/j.jhep.2006.04.010

[79] Derynck R, Zhang YE. Smad-dependent and Smad-independent pathways in TGF-β family signalling. Nature. 2003;**425**(6958):577-584. DOI:10.1038/nature02006

[80] Wang C, Song X, Li Y, Han F, Gao S, Wang X, et al. Low-dose paclitaxel ameliorates pulmonary fibrosis by suppressing TGF-β1/Smad3 pathway via miR-140 upregulation. PLoS ONE. 2013;**8**(8):e70725. DOI: 10.1371/journal.pone.0070725

[81] Wells RG, Kruglov E, Dranoff JA. Autocrine release of TGF-beta by portal fibroblasts regulates cell growth. FEBS Letters. 2004;**559**(1-3):107-110. DOI: 10.1016/S0014-5793(04)00037-7

[82] Cui X, Shimizu I, Lu G, Itonaga M, Inoue H, Shono M, et al. Inhibitory effect of a soluble transforming growth factor beta type II receptor on the activation of rat hepatic stellate cells in primary culture. Journal of Hepatology. 2003;**39**(5):731-737. DOI: 10.1016/s0168-8278(03)00216-2

[83] De Bleser PJ, Niki T, Rogiers V, Geerts A. Transforming growth factor beta gene expression in normal and fibrotic rat liver. Journal of Hepatology. 1997;**26**(4):886-893. DOI: 10.1016/s0168-8278(97)80257-7

[84] Liu X, Hu H, Yin JQ. Therapeutic strategies against TGF-beta signaling pathway in hepatic fibrosis. Liver International. 2006;**26**(1):8-22. DOI: 10.1111/j.1478-3231.2005.01192.x

[85] Cui Q, Wang Z, Jiang D, Qu L, Guo J, Li Z. HGF inhibits TGF-β1-induced myofibroblast differentiation and ECM deposition via MMP-2 in Achilles tendon in rat. European Journal of Applied Physiology. 2011;**111**(7):1457-1463. DOI: 10.1007/s00421-010-1764-4

[86] Kirmaz C, Terzioglu E, Topalak O, Bayrak P, Yilmaz O, Ersoz G, Sebik F. Serum transforming growth factor beta1(TGF-beta1) in patients with cirrhosis, chronic hepatitis B and chronic hepatitis C [corrected]. European Cytokine Network. 2004;**15**(2):112-116. [PMID: 15319169]

[87] Oberhammer F, Pavelka M, Sharma S, Tiefenbacher R, Purchio A, Bursch W, et al. Induction of apoptosis in cultured hepatocytes and in recessing liver by transforming growth factor-beta1. Proceedings of the National Academy of Science of the United States of America. 1992;**89**(12):5408-5412. DOI: 10.1073/pnas.89.12.5408

[88] Lin JK, Chou CK. In vitro apoptosis in the human hepatoma cell line induced by transforming growth factor-beta1. Cancer Research. 1992;**52**(2):385-388. PMID: 1309441

[89] McClain CJ, Song Z, Barve SS, Hill DB, Deaciuc I. Recent advances in alcoholic liver diseases IV. Dysregulated cytokine metabolism in alcoholic liver disease. AJP: Gastrointestinal and Liver Physiology. 2004;**287**(3):G497-G502. DOI: 10.1152/ajpgi.00171.2004

[90] Canbay A, Feldstein AE, Higuchi H, Werneburg N, Grambihler A, Bronk SF, et al. Kupffer cell engulfment of apoptotic bodies stimulates death ligand and cytokine expression. Hepatology. 2003;**38**(5):1188-1198. DOI: 10.1053/jhep.2003.50472

[91] Connolly MK, Bedrosian AS, Mallen-St Clair J, Mitchell AP, Ibrahim J, Stroud A, et al. In liver fibrosis, dendritic cells govern hepatic inflammation in mice via TNF-alpha. Journal of Clinical Investigation. 2009;**119**(11):3213-3225. DOI: 10.1172/JCI37581

[92] Crespo J, Rivero M, Fábrega E, Cayón A, Amado JA, García-Unzeta MT, et al. Plasma leptin and TNF-alpha levels in chronic hepatitis C patients and their relationship to hepatic fibrosis. Digestive Diseases and Sciences. 2002;**47**(7):1604-1610. PMID: 12141823

[93] Saile B, Matthes N, El Armouche H, Neubauer K, Ramadori G. The bcl, NFkappaB and p53/p21WAF1 systems are involved in spontaneous apoptosis and in the anti-apoptotic effect of TGF-beta or TNF-alpha on activated hepatic stellate cells. European Journal of Cell Biology. 2001;**80**(8):554-561. DOI: 10.1078/0171-9335-00182

[94] Varela-Rey M, Fontán-Gabás L, Blanco P, López-Zabalza MJ, Iraburu MJ. Glutathione depletion is involved in the inhibition of procollagen alpha1(I) mRNA levels caused by TNF-alpha on hepatic stellate cells. Cytokine. 2007;**37**(3):212-217. DOI: 10.1016/j.cyto.2007.03.013

[95] Shiratori Y1, Imazeki F, Moriyama M, Yano M, Arakawa Y, Yokosuka O, Kuroki T, Nishiguchi S, Sata M, Yamada G, Fujiyama S, Yoshida H, Omata M. Histologic improvement of fibrosis in patients with hepatitis C who have sustained response to interferon therapy. Annals of Internal Medicine. 2000;**132**(7):517-524. DOI: 10.7326/0003-4819-132-7-200004040-00002

[96] Ogawa T, Kawada N, Ikeda K. Effect of natural interferon α on proliferation and apoptosis of hepatic stellate cells. Hepatology International. 2009;**3**(3):497-503. DOI: 10.1007/s12072-009-9129-y

[97] Rao HY, Wei L, Wang JH, Fei R, Jiang D, Zhang Q, et al. Inhibitory effect of human interferon-beta-1a on activated rat and human hepatic stellate cells. Journal of Gastroenterology and Hepatology. 2010;**25**(11):1777-1784. DOI: 10.1111/j.1440-1746.2010.06264.x

[98] Baroni GS, D'Ambrosio L, Curto P, Casini A, Mancini R, Jezequel AM, et al. Interferon gamma decreases hepatic stellate cell activation and extracellular matrix deposition in rat liver fibrosis. Hepatology. 1996;**23**(5):1189-1199. DOI: 10.1002/hep.510230538

[99] Du S, Li H, Cui Y, Yang L, Wu J, Huang H, et al. Houttuynia cordata inhibits lipopoly-saccharideinduced rapid pulmonary fibrosis by up-regulating IFN-γ and inhibiting the TGF-β1/Smad pathway. International Immunopharmacology. 2012;**13**(3):331-340. DOI: 10.1016/j.intimp.2012.03.011

[100] Saile B, Eisenbach C, Dudas J, El-Armouche H, Ramadori G. Interferon-gamma acts proapoptotic on hepatic stellate cells (HSC) and abrogates the antiapoptotic effect of interferon alpha by an HSP70-dependant pathway. European Journal of Cell Biology. 2004;**83**(9):469-476. DOI: 10.1078/0171-9335-00409

[101] Hammerich L, Tacke F. Interleukins in chronic liver disease: Lessons learned from experimental mouse models. Clinical and Experimental Gastroenterology. 2014;**7**:297-306. DOI: 10.2147/ceg.s43737

[102] Gieling RG, Wallace K, Han YP. Interleukin-1 participates in the progression from liver injury to fibrosis. AJP: Gastrointestinal and Liver Physiology. 2009;**296**(6):G1324-G1331. DOI: 10.1152/ajpgi.90564.2008

[103] Mancini R, Benedetti A, Jezequel AM. An interleukin-1 receptor antagonist decreases fibrosis induced by dimethylnitrosamine in rat liver. Virchows Archive. 1994;**424**(1):25-31. DOI: 10.1007/BF00197389

[104] Kamari Y, Shaish A, Vax E, Shemesh S, Kandel-Kfir M, Arbel Y, et al. Lack of interleukin-1α or interleukin-1β inhibits transformation of steatosis to steatohepatitis and liver fibrosis in hypercholesterolemic mice. Journal of Hepatology. 2011;**55**(5):1086-1094. DOI: 10.1016/j.jhep.2011.01.048

[105] Petrasek J, Bala S, Csak T, Lippai D, Kodys K, Menashy V, et al. IL-1 receptor antagonist ameliorates inflammasome-dependent alcoholic steatohepatitis in mice. Journal of Clinical Investigation. 2012;**122**(10):3476-3489. DOI: 10.1172/JCI60777

[106] Du WJ, Zhen JH, Zeng ZQ, Zheng ZM, Xu Y, Qin LY, et al. Expression of interleukin-17 associated with disease progression and liver fibrosis with hepatitis B virus infection: IL-17 in HBV infection. Diagnostic Pathology. 2013;**8**:40. DOI: 10.1186/1746-1596-8-40

[107] Hara M, Kono H, Furuya S, Hirayama K, Tsuchiya M, Fujii H. Interleukin-17A plays a pivotal role in cholestatic liver fibrosis in mice. Journal of Surgical Research. 2013;**183**(2):574-582. DOI: 10.1016/j.jss.2013.03.025

[108] Meng F, Wang K, Aoyama T, Grivennikov SI, Paik Y, Scholten D, Cong M, et al. Interleukin-17 signaling in inflammatory, Kupffer cells, and hepatic stellate cells exacerbates liver fibrosis in mice. Gastroenterology. 2012;**143**(3):765-776.e1-3. DOI: 10.1053/j.gastro.2012.05.049

[109] Zheng L, Chu J, Shi Y, Zhou X, Tan L, Li Q, et al. Bone marrow-derived stem cells ameliorate hepatic fibrosis by down-regulating interleukin-17. Cell and Bioscience. 2013;**3**(1):46. DOI: 10.1186/2045-3701-3-46

[110] Shahar I, Fireman E, Topilsky M, Grief J, Kivity S, Spirer Z, et al. Effect of IL-6 on alveolar fibroblast proliferation in interstitial lung diseases. Clinical Immunology and Immunopathology. 1996;**79**(3):244-251. DOI: 10.1006/clin.1996.0075

[111] Wynn TA. Cellular and molecular mechanisms of fibrosis. Journal of Pathology. 2008;**214**(2):199-210. DOI: 10.1002/path.2277

[112] Kovalovich K, DeAngelis RA, Li W, Furth EE, Ciliberto G, Taub R. Increased toxin-induced liver injury and fibrosis in interleukin-6-deficient mice. Hepatology. 2000;**31**(1):149-159. DOI: 10.1002/hep.510310123

[113] Klein C, Wüstefeld T, Assmus U, Roskams T, Rose-John S, Müller M, et al. The IL-6-gp130-STAT3 pathway in hepatocytes triggers liver protection in T cell-mediated liver injury. Journal of Clinical Investigation. 2005;**115**(4):860-869. DOI: 10.1172/JCI23640

[114] Nasir GA, Mohsin S, Khan M, Shams S, Ali G, Khan SN, et al. Mesenchymal stem cells and Interleukin-6 attenuate liver fibrosis in mice. Journal of Translational Medicine. 2013;**11**:78. DOI: 10.1186/1479-5876-11-78

[115] Chou WY, Lu CN, Lee TH, Wu CL, Hung KS, Concejero AM, et al. Electroporative interleukin-10 gene transfer ameliorates carbon tetrachloride-induced murine liver

fibrosis by MMP and TIMP modulation. Acta Pharmacologica Sinica. 2006;**27**(4):469-476. DOI: 10.1111/j.1745-7254.2006.00304.x

[116] Nelson DR, Lauwers GY, Lau JY, Davis GL. Interleukin 10 treatment reduces fibrosis in patients with chronic hepatitis C: A pilot trial of interferon nonresponders. Gastroenterology. 2000;**1188**(4):655-660. DOI: 10.1016/S0016-5085(00)70134-X

[117] Zhang LJ, Zheng WD, Chen YX, Huang YH, Chen ZX, Zhang SJ, et al. Antifibrotic effects of interleukin-10 on experimental hepatic fibrosis. Hepatogastroenterology. 2007;**54**(79):2092-2098. PMID: 18251166

[118] Thompson K, Maltby J, Fallowfield J, McAulay M, Millward-Sadler H, Sheron N. Interleukin-10 expression and function in experimental murine liver inflammation and fibrosis. Hepatology. 1998;**28**(6):1597-1606. DOI: 10.1002/hep.510280620

[119] Louis H, Van Laethem JL, Wu W, Quertinmont E, Degraef C, Van den Berg K, et al. Interleukin-10 controls neutrophilic infiltration, hepatocyte proliferation, and liver fibrosis induced by carbon tetrachloride in mice. Hepatology. 1998;**28**(6):1607-1615. DOI: 10.1002/hep.510280621

[120] Hung KS, Lee TH, Chou WY, Wu CL, Cho CL, Lu CN, et al. Interleukin-10 gene therapy reverses thioacetamide-induced liver fibrosis in mice. Biochemical and Biophysical Research Communications. 2005;**336**(1):324-331. DOI: 10.1016/j.bbrc.2005.08.085

[121] Radaeva S, Sun R, Pan HN, Hong F, Gao B. Interleukin 22 (IL-22) plays a protective role in T cell-mediated murine hepatitis: IL-22 is a survival factor for hepatocytes via STAT3 activation. Hepatology. 2004;**39**(5):1332-1342. DOI: 10.1002/hep.20184

[122] Ki SH, Park O, Zheng M, Morales-Ibanez O, Kolls JK, Bataller R, et al. Interleukin-22 treatment ameliorates alcoholic liver injury in a murine model of chronic-binge ethanol feeding: Role of signal transducer and activator of transcription 3. Hepatology. 2010;**52**(4):1291-1300. DOI: 10.1002/hep.23837

[123] Kong X, Feng D, Wang H, Hong F, Bertola A, Wang FS, et al. Interleukin-22 induces hepatic stellate cell senescence and restricts liver fibrosis in mice. Hepatology. 2012;**56**(3):1150-1159. DOI: 10.1002/hep.25744

[124] Feng D, Kong X, Weng H, Park O, Wang H, Dooley S, et al. Interleukin-22 promotes proliferation of liver stem/progenitor cells in mice and patients with chronic hepatitis B virus infection. Gastroenterology. 2012;**143**(1):188-198.e7. DOI: 10.1053/j.gastro.2012.03.044

[125] Li S, Tan HY, Wang N, Zhang ZJ, Lao L, Wong CW, et al. The role of oxidative stress and antioxidants in liver diseases. International Journal of Molecular Sciences. 2015;**16**(11):26087-26124. DOI: 10.3390/ijms161125942

[126] Sanchez-Valle V, Chavez-Tapia NC, Uribe M, Mendez-Sanchez N. Role of oxidative stress and molecular changes in liver fibrosis: A review. Current Medicinal Chemistry. 2012;**19**(28):4850-4860. DOI: 10.2174/092986712803341520

[127] Heeba GH, Mahmoud ME. Therapeutic potential of morin against liver fibrosis in rats: Modulation of oxidative stress, cytokine production and nuclear factor kappa

B. Environmental Toxicology and Pharmacology. 2014;**37**(2):662-671. DOI: 10.1016/j. etap.2014.01.026

[128] Li S, Hong M, Tan HY, Wang N, Feng Y. Insights into the role and interdependence of oxidative stress and inflammation in liver diseases. Oxidative Medicine and Cellular Longevity. 2016;**2016**:1-21. DOI: 10.1155/2016/4234061

[129] Ambros V. The functions of animal microRNAs. Nature. 2004;**431**:350-355 [PMID: 15372042 DOI: 10.1038/nature02871]

[130] He Y, Huang C, Zhang SP, Sun X, Long XR, Li J. The potential of microRNAs in liver fibrosis. Cellular Signalling. 2012;**24**(12):2268-2272. DOI: 10.1016/j.cellsig.2012.07.023

[131] Trebicka J, Anadol E, Elfimova N, Strack I, Roggendorf M, Viazov S, et al. Hepatic and serum levels of miR-122 after chronic HCV-induced fibrosis. Journal of Hepatology. 2013;**58**(2):234-239. DOI: 10.1016/j.jhep.2012.10.015

[132] Murakami Y, Kawada N. MicroRNAs in hepatic pathophysiology. Hepatology Research. 2017;**47**(1):60-69. DOI: 10.1111/hepr.12730

[133] Zhang Z, Gao Z, Hu W, Yin S, Wang C, Zang Y, et al. 3,3'-Diindolylmethane ameliorates experimental hepatic fibrosis via inhibiting miR-21 expression. British Journal of Pharmacology. 2013;**170**(3):649-660. DOI: 10.1111/bph.12323

[134] Zhang J, Jiao J, Cermelli S, Muir K, Jung KH, Zou R, et al. miR-21 inhibition reduces liver fibrosis and prevents tumor development by inducing apoptosis of CD24+ progenitor cells. Cancer Research. 2015;**75**(9):1859-1867. DOI: 10.1158/0008-5472.CAN-14-1254

[135] Murakami Y, Toyoda H, Tanaka M, Kuroda M, Harada Y, Matsuda F, et al. The progression of liver fibrosis is related with overexpression of the miR-199 and 200 families. PLoS ONE. 2011;**6**(1):e16081. DOI: 10.1371/journal.pone.0016081

[136] Ogawa T, Enomoto M, Fujii H, Sekiya Y, Yoshizato K, Ikeda K, et al. MicroRNA-221/222 upregulation indicates the activation of stellate cells and the progression of liver fibrosis. Gut 2012;**61**(11):1600-1609. DOI: 10.1136/gutjnl-2011-300717

[137] Roderburg C, Mollnow T, Bongaerts B, Elfimova N, Vargas Cardenas D, Berger K, et al. Micro-RNA profiling in human serum reveals compartment-specific roles of miR-571 and miR-652 in liver cirrhosis. PLoS ONE. 2012;**7**(3):e32999. DOI: 10.1371/journal. pone.0032999

[138] Okada H, Honda M, Campbell JS, Takegoshi K, Sakai Y, Yamashita T, et al. Inhibition of microRNA-214 ameliorates hepatic fibrosis and tumor incidence in platelet-derived growth factor C transgenic mice. Cancer Science. 2015;**106**(9):1143-1152. DOI: 10.1111/cas.12730

[139] Iizuka M, Ogawa T, Enomoto M, Motoyama H, Yoshizato K, Ikeda K, et al. Induction of microRNA-214-5p in human and rodent liver fibrosis. Fibrogenesis Tissue Repair. 2012;**5**(1):12. DOI: 10.1186/1755-1536-5-12

[140] Venugopal SK, Jiang J, Kim TH, Li Y, Wang SS, Torok NJ, et al. Liver fibrosis causes downregulation of miRNA-150 and miRNA-194 in hepatic stellate cells, and their over-expression causes decreased stellate cell activation. AJP: Gastrointestinal and Liver Physiology. 2010;**298**(1):G101-G106. DOI: 10.1152/ajpgi.00220.2009

[141] Roderburg C, Urban GW, Bettermann K, Vucur M, Zimmermann H, Schmidt S, et al. Micro-RNA profiling reveals a role for miR-29 in human and murine liver fibrosis. Hepatology. 2011;**53**(1):209-218. DOI: 10.1002/hep.23922

[142] Roderburg C, Luedde M, Vargas Cardenas D, Vucur M, Mollnow T, Zimmermann HW, et al. miR-133a mediates TGF-β-dependent derepression of collagen synthesis in hepatic stellate cells during liver fibrosis. Journal of Hepatology. 2013;**58**(4):736-742. DOI: 10.1016/j.jhep.2012.11.022

[143] Tu T, Calabro SR, Lee A, Maczurek AE, Budzinska MA, Warner FJ, et al. Hepatocytes in liver injury: Victim, bystander, or accomplice in progressive fibrosis? Journal of Gastroenterology and Hepatology. 2015;**30**(12):1696-1704. DOI:10.1111/jgh.13065

[144] Martínez-Esparza M, Tristán-Manzano M, Ruiz-Alcaraz AJ, García-Peñarrubia P. Inflammatory status in human hepatic cirrhosis. World Journal of Gastroenterology. 2015;**21**(41):11522-15411. DOI: 10.3748/wjg.v21.i41.11522

[145] Schuppan D, Cramer T, Bauer M, Strefeld T, Hahn EG, Herbst H. Hepatocytes as a source of collagen type XVIII endostatin. Lancet. 1998;**352**(9131):879-880. DOI: 10.1016/S0140-6736(05)60006-2

[146] Schuppan D, Ruehl M, Somasundaram R, Hahn EG. Matrix as a modulator of hepatic fibrogenesis. Seminars in Liver Disease. 2001;**21**(3): 351-372. DOI: 10.1055/s2001-17556

[147] Myers JC, Li D, Bageris A, Abraham V, Dion AS, Amenta PS. Biochemical and immu-nohistochemical characterization of human type XIX defines a novel class of base-ment membrane zone collagens. American Journal of Pathology. 1997;**151**(6):1729-1740 PMID: 9403723

[148] Schuppan D. Structure of the extracellular matrix in normal and fibrotic liver: Collagens and glycoproteins. Seminars in Liver Disease. 1990;**10**(1):1-10. DOI: 10.1055/s-2008-1040452

[149] Benyon RC, Arthur MJ. Extracellular matrix degradation and the role of hepatic stellate cells. Seminars in Liver Disease. 2001;**21**(3):373-384. DOI: 10.1055/s-2001-17552

[150] Baiocchini A, Montaldo C, Conigliaro A, Grimaldi A, Correani V, Mura F, et al. Extracellular matrix molecular remodeling in human liver fibrosis evolution. PLoS ONE. 2016;**11**(3):e0151736. DOI: 10.1371/journal.pone.0151736

[151] van Dijk F, Olinga P, Poelstra K, Beljaars L. Targeted therapies in liver fibrosis: Combining the best parts of platelet-derived growth factor BB and interferon gamma. Frontiers in Medicine (Lausanne). 2015;**2**:72. DOI: 10.3389/fmed.2015.00072

[152] Toosi AE. Liver fibrosis: Causes and methods of assessment, a review. Romanian Journal of Internal Medicine. 2015;**53**(4):304-314. 10.1515/rjim-2015-0039

[153] Sun M, Kisseleva T. Reversibility of liver fibrosis. Clinics and Research in Hepatology and Gastroenterology. 2015;**39**(Suppl 1):S60–S63. DOI: 10.1016/j.clinre.2015.06.015

[154] Friedman SL. Hepatic stellate cells: Protean, multifunctional, and enigmatic cells of the liver. Physiological Reviews. 2008;**88**(1):125-172. DOI: 10.1152/physrev.00013.2007

[155] Cohen-Naftaly M, Friedman SL. Current status of novel antifibrotic therapies in patients with chronic liver disease. Therapeutic Advances in Gastroenterology. 2011;**4**(6):391-417. DOI: 10.1177/1756283X11413002

[156] Yin C, Evason KJ, Asahina K, Stainier DY. Hepatic stellate cells in liver development, regeneration, and cancer. Journal of Clinical Investigation. 2013;**123**(5):1902-1910. DOI: 10.1172/jci66369

[157] Friedman SL. Mechanisms of hepatic fibrogenesis. Gastroenterology. 2008;**134**(6):1655-1669. DOI:10.1053/j.gastro.2008.03.003

[158] Trautwein C, Friedman SL, Schuppan D, Pinzani M. Hepatic fibrosis: Concept to treatment. Journal of Hepatology. 2015;**62**(1):S15–S24. DOI: 10.1016/j.jhep.2015.02.039

[159] Canbay A, Higuchi H, Bronk SF, Taniai M, Sebo TJ, Gores GJ. Fas enhances fibrogenesis in the bile duct ligated mouse: A link between apoptosis and fibrosis. Gastroenterology. 2002;**123**(4):1323-1330. DOI: 10.1053/gast.2002.35953

[160] Cassiman D, Libbrecht L, Desmet V, Denef C, Roskams T. Hepatic stellate cell/myofibroblast subpopulations in fibrotic human and rat livers. Journal of Hepatology. 2002;**36**(2):200-209. DOI: 10.1016/s0168-8278(01)00260-4

[161] Pinzani M, Marra F. Cytokine receptors and signaling in hepatic stellate cells. Seminars in Liver Disease. 2001;**21**(3):397-416. DOI: 10.1055/s-2001-17554

[162] Maher JJ, Lozier JS, Scott MK. Rat hepatic stellate cells produce cytokine-induced neutrophil chemoattractant in culture and in vivo. American Journal of Physiology. 1998;**275**(4pt1):G847–G853. PMID: 9756517

[163] Zhang CY, Yuan WG, He P, Lei JH, Wang CX. Liver fibrosis and hepatic stellate cells: Etiology, pathological hallmarks and therapeutic targets. World Journal of Gastroenterology. 2016;**22**(48):10512-10522. DOI: 10.3748/wjg.v22.i48.10512

[164] Pradere JP, Kluwe J, De Minicis S, Jiao JJ, Gwak GY, Dapito DH, et al. Hepatic macrophages but not dendritic cells contribute to liver fibrosis by promoting the survival of activated hepatic stellate cells in mice. Hepatology. 2013;**58**(4):1461-1473. DOI: 10.1002/hep.26429

[165] Barnes MA, McMullen MR, Roychowdhury S, Madhun NZ, Niese K, Olman MA, et al. Macrophage migration inhibitory factor is required for recruitment of scar-associated macrophages during liver fibrosis. Journal of Leukocyte Biology. 2015;**97**(1):161-169. DOI: 10.1189/jlb.3A0614-280R

[166] Ehling J, Bartneck M, Wei X, Gremse F, Fech V, Möckel D, et al. CCL2-dependent infiltrating macrophages promote angiogenesis in progressive liver fibrosis. Gut. 2014;**63**(12):1960-1971. DOI: 10.1136/gutjnl-2013-306294

[167] Radaeva S, Sun R, Jaruga B, Nguyen VT, Tian Z, Gao B. Natural killer cells ameliorate liver fibrosis by killing activated stellate cells in NKG2D-dependent and tumor necrosis factor-related apoptosis-inducing ligand-dependent manners. Gastroenterology. 2006;**130**(2):435-452. DOI: 10.1053/j.gastro.2005.10.055

[168] Gores GJ, Kaufmann SH. Is TRAIL hepatotoxic? Hepatology. 2001;**34**(1):3-6. DOI: 10.1053/jhep.2001.25173

[169] Ebrahimi H, Naderian M, Sohrabpour AA. New concepts on pathogenesis and diagnosis of liver fibrosis; a review article. Middle East Journal of Digestive Diseases. 2016;**8**(3):166-178. DOI: 10.15171/mejdd.2016.29

[170] Choi ET, Callow AD, Sehgal NL, Brown DM, Ryan US. Halofuginone, a specific collagen type I inhibitor, reduces anastomotic intima hyperplasia. Archives of Surgery. 1995;**130**(3):257-261. DOI: 10.1001/archsurg.1995.01430030027004

[171] Pines M, Spector I. Halofuginone—The multifaceted molecule. Molecules. 2015;**20**(1): 573-594. DOI: 10.3390/molecules20010573

[172] Giannelli G, Mikulits W, Dooley S, Fabregat I, Moustakas A, ten Dijke P, et al. The rationale for targeting TGF-β in chronic liver diseases. European Journal of Clinical Investigation. 2016;**46**(4):349-361. DOI: 10.1111/eci.12596

[173] Roberts AB, Russo A, Felici A, Flanders KC. Smad3: A key player in pathogenetic mechanisms dependent on TGF-β. Annals of the New York Academy of Sciences. 2003;**995**(1):1-10. DOI: 10.1111/j.1749-6632.2003.tb03205.x

[174] Uemura M, Swenson ES, Gaca MD, Giordano FJ, Reiss M, Wells RG. Smad2 and Smad3 play different roles in rat hepatic stellate cell function and {alpha}-smooth muscle actin organization. Molecular Biology of the Cell. 2005;**16**(9):4214-4224. DOI: 10.1091/mbc. e05-02-0149

[175] Ghosh AK. Factors involved in the regulation of type I collagen gene expression: Implication in fibrosis. Experimental Biology and Medicine (Maywood). 2002;**227**(5): 301-314. PMID: 11976400

[176] Turgeman T, Hagai Y, Huebner K, Jassal DS, Anderson JE, Genin O, et al. Prevention of muscle fibrosis and improvement in muscle performance in the mdx mouse by halofuginone. Neuromuscular Disorders. 2008;**18**(11):857-868. DOI: 10.1016/j. nmd.2008.06.386

[177] McGaha TL, Phelps RG, Spiera H, Bona C. Halofuginone, an inhibitor of type-I collagen synthesis and skin sclerosis, blocks transforming-growth-factor-beta-mediated Smad3 activation in fibroblasts. Journal of Investigative Dermatology. 2002;**118**(3):461-470. DOI: 10.1046/j.0022-202x.2001.01690

[178] Zion O, Genin O, Kawada N, Yoshizato K, Roffe S, Nagler A, et al. Inhibition of transforming growth factor beta signaling by halofuginone as a modality for pancreas fibrosis prevention. Pancreas. 2009;38(4):427-435. DOI: 10.1097/MPA.0b013e3181967670

[179] Xavier S, Piek E, Fujii M, Javelaud D, Mauviel A, Flanders KC, et al. Amelioration of radiation induced fibrosis: Inhibition of transforming growth factor-beta signaling by halofuginone. Journal of Biological Chemistry. 2004;279(15):15167-15176. DOI: 10.1074/jbc.M309798200

[180] Yee KO, Connolly CM, Pines M, Lawler J. Halofuginone inhibits tumor growth in the polyoma middle T antigen mouse via a thrombospondin-1 independent mechanism. Cancer Biology & Therapy. 2006;5(2):218-224. DOI: 10.4161/cbt.5.2.2419

[181] Gnainsky Y, Kushnirsky Z, Bilu G, Hagai Y, Genina O, Volpin H, et al. Gene expression during chemically induced liver fibrosis: Effect of halofuginone on TGF-beta signaling. Cell and Tissue Research. 2007;328(1):153-166. DOI: 10.1007/s00441-006-0330-1

[182] Roffe S, Hagai Y, Pines M, Halevy O. Halofuginone inhibits Smad3 phosphorylation via the PI3K/Akt and MAPK/ERK pathways in muscle cells: Effect on myotube fusion. Experimental Cell Research. 2010;316(6):1061-1069. DOI: 10.1016/j.yexcr.2010.01.003

[183] Zeplin PH. Halofuginone down-regulates Smad3 expression and inhibits the TGFbeta-induced expression of fibrotic markers in human corneal fibroblasts. Annals of Plastic Surgery. 2014;72(4):489. DOI: 10.1097/SAP.0b013e31828a49e3

[184] Nagler A, Genina O, Lavelin I, Ohana M, Pines M. Halofuginone: An inhibitor of collagen type I synthesis: Prevents formation of post-operative adhesions formation in the rat uterine horn model. American Journal of Obstetrics and Gynecology. 1999;180(3):558-563. DOI: 10.1016/s0002-9378(99)70254-1

[185] Nagler A, Katz A, Aingorn H, Miao HQ, Condiotti R, Genina O, Pines M, et al. Inhibition of glomerular mesangial cell proliferation and extracellular matrix deposition by halofuginone. Kidney International. 1997;52(6):1561-1569. DOI: 10.1038/ki.1997.486

[186] Pines M. Targeting TGFβ signaling to inhibit fibroblasts activation as a therapy for fibrosis and cancer. Expert Opinion on Drug Discovery. 2008;3(1):11-20. DOI: 10.1517/17460441.3.1.11

[187] Pines M. Halofuginone for fibrosis, regeneration and cancer in the gastrointestinal tract. World Journal of Gastroenterology. 2014;20(40):14778-14786. DOI: 10.3748/wjg.v20.i40.14778

[188] Sundrud MS, Koralov SB, Feuerer M, Calado DP, Kozhaya AE, Rhule-Smith A, et al. Halofuginone inhibits TH17 cell differentiation by activating the amino acid starvation response. Science. 2009;324(5932):1334-1338. DOI: 10.1126/science.1172638

[189] Pietrella D, Rachini A, Pines M, Pandey N, Mosci P, Bistoni F, et al. Th17 cells and IL-17 in protective immunity to vaginal candidiasis. PLoS ONE. 2011;6(7):e22770. DOI: 10.1371/journal.pone.0022770

[190] Keller TL, Zocco D, Sundrud MS, Hendrick M, Edenius M, Yum J, et al. Halofuginone and other febrifugine derivatives inhibit prolyl-tRNA synthetase. Nature Chemical Biology. 2012;8(3):311-317. DOI: 10.1038/nchembio.790

[191] Mangan PR, Harrington LE, O'Quinn DB, Helms WS, Bullard DC, Elson CO, et al. Transforming growth factor-beta induces development of the T(H)17 lineage. Nature. 2006;441(7090):231-234. DOI: 10.1038/nature04754

[192] Gnainsky Y, Spira G, Paizi M, Bruck R, Nagler A, Abu-Amara SN, et al. Halofuginone, an inhibitor of collagen synthesis by rat stellate cells, stimulates insulin-like growth factor binding protein-1 synthesis by hepatocytes. Journal of Hepatology. 2004;40(2):269-277. PMID: 14739098

[193] Gnainsky Y, Spira G, Paizi M, Bruck R, Nagler A, Genina O, et al. The involvement of the tyrosine phosphatase early gene of liver regeneration (PRL-1) in cell cycle and in liver regeneration and fibrosis–effect of halofuginone. Cell and Tissue Research. 2006;324(3):385-394. DOI: 10.1007/s00441-005-0092-1

[194] Hernandez-Gea V, Toffanin S, Friedman SL, Llovet JM. Role of the microenvironment in the pathogenesis and treatment of hepatocellular carcinoma. Gastroenterology. 2013;144(3):512-527. DOI: 10.1053/j.gastro.2013.01.002

[195] Nissen NN, Martin P. Hepatocellular carcinoma: The high-risk patient. Journal of Clinical Gastroenterology. 2002;35(5 Suppl 2):S79–S85. DOI: 10.1097/00004836-200211002-00003

[196] Nagler A, Ohana M, Shibolet O, Shapira MY, Alper R, Vlodavsky I, et al. Suppression of hepatocellular carcinoma growth in mice by the alkaloid coccidiostat halofuginone. European Journal of Cancer. 2004;40(9):1397-1403. DOI: 10.1016/j.ejca.2003.11.036

[197] Taras D, Blanc JF, Rullier A, Dugot-Senant N, Laurendeau I, Bièche I, et al. Halofuginone suppresses the lung metastasis of chemically induced hepatocellular carcinoma in rats through MMP inhibition. Neoplasia. 2006;8(4):312-318. DOI: 10.1593/neo.05796

11

Non-Alcoholic Steatohepatitis, Liver Cirrhosis and Hepatocellular Carcinoma: The Molecular Pathways

Dzeina Mezale, Ilze Strumfa, Andrejs Vanags,
Matiss Mezals, Ilze Fridrihsone, Boriss Strumfs and
Dainis Balodis

Abstract

Non-alcoholic steatohepatitis (NASH) is growing into global problem, mainly due to NASH-induced cirrhosis and hepatocellular carcinoma (HCC), that can develop either subsequently to cirrhosis or preceding it. In addition, NASH-induced cirrhosis constitutes a significant fraction of cases diagnosed as cryptogenic cirrhosis. Thus, there is a need for deeper understanding of the molecular basis, leading to liver steatosis, then—to the associated inflammation seen in NASH, loss of liver architecture and cirrhosis, followed or paralleled by carcinogenesis and HCC. Insulin resistance, increased hepatic iron level, and certain cytokines, including TNF-α and IL-6 derived from extrahepatic adipose tissues, can trigger the chain of events. The imbalance between leptin and adiponectin is important as well. These markers remain important during the whole course from NASH through liver cirrhosis to HCC. The molecular pathogenesis substantiates treatment: hypertriglyceridemia can be lowered by low calorie diet; mTOR complex can become inhibited by physical activity and metformin; cholesterol synthesis, RAF/MAPK1/ERK and p21 pathway by statins; inflammation by pentoxyfillin, and kinases (in HCC) by sorafenib. Bidirectional regulation of telomere attrition, senescence and p21 pathway, restoration of wild-type p53 activity and regulation of miRNA network represent attractive future treatment options. Focusing on relevant molecular pathways allows deeper understanding of NASH pathogenesis, leading to identification of predictive markers and treatment targets.

Keywords: non-alcoholic fatty liver disease, non-alcoholic steatohepatitis, liver cirrhosis, cryptogenic cirrhosis, hepatocellular carcinoma

1. Introduction

Non-alcoholic fatty liver disease (NAFLD) is a clinical and pathological entity with features that resemble alcohol-induced liver steatosis, but, by the definition, it occurs in patients with little or no history of alcohol consumption. NAFLD is subdivided into non-alcoholic fatty liver (NAFL) and non-alcoholic steatohepatitis (NASH). It encompasses a histological spectrum that ranges from fat accumulation in hepatocytes without concomitant inflammation or fibrosis (simple hepatic steatosis, NAFL) to hepatic steatosis with a necroinflammatory component (inflammation-induced apoptosis in hepatocytes) that may or may not have associated fibrosis. The latter condition, referred to as non-alcoholic steatohepatitis (NASH), can lead to NASH-induced liver cirrhosis (**Figure 1**). In addition, NASH is now recognised as the main cause of cryptogenic cirrhosis [1], as sequential association has been demonstrated in up to 75% of cryptogenic cirrhosis cases (see also Section 3 for detailed discussion of the relationships between NASH and cryptogenic cirrhosis). Liver cirrhosis may further lead to hepatocellular carcinoma (HCC), the most common primary liver cancer known for its poor clinical outcome and limited therapeutic options. Although previously it was considered that risk of HCC is limited to cirrhotic patients [2], a significant fraction of NASH-associated HCC develops in liver showing none or mild fibrosis. The association between NAFLD/NASH and increased HCC risk is supported by strong epidemiologic evidence.

In the year 2010, the annual incidence of HCC in the population of the USA was at least 6 per 100,000. The mortality rate was almost identical to the incidence underscoring the serious prognosis [3]. Patients with NAFLD/NASH are subjected to an increased lifetime risk of HCC. In a 16-year follow-up study, the standardised incidence ratio of HCC in patients with NAFLD/NASH was 4.4 [4]. In a recent global meta-analysis, the HCC incidence among NAFLD patients reached 0.44 (range, 0.29–0.66) per 1000 person-years [5]. The HCC-related mortality rates among NAFLD patients range from 0.25 to 2.3% over 8.3 and 13.7 years of follow-up, respectively [5, 6]. NAFLD/NASH-associated HCC is believed to be the leading cause of obesity-related cancer deaths in middle-aged men in the USA [4]. Consistently, the proportion of HCC related to NAFLD/NASH is increasing worldwide and is reported to range between 4 and 22% in Western countries [7]. Although the exact burden of HCC associated with NAFLD/NASH still remains uncertain, it seems evident that NAFLD and NASH will become the most common causative/risk factors for HCC, surpassing viral or alcohol-related cirrhosis in the future [7]. In the USA, the number of NAFLD-associated HCC cases is annually growing (2004–2009) for 9% [8], while decreased burden of viral hepatitis-induced HCC might be expected due to the achievements in antiviral treatment targeting hepatitis C virus [9].

NAFLD is the major hepatic manifestation of obesity and associated metabolic conditions. The epidemiology of NAFLD mirrors the recent spread of obesity and diabetes. With increasing prevalence of these conditions, NAFLD has become the most common liver disorder in USA [10] and other Western industrialised countries, facing high occurrence of the major risk factors for NAFLD, namely, central obesity, type 2 diabetes mellitus, dyslipidemia and metabolic syndrome [11]. In a recent meta-analysis of 86 studies, comprising 8,515,431 persons from 22 countries, the global prevalence of NAFLD was 25.24% (95% confidence interval [CI], 22.10–28.65) showing the highest occurrence in the Middle East and South America and the lowest in Africa [5].

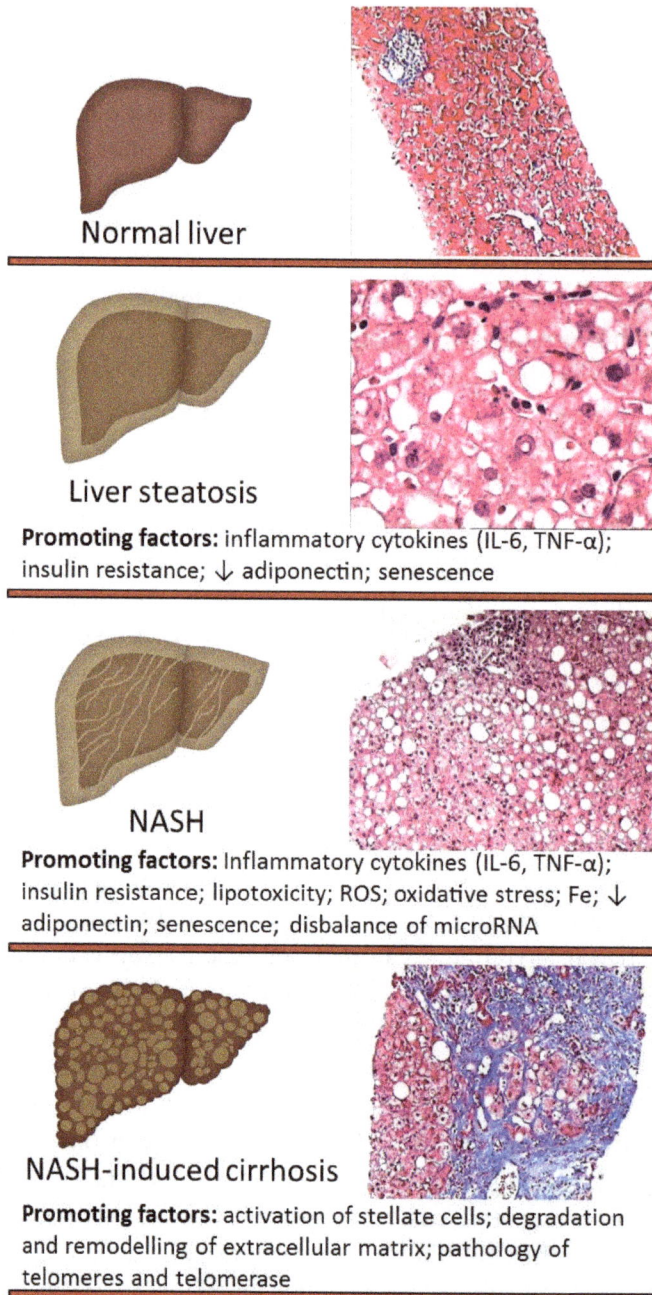

Normal liver

Liver steatosis

Promoting factors: inflammatory cytokines (IL-6, TNF-α); insulin resistance; ↓ adiponectin; senescence

NASH

Promoting factors: Inflammatory cytokines (IL-6, TNF-α); insulin resistance; lipotoxicity; ROS; oxidative stress; Fe; ↓ adiponectin; senescence; disbalance of microRNA

NASH-induced cirrhosis

Promoting factors: activation of stellate cells; degradation and remodelling of extracellular matrix; pathology of telomeres and telomerase

Figure 1. Progression of NAFLD. Abbreviations: IL, interleukin; TNF, tumour necrosis factor; ROS, reactive oxygen species; Fe, accumulation of iron compounds.

Thus, 90% of patients suffering from morbid obesity (defined as having body mass index 40 kg/m² or higher) and 74% patients affected by diabetes mellitus develop NAFLD. In addition, NAFLD has been observed even in non-obese, non-diabetic patients who have increased insulin levels in blood and resistance to insulin action. Consequently, NAFLD affects up to 20–30% of adults in Europe and 46% in the USA: a tremendously high prevalence for a condition that can cause any significant complications [9, 10].

Most patients are diagnosed with NAFLD in their 40s or 50s. Studies vary in regard to the gender distribution of NAFLD, with some suggesting that it is more common in women and others suggesting more frequent occurrence in men [11, 12].

Since 1998, non-alcoholic fatty liver disease has been considered a condition with a "two-hit" course of pathogenesis, first proposed by Day and James [13], describing the role of lipid peroxidation in liver injury. The "first hit" is the development of hepatic steatosis. It was suggested that hepatic triglyceride accumulation increased the susceptibility of the liver to the "second injury hit" by inflammatory cytokines and/or adipokines, mitochondrial dysfunction and elevated oxidative stress that together promote steatohepatitis and fibrosis [14]. Alternatively, many factors may act simultaneously leading to the development of NAFLD: this hypothesis corresponds to the multihit model proposed by Tilg and Moschen [15].

Experimental and population studies have shown the links between NAFLD/NASH and development of HCC. However, the mechanisms by which NASH progresses to HCC are only beginning to be elucidated [14]. NASH is the most rapidly growing risk for liver transplantation because of HCC. Wong et al. in their study included 61,868 patients over the period 2002–2012 and found that the proportion of NASH-related HCC increased from 8.3 to 13.5%, an increase of near 63% [16].

This increase is alarming as HCC already is the fifth most frequently diagnosed cancer and the second leading oncologic death cause worldwide [17], with increasing incidence and mortality rates in Europe [18]. Thus it is crucial to analyse molecular pathways involved in NASH-induced cirrhosis and HCC carcinogenesis. Focusing on the molecular events involved in pathogenetic chain of events from NASH to liver cirrhosis and HCC would provide not only better theoretical understanding of liver diseases preceding and following cirrhosis but would also allow to recognise predictive markers and treatment targets before HCC development.

2. Common pathogenetic mechanisms of NAFLD

Hepatic steatosis or excessive triglyceride accumulation in the liver is a prerequisite to the histological diagnosis of NAFLD. Several mechanisms may lead to steatosis, including (1) increased fat supply because of high-fat diet or excess lipolysis in adipose tissues, which increase free fatty acid (FFA) level; (2) decreased fat export in the form of very low density lipoprotein-triglyceride complex, secondary to either reduced synthesis of the relevant proteins or compromised excretion; (3) decreased or impaired β-oxidation of FFA to adenosine triphosphate and (4) increased hepatic synthesis of fatty acids through *de novo* lipogenesis [1, 19]. Free fatty acid delivery to the liver accounts for almost two-thirds of its lipid accumulation. *De novo* lipogenesis therefore only contributes to the accumulation of hepatic fat in case of NAFLD [15].

The molecular mechanisms responsible for the accumulation of fat in the liver are complex (**Figure 2**). Certain inflammatory cytokines, particularly those derived from extrahepatic

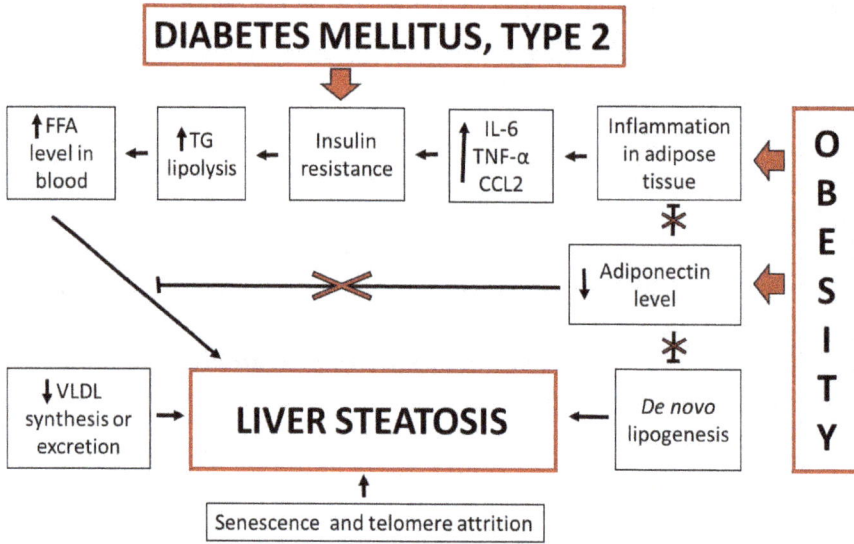

Figure 2. Pathogenesis of liver steatosis. Abbreviations: FFA, free fatty acids; TG, triglycerides; IL, interleukin; TNF, tumour necrosis factor; CCL2, CC motif chemokine ligand 2; VLDL, very low density lipoproteins.

adipose tissues, can trigger this process. Insulin resistance appears to be at the centre for the massive metabolic dysregulations that initiate and aggravate hepatic steatosis. At a certain point, the simple steatosis transforms to steatohepatitis in about 20–30% of NAFLD patients [19]. A major feature in the transition from NAFLD to NASH is the appearance of hepatic inflammation [14]. This breakthrough-like process is mediated by the interplay of multiple hit factors and is orchestrated by rich network of miRNAs [20]. Currently, a number of common pathogenetic mechanisms have been proposed and characterised for the transition from simple steatosis to NASH [19]. A summary of these mechanisms is shown in **Figure 3**.

2.1. Inflammation in peripheral adipose tissue

Hypoxia and death of rapidly expanding adipocytes are considered important initiating factors of adipose tissue inflammation in obesity [19]. During inflammation, typical cytokines like tumour necrosis factor (TNF)-α, interleukin (IL)-6 and CC motif chemokine ligand 2 (CCL2) are secreted by inflammatory cells infiltrating adipose tissue [21]. TNF-α was the first pro-inflammatory cytokine detected in adipose tissue. TNF-α and IL-6 are involved in the regulation of insulin resistance [19]. TNF-α and IL-6 induce insulin resistance in adipocytes, stimulating triglyceride lipolysis and fatty acid release into the circulation. CCL2 recruits macrophages to the adipose tissue, resulting in even higher local cytokine production and perpetuating the inflammatory cycle [19]. In the liver, increased expression of hepatic IL-6 correlates with higher degree of insulin resistance in patients with suspected NAFLD [1].

At the same time, extrahepatic adipocytes are compromised in their natural ability to secrete adiponectin, an anti-inflammatory adipokine that facilitates the normal partitioning of lipid

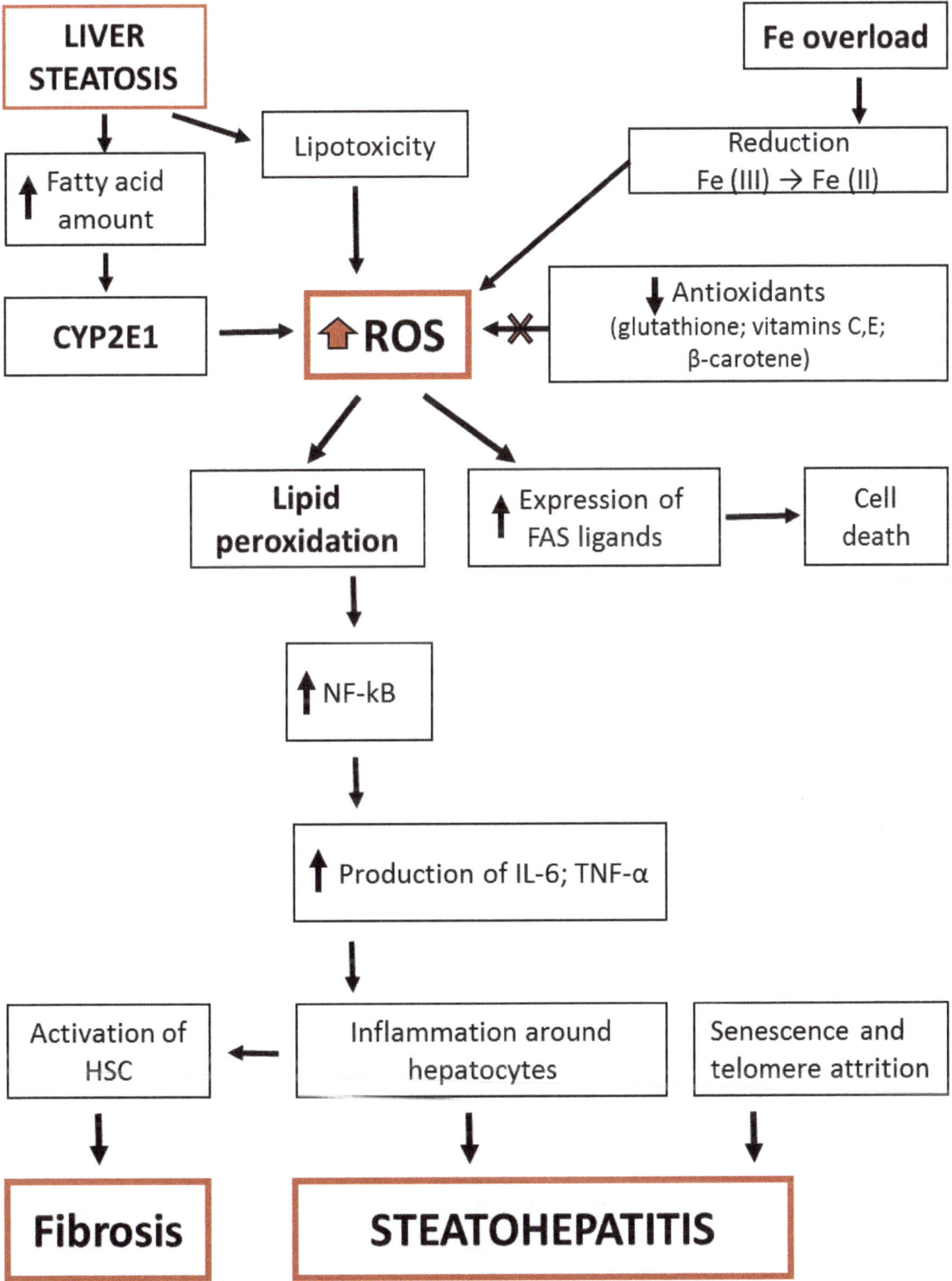

Figure 3. Pathogenesis of non-alcoholic steatohepatitis. Abbreviations: CYPE1, cytochrome CYP2E1; ROS, reactive oxygen species; Fe, iron; NF-κB, nuclear factor kappaB; IL, interleukin; TNF, tumour necrosis factor; HSC, hepatic stellate cells.

to adipocytes for storage [19]. Adiponectin is a hormone secreted exclusively by adipose tissue. It has beneficial effects on lipid metabolism. In the liver, adiponectin is considered to have insulin-sensitising, anti-fibrogenic and anti-inflammatory properties by acting on hepatocytes, liver stellate cells and hepatic macrophages (Kupffer cells), respectively. Adiponectin suppresses the transportation of free fatty acids to the liver as well as gluconeogenesis and *de novo* synthesis of fats but enhances oxidisation of FFAs [21]. The adiponectin-induced suppression of aldehyde oxidase and transforming growth factor has net anti-fibrotic effect [21], while decreased release of pro-inflammatory cytokines including TNF-α reduces inflammation [1]. Decreased levels of adiponectin result in loss of these protective metabolic, anti-fibrotic and anti-inflammatory effects.

Together, these abnormalities accentuate fat loss from adipocytes and promote ectopic fat accumulation [19].

2.2. Insulin resistance

Obesity and type 2 diabetes mellitus, both conditions associated with peripheral insulin resistance, are frequently diagnosed in patients affected by non-alcoholic fatty liver disease [12]. Evaluating patients suffering from diabetes mellitus, NAFLD was found in 74% of them in North American study, 70% in Italian population and 35–56% in Eastern countries. In Mexico, prevalence of NASH in diabetics was 18.5%. The prevalence of NAFLD in obese patients is 57–90% in Western and 10–80% in Eastern populations. NASH is present in 15–20% patients affected by obesity. The frequency of NASH is higher in those undergoing bariatric surgery and can reach 48–60% in USA men, 20–31% in USA females and up to 80% in Taiwan patients [9, 10, 12].

Insulin resistance has also been observed in NASH patients who are not obese and those who have normal glucose tolerance [1]; however, not all people with NAFLD have increased insulin resistance. NAFLD also cannot be considered as a cause for insulin resistance but rather as a consequence [19].

Resistance to the action of insulin results in important metabolic changes, including the turnover of lipids. It is characterised not only by increased circulating insulin levels but also by increased hepatic gluconeogenesis, impaired glucose uptake by muscle, enhanced peripheral lipolysis, increased triglyceride synthesis and increased hepatic uptake of fatty acids, as well as increased release of inflammatory cytokines from peripheral adipose tissues, which are the key factors promoting accumulation of liver fat and progression of hepatic steatosis [1, 19].

2.3. Lipotoxicity

The term "lipotoxicity" describes the deleterious effects of excess FFA and ectopic fat accumulation resulting in organ dysfunction and/or cellular death. In obesity, excessive food intake combined with high FFA output from insulin-resistant adipose tissue surpasses the storage and oxidative capacity of tissues such as skeletal muscle, liver, or pancreatic β-cells [22]. Long-chain saturated fatty acids, as well as free cholesterol derived from *de novo* synthesis can be harmful to hepatocytes. Free cholesterol accumulation leads to liver injury through the activation of intracellular signalling pathways in Kupffer cells, liver stellate cells, and hepatocytes [19], ultimately promoting inflammation and fibrosis [23]. FFAs are redirected into noxious pathways of nonoxidative metabolism with intracellular accumulation of toxic metabolites. It is not TG accumulation *per se* that is uniquely hazardous, but rather the lipid-derived metabolites that trigger the development of reactive oxygen species (ROS) and activation of inflammatory pathways [22], including up-regulation of nuclear factor kappaB, production of TNF-α and IL-6 [24], and the subsequent inflammatory reaction in the liver [1].

2.4. Oxidative stress

In the context of increased supply of fatty acids to hepatocytes, oxidative stress can occur. It is attributable to the raised levels of reactive oxygen/nitrogen species and lipid peroxidation that are generated during free fatty acid metabolism in microsomes, peroxisomes, and mitochondria [19]. NAFLD and NASH-induced oxidative stress is partly regulated through cytochrome P450 2E1 (CYP2E1) as it metabolises C10–C20 fatty acids [14] that in turn produce hepatotoxic free oxygen radical species [1]. Peroxidation of plasma and intracellular membranes may cause direct cell necrosis/apoptosis and development of megamitochondria, while ROS-induced expression of Fas-ligand on hepatocytes may induce fratricidal cell death [19]. Recent studies support the idea that oxidative stress may be a primary cause of liver fat accumulation and subsequent liver injury [25], as well as ROS may play a part in fibrosis development. Lipid peroxidation and free oxygen radical species can also deplete antioxidant stores such as glutathione, vitamin E, beta-carotene, and vitamin C, rendering the liver susceptible to oxidative injury [1].

2.5. Increased hepatic iron concentration

The degree of liver fibrosis in nonalcoholic steatohepatitis shows correlation with the concentration of iron compounds in the hepatocytes. The underlying mechanism might involve the ferric-to-ferrous reduction (switch of trivalent Fe(III) to divalent Fe(II) compounds), resulting in simultaneous production of free oxygen radicals [1]. In addition, sinusoidal iron accumulation might also have a pathogenetic role in the progression of chronic liver diseases and development of hepatocellular carcinoma [26]. However, at least in Eastern populations, disturbances of iron metabolism are rarely observed in NAFLD patients [12]. In patients without iron overload, increased ferritin level in the blood may still be associated with insulin resistance and fatty liver [27].

2.6. MicroRNAs in NAFLD

MicroRNAs are small molecules of non-coding RNA that act as large-scale molecular switches. The pathogenetic chain of events in the transition to NAFL, NASH, and liver cirrhosis is richly regulated by miRNA network: it has been estimated that approximately 54 miRNAs regulate 107 genes involved in the development of NAFLD. The up-regulation of miR-26b and down-regulation of miR-26a decrease insulin sensitivity, while lower levels of miR-451 are associated with pro-inflammatory background. The up-regulation of miR-155 and miR-107 promotes fat accumulation in liver cells. Enhanced fibrosis is mediated by miR-21. Assessing patients with NAFLD-associated liver fibrosis, at least 9 miRNAs are expressed in modified levels, including higher expression of miR-31, miR-182, miR-183, miR-224, and miR-150 as well as down-regulated levels of miR-17, miR-378i, miR-219a, and miR-590. In the progression of liver fibrosis, the normally high levels of miR-22 and miR-125b are suppressed. The miR-29 family showing anti-fibrotic action in many organs is also suppressed [20].

3. NASH-induced liver cirrhosis

Liver cirrhosis develops (**Table 1**) when simple steatosis progresses to steatohepatitis and then fibrosis [11]. The composition of the hepatic fibrosis is similar regardless of the cause of injury as it follows the paradigm for wound healing in other tissues, including skin, lung and kidney. Fibrosis occurs first in regions of most severe injury over several months to years of ongoing tissue damage [23, 28, 29].

Targets	Involved cells or molecules	Result
Stellate cells	Activated stellated cells are transformed to proliferating, fibrogenic and contractile myofibroblasts	Remodelling of the matrix
Macromolecules in the extracellular matrix	Collagens: the total collagen content increases 3- to 10-fold including an increase in fibril-forming collagens (i.e., types I, III, and IV) and some non-fibril forming collagens (types IV and VI).	The extracellular matrix switches from the normal low-density basement membrane-like matrix to the interstitial type
	Glycoproteins: fibronectin, laminin, SPARC, osteonectin, tenascin, and von Willebrand factor	
	Matrix-bound growth factors	
	Glycosaminoglycans: perlecan, decorin, aggrecan, lumican, and fibromodulin	
	Proteoglycans: shift from heparan sulphate-containing proteoglycans to those containing chondroitin and dermatan sulphates	
Degradation of extracellular matrix	Matrix metalloproteinase 2	Disruption of normal matrix facilitates replacement by desmoplastic matrix
	Matrix metalloproteinase 9	
	Membrane-type metalloproteinase 1 and/or 2	
	Stromelysin 1	

Table 1. The key structures in the development of liver cirrhosis.

Cryptogenic cirrhosis is the end stage of a chronic liver disease in which the underlying aetiology remains unknown after extensive clinical, serological and pathological evaluation [30, 31]. In different studies, 3–30% of liver cirrhosis cases have been attributed to the cryptogenic group [9]. Naturally, occasionally the diagnosis of cryptogenic cirrhosis is issued just due to lack of information despite the definition demanding complete investigation. Studying explanted livers of cirrhotic patients undergoing liver transplantation and having preoperative diagnosis of cryptogenic cirrhosis, specific cause was identified in 28.6% of cases. The relevant diagnoses included autoimmune hepatitis, sarcoidosis, primary biliary cirrhosis, sclerosing cholangitis, congenital hepatic fibrosis and Wilson's disease [32]. Other data/investigational methods can yield significant information as well. For instance, a significant fraction of cases initially diagnosed as cryptogenic liver cirrhosis can be associated with occult hepatitis B infection [33].

Recent evidence suggests that cryptogenic cirrhosis is strongly associated with development of HCC, while in a varying percentage (6.9–50%) of HCC, the underlying aetiology of liver disease cannot be determined. In a retrospective study of 641 HCC patients, cryptogenic cirrhosis was found in 44 (6.9%) cases, characterised also by more frequent occurrence of obesity and diabetes mellitus than in patients having history of chronic viral hepatitis and alcohol abuse. Considering the known association between obesity, diabetes and NASH, it was hypothesised that NASH is the precursor of cryptogenic cirrhosis and hepatocellular carcinoma [34].

At present, there is strong evidence that cryptogenic cirrhosis represents the end state of NASH at least in a fraction of patients. First, the progression of fibrosis in NASH is associated with gradual loss of fat vacuoles. Thus, the specific morphological changes would be burned out when the cirrhosis develops. Second, patients diagnosed with cryptogenic cirrhosis have high prevalence of metabolic changes as type 2 diabetes mellitus, obesity, or history of those disorders. If the history of preceding diabetes mellitus or obesity or liver biopsy revealing NAFLD is considered as the diagnostic criteria, 30–75% of cryptogenic cirrhosis cases can be retrospectively associated with NASH [9]. Third, due to growing awareness of the entity of NASH-induced cirrhosis, direct evidence has been brought by data obtained in explanted livers. Cases that were clinically diagnosed as cryptogenic cirrhosis were reclassified as NAFLD (either cirrhosis or pre-cirrhotic stage) in 78.6% of cases [12, 35, 36].

In comparison with liver cirrhosis due to other aetiologies, NASH-induced cirrhosis is diagnosed in older patients. Higher cardiovascular mortality is observed, in addition to the classic complications of liver cirrhosis attributable to portal hypertension and oesophageal variceal bleeding, infections and renal failure [9].

In a population-based, large study, carried out in the United Kingdom, the following distribution of cirrhosis by the cause was found (in patients, diagnosed in 1987–2006): alcohol-induced, 56.1%; cryptogenic, 20.8%; attributable to viral hepatitis, 12.0%; autoimmune or metabolic (i.e., in this study—haemochromatosis or alpha-1-antitrypsin deficiency), 11.0% [37]. In a nationwide Danish study regarding 11,605 patients diagnosed with liver cirrhosis in 1977–1989, 61.7% of cases were alcohol-induced, 2.8%—attributable to primary biliary cirrhosis, 14.6%—related to chronic hepatitis (including autoimmune inflammation) and 20.9%—

non-specified [38]. Regarding the cause of cirrhosis in explanted livers, 48.6% were related to chronic viral hepatitis (31.1% to HCV and 15.9% to HBV, 1.6% to HCV and HBV coinfection), 23.1% to alcohol-induced liver damage and 16.7% to NAFLD [36]. The data on explanted livers may not reflect the true incidence of NASH-induced cirrhosis as NAFLD patients are less likely to receive transplant. The probability to receive liver transplant within 1 year is 40.5% in NAFLD, contrasting with 47% for hepatitis C or alcohol-induced cirrhosis. The difference is the result of several factors: contraindications due to morbid obesity, comorbidities, older physiologic age, impaired renal function as well as slower disease progression [9].

Thus, cryptogenic cirrhosis is a significant burden for health care systems. Patients undergoing liver transplantation for cryptogenic cirrhosis are subjected to higher postoperative mortality, lower cumulative 5- and 10-year survival and higher rate of chronic rejection [32]. NASH is the most rapidly growing indication for simultaneous liver and kidney transplantation. NASH and cryptogenic cirrhosis in patients having body mass index greater than 30 kg/m^2 constituted 6.3% in the years 2002–2003 but 19.2% in the years 2010–2011 [39].

As the liver becomes fibrotic, significant changes occur in the extracellular matrix (ECM) quantitatively and qualitatively. ECM refers to macromolecules that comprise the scaffolding of either normal or fibrotic liver. These include collagens, non-collagen glycoproteins, matrix-bound growth factors, glycosaminoglycans, proteoglycans and matricellular proteins. In case of fibrosis, the total collagen content increases 3- to 10-fold including an increase in fibril-forming collagens (i.e., types I, III and IV) and some non-fibril forming collagens (types IV and VI). Glycoproteins (fibronectin; laminin; secreted protein, acidic and rich in cysteine: SPARC; osteonectin; tenascin, and von Willebrand factor), proteoglycans and glycosaminoglycans (perlecan, decorin, aggrecan, lumican, and fibromodulin) also accumulate in cirrhotic liver. Particularly notable is the shift from heparan sulphate-containing proteoglycans to those containing chondroitin and dermatan sulphates. These processes represent a change in the type of ECM in subendothelial space from the normal low-density basement membrane-like matrix to the interstitial type.

The replacement of the low-density matrix with the interstitial type influences the function of hepatocytes, liver stellate cells, and endothelium of blood vessels: the microvilli disappear on the surface of liver parenchymal cells, and endothelium loses fenestrations precluding effective molecule exchange between blood and liver parenchyma. In addition, stellate cells undergo activation [23].

The hepatic stellate cell is the primary source of ECM in normal and fibrotic liver. Hepatic stellate cells, located in subendothelial space of Disse between hepatocytes and sinusoidal endothelial cells, represent one-third of the non-parenchymal population or approximately 15% of the total number of resident cells in normal liver. Stellate cells comprise a heterogeneous group of cells that are functionally and anatomically similar but differ in their expression of cytoskeletal filaments, retinoid content, and potential for activation. Stellate cells with fibrogenic potential are not confined to liver and have been identified in other organs such as the pancreas, where they contribute to desmoplasia in chronic pancreatitis and carcinoma. Hepatic stellate cell activation is the common pathway leading to hepatic fibrosis. During activation, stellate cells undergo a transition from a quiescent vitamin A-rich cell into proliferating, fibrogenic, and contractile myofibroblasts [23], which have strong ability to secrete collagen and migrate to the area of necrosis and inflammation [40]. Proliferation of stellate cells occurs predominantly in regions of greatest injury.

Considering liver fibrosis, the balance between synthesis and degradation of extracellular matrix also is of importance as enhanced destruction of the normal matrix in the space between hepatocytes and endothelial cells leads to accumulation of dense scar tissue. Degradation occurs through the actions of at least four enzymes: matrix metalloproteinase (MMP) 2 and MMP9, which degrade type IV collagen; membrane-type metalloproteinase 1 or 2, which activate latent MMP2 and stromelysin 1, which degrades proteoglycans and glycoproteins and activates latent collagenases. Stellate cells are the principal source of MMP2 and stromelysin. Activation of latent MMP2 may require interaction with hepatocytes. Markedly increased expression of MMP2 is a characteristic of cirrhosis. MMP9 is secreted locally by Kupffer cells. Disruption of the normal liver matrix is also a prerequisite for tumour invasion and stromal desmoplasia.

The cytochrome CYP2E1 may have an important role in the generation of reactive oxygen species that stimulate liver stellate cells. Cultured hepatic stellate cells grown in the presence of CYP2E1-expressing cells increase the production of collagen, an effect prevented by antioxidants or a CYP2E1 inhibitor. These data suggest that the CYP2E1-derived reactive oxygen species are responsible for the increased collagen production. Such findings may help to explain the pathogenesis of liver injury in alcoholic liver disease since CYP2E1 is alcohol inducible. As noted above, reactive oxygen species are generated through lipid peroxidation from hepatocytes, macrophages, stellate cells, and inflammatory cells. In alcoholic or non-alcoholic steatohepatitis, ROS generation in hepatocytes results from induction of cytochrome P450 2E1, leading to pericentral (zone 3) injury. Also, oxidase of the reduced nicotinamide adenine dinucleotide phosphate (NADPH) mediates fibrogenic activation of hepatic stellate cells, as well as of Kupffer cells or resident liver macrophages through generation of oxidative stress. Increasing knowledge about NADPH oxidase isoforms and their cell-specific activities is leading to their emergence as a therapeutic target [23].

Pathology of telomeres and the related molecular events represent another key mechanism that is associated both with induction of liver steatosis and progression of NAFLD [41]. Telomerase mutations can accelerate progression of chronic liver disease to cirrhosis [42]. Missense mutations in telomerase reverse transcriptase hTERT are found more frequently in cirrhosis regardless of aetiology [41]. Thus, missense mutations were observed in 7% of cirrhotic patients in USA [43]. Functional mutations were identified in 3% of German patients affected by cirrhosis [44].

Telomeres are repeated, short DNA sequences (in humans—TTAGGG) located at the chromosome end. These structures prevent chromosomal end-to-end fusion as well as protect the coding DNA from progressive loss at mitosis. During each mitosis, the DNA polymerase complex cannot replicate the terminal 5' end of the lagging strand. Consequently, the chromosomal end is lost. Due to the presence of telomeres, this loss is limited to telomeres. However, the telomeres shorten in each mitosis. Telomere attrition is especially marked in chronic diseases associated with increased cell loss and proliferation. When they become critically short, cellular ageing s. senescence and apoptosis follows. To ensure the unlimited proliferation of cancer, malignant cells maintain telomere length via different mechanisms. The most significant ones include telomerase reverse transcriptase hTERT, its RNA template: telomerase RNA component hTERC, the hTERC-protecting and stabilising dyskerin complex (consisting of four nucleolar proteins) and shelterin complex, including six proteins [41].

NAFLD is characterised by telomere shortening and increased cellular senescence in comparison to healthy controls [45]. The changes in telomeres represent an important mechanism in the transition to liver cirrhosis. However, dual effects are observed. In progressing chronic liver disease, cellular senescence enhances the loss of parenchyma, limiting the replicative potential of hepatocytes. In contrast, in advanced liver damage, the ageing of stellate cells stops the remodelling and thus, the further progression of fibrosis. Still another prognostic aspect can be involved regarding HCC development: senescent stellate cells can promote carcinogenesis by secreting pro-carcinogenic mediators. These changes are described as the senescence-associated secretory program [41]. The extent of fibrosis in NAFLD is associated with p21 protein representing another molecular regulator of cellular senescence [41].

Although shorter telomeres are considered a hallmark of liver cirrhosis regardless of aetiology [41], the telomeres in NAFLD patients are shorter than in those affected by cryptogenic cirrhosis. In NAFLD, telomere length correlates with the level of hTERT mRNA, while hTERT-independent mechanisms already start to operate in cryptogenic cirrhosis [45].

4. NASH-induced HCC

Although the association between NAFLD and HCC was first observed more than two decades ago, mostly through NASH-induced cirrhosis [11], the molecular events that link NAFLD and HCC are still incompletely understood. Following the general principles of cancerogenesis, HCC in cirrhotic liver develops by dysplasia—carcinoma pathway: from a dysplastic cirrhotic nodule. The process is slow and can last for several decades [34]. The genetic events that are prerequisite for malignant change develop in the background of increased cellular proliferation. Hypothetically, it is possible that the molecular portrait of HCC in DNA, mRNA, microRNA and protein level is different in accordance to the inciting factor of the underlying liver disease. If this is true, specific molecular targets may exist for the diagnostics, prevention or treatment of NASH-induced HCC or HCC arising in diabetic and/or obese patients [10].

The course of HCC that is associated with cryptogenic cirrhosis differs from HCC developing in other clinical settings [46]. HCC also varies by epigenetic signature in accordance to the cause [47].

The risk of hepatocellular carcinoma differs by the aetiology of cirrhosis. To estimate this, a large population-based study was carried out in the United Kingdom. All patients diagnosed with liver cirrhosis were identified, and the results were compared to national cancer registry identifying those diagnosed with HCC. The 10-year cumulative incidence of HCC was 4% in cirrhosis induced by chronic viral hepatitis, 3.2% in cirrhosis due to autoimmune or metabolic (in this study—haemochromatosis, alpha-1-antitrypsin deficiency) diseases, 1.2%

in alcohol-induced cirrhosis and 1.1% in cryptogenic cirrhosis, while the same estimates at 1 year were 1.0, 0.8, 0.3 and 0.3%, respectively. This study has the significant benefit of exploring HCC risk in patients that differ by aetiology of cirrhosis but belong to the same population [37]. Considering patients referred for liver transplantation, the frequency of hepatocellular carcinoma in cryptogenic cirrhosis is lower (8%) than in cirrhosis related to chronic hepatitis B (29%) or C (19%) as reported by Alamo et al. [32]. For the epidemiological estimates of HCC in different liver pathology, see also **Table 2** [37, 38].

The causal distribution of HCC shows geographic variations. Thus, in Canadian patients, 45% of cases were attributable to alcohol-induced cirrhosis, 26% to cryptogenic cirrhosis and 13% to hepatitis C. In patients from Saudi Arabia, 47% of HCC were caused by hepatitis C, 27% by cryptogenic cirrhosis and 21% to hepatitis B [48]. In USA, regarding the HCC cause, 54.9% of cases were induced by HCV, 16.4% by alcohol, 14.1% by NAFLD and 9.5% by HBV [10]. In explanted livers, 81.8% of HCC were associated with viral hepatitis, 9.1% with alcohol-induced liver damage and 9.1% with NAFLD [36].

In the USA, the number of NAFLD-associated HCC cases is annually growing for 9%, if the time span 2004–2009 is evaluated [10]. In Europe, NAFLD-related HCC comprised 35% of all HCC cases in 2010. HCC that is not related to hepatitis B or C is becoming increasingly frequent in Japan as well; however, here, it comprises only 10% of all HCC cases [53]. NASH is responsible for higher percentage of HCC in Western than in Eastern societies [12].

Hepatocellular carcinoma in patients affected by metabolic syndrome has distinct morphology [49]. NAFLD-associated HCC is characterised by larger size [34] and moderate or high differentiation degree [34], showing high differentiation as frequently as in 65% of cases [49]. However, the tumours lack capsule thus confirming the true malignant biological potential [34]. This is an important diagnostic trait considering the association between NAFLD, low-grade HCC [49], and liver adenomatosis [50].

The prognostic estimates are somewhat controversial. The NAFLD-associated hepatocellular carcinomas are diagnosed as more advanced tumours in older patients showing higher cardiovascular morbidity. The patients are less likely to receive liver transplant and have higher

Estimate	Alcohol-induced cirrhosis	Autoimmune and genetic diseases	Chronic hepatitis	Cryptogenic cirrhosis	Reference
SIR; 95% CI	70.6; 59.5–83.2	47.0;[1] 12.6–120.2	42.7;[2] 25.2–67.3	43.4; 30.3–60.4	Sorensen et al. [38]
Incidence rate per 1000 person years; 95% CI	3.2; 2.1–4.8	5.3; 2.6–10.5	7.6;[3] 4.3–13.4	3.1; 1.6–5.9	West et al. [37]

Abbreviations: SIR, standardised incidence ratio; CI, confidence interval.
[1]Primary biliary cirrhosis.
[2]Including viral and autoimmune causes.
[3]Viral hepatitis.

Table 2. Epidemiological estimates of hepatocellular carcinoma by the cause of chronic advanced liver pathology.

tumour-specific mortality [10]. HCC associated with cryptogenic cirrhosis is larger than can-cers related to HCV even in patients who correspond to Milan criteria [51]. However, after curative treatment, the recurrence risk and mortality are lower for HCC arising in cryptogenic cirrhosis—finding that is in accordance with the grade difference [52].

Although previously it was considered that HCC risk is limited to cirrhotic patients, currently at least 25–30% of NAFLD-related hepatocellular carcinomas develop in the absence of cirrho-sis [9]. In Japanese group, 33% of NAFLD-related HCC occurred in the background of none or mild fibrosis contrasting with only 16% in alcohol-induced HCC [53]. According to other researchers, up to 65% of NAFLD-associated HCC evolve in the absence of fibrosis [49]. The proportion of NAFLD-associated HCC developing in non-cirrhotic liver has been variably estimated as 15, 38, or 49% [54–57]. These tumours tend to be larger [57].

The development of HCC in noncirrhotic liver has been associated with malignant transfor-mation in liver cell adenoma [34, 49]. Malignant change in hepatic adenoma correlates with metabolic syndrome [58]. Inflammatory molecular type of liver cell adenoma shows clinical correlation with obesity. The underlying molecular basis could include either activated IL-6 signalling or hyperoestrogenemia associated with obesity. However, a controversy exists here as inflammatory type of liver adenoma is not prone to malignisation [50].

Several pathogenetic ways account for a tumour-promoting environment in obesity and dia-betes, allowing to distinguish the pathogenesis of HCC linked to NAFLD from that of viral and other aetiologies.

Obesity has been linked to higher frequency of cancers in a variety of tissues [59, 60] including the liver (**Table 3**). HCC is increasingly diagnosed among obese individuals. In a prospec-tive cohort of the Cancer Prevention Study with more than 900,000 North American subjects, the relative risk of dying from liver cancer among men with a body mass index reaching or exceeding 35 kg/m² was remarkably higher (4.5 fold) compared to a reference group with nor-mal body weight. In a large cohort involving 362,552 Swedish men, the relative risk of HCC in individuals with a body mass index reaching or exceeding 30 kg/m² was 3.1 fold higher than in controls having normal weight. Studies from other parts of the world indicate that the link between obesity and increased incidence of HCC has been globally recognised [61].

Obesity has a significant tumour-promoting effect regarding HCC. This effect largely depends on the chronic general low-grade inflammatory response it induces, which involves production of TNF-α and IL-6. Both these molecular mediators are tumour-promoting cyto-kines [62] and major drivers of cell proliferation in NAFLD and NASH [21]. TNF-α and other mediators produced by activated inflammatory macrophages stimulate compensatory hepa-tocyte proliferation and expand HCC progenitors. TNF-α further reinforces the inflammatory microenvironment and induces expression of chemokines (CCL2, CCL7 and CXCL13) and growth factors/cytokines (IL-1β, IL-6, TNF–α itself and hepatocyte growth factor) both by progenitors of hepatocellular carcinoma and surrounding cells [63]. TNF-α up-regulates the cellular proliferation through the molecular pathways of nuclear factor kappaB, mTOR and wide spectrum of kinases. The proliferative and anti-apoptotic activities of IL-6 are largely mediated through the signal transducer and activator of transcription 3, STAT3 [10]. IL-6 also

Location	Level of evidence
Oesophageal adenocarcinoma	Strong
Colorectal cancer in males	Strong
Pancreatic cancer	Strong
Breast cancer	Strong
Endometrial cancer	Strong
Renal cancer	Strong
Multiple myeloma	Strong
Liver cancer	Highly suggestive
Colonic cancer in females	Suggestive
Ovarian cancer	Suggestive
Prostate cancer	Suggestive
Thyroid cancer	Suggestive
Melanoma in males	Weak

Table 3. Obesity-related human cancers [60].

contributes to the metabolic background of cancer sustaining insulin resistance that can be improved by systemic neutralization of IL-6 [64].

Another mechanism involved in the progression of NAFLD to HCC in obese individuals is the imbalance between leptin and adiponectin. Particularly, obesity is linked to increased levels of leptin [34]. Apart from its role in obesity-associated insulin resistance and inflammation, leptin is a pro-inflammatory, pro-angiogenic, and pro-fibrogenic cytokine with a growth-promoting effect by activating the Janus kinase/STAT, phosphoinositide 3-kinase (PI3K)/Akt, and extracellular signal-regulated kinase (ERK) signalling pathways [61]. The up-regulation of PI3K/Akt pathway leads to activation of downstream molecular mediator mTOR that is found in 40% of HCC cases. Leptin-induced up-regulation of mTOR also inhibits autophagy—a process that normally would limit oxidative stress by removing damaged mitochondria. Suppression of autophagy, in turn, increases oxidative tissue damage and subsequent inflammation [21]. Since leptin exerts pro-inflammatory and pro-fibrogenic effects by activating Kupffer cells and stellate cells, it has been associated to disease progression in fibrotic NAFLD [10]. Leptin can also promote invasion and migration of hepatocellular carcinoma cells [65].

Adiponectin, another major adipokine with potent anti-inflammatory, antiangiogenic and tumour growth-limiting properties, is suppressed in obesity [15, 24]. Adiponectin activates 5′-adenosine monophosphate–activated protein kinase, which can suppress tumour growth and increase apoptosis by regulating the mTOR and c-Jun N-terminal kinase/caspase 3 pathways. Moreover, adiponectin opposes the effects of leptin by inhibiting activation of Akt and STAT3, as well as by increasing the expression of SOCS3: the suppressor of cytokine signalling 3 [61].

Thus, low adiponectin levels may be insufficient to suppress endotoxin-mediated inflammatory signalling in Kupffer cells and other macrophages, as well as control angiogenesis, a pivotal mechanism of tumour growth [10]. Microarray analysis of tissue adiponectin levels in HCC patients revealed that adiponectin expression was inversely correlated with tumour size, supporting the hypothesis that adiponectin may inhibit proliferation and dedifferentiation [66].

HCC can show marked accumulation of fat within the neoplastic cells (**Figure 4**). In a study by Salomao et al., 36% of patients who developed HCC in the setting of steatohepatitis were diagnosed as having a steatohepatitic variant of HCC as compared to 1.3% of HCC patients without steatohepatitis [67]. Increased intensity of fatty acid synthesis and characteristic pattern of perilipin proteins has been demonstrated in HCC. Regarding gene expression pattern, activated lipogenesis is associated with higher cell proliferation and worse prognosis in HCC [10]. Hypothetically, HCC cells might benefit from the energetic value of fat compounds or use lipids as building blocks of new cells.

Lipotoxicity, defined as the cellular dysfunction caused by ectopic deposition of fat in non-adipose tissues, may contribute to the development of HCC in NAFLD. Activated oxidation of fatty acids generates high burden of free radicals and lipid peroxide compounds that oxidise and damage large molecules and cell organoids, e.g., mitochondria and endoplasmic reticulum. The damaged cells are subjected to apoptosis, leading to higher activity in liver destruction and progression towards cirrhosis that in turn is closely associated with enhanced proliferation and accumulation of genetic damage. Accumulation of fatty acids may interfere with cellular signalling and promote oncogenesis through altered regulation of gene transcription [10]. Oxidative stress can induce mutations in the tumour suppressor gene *TP53* in a pattern observed in HCC [68].

Adipose tissue expansion, release of pro-inflammatory cytokines, and lipotoxicity collectively promote systemic and hepatic insulin resistance, resulting in hyperinsulinemia [34]. The risk of HCC in patients affected by diabetes mellitus is 2.31 [57]. Insulin resistance and hyperinsulinemia are the most common metabolic features of NAFLD, which correlate with impaired hepatic clearance of insulin and have been linked to tumour development [69]. Deregulated metabolic effects of insulin result in excessive activation of proliferative signalling cascades.

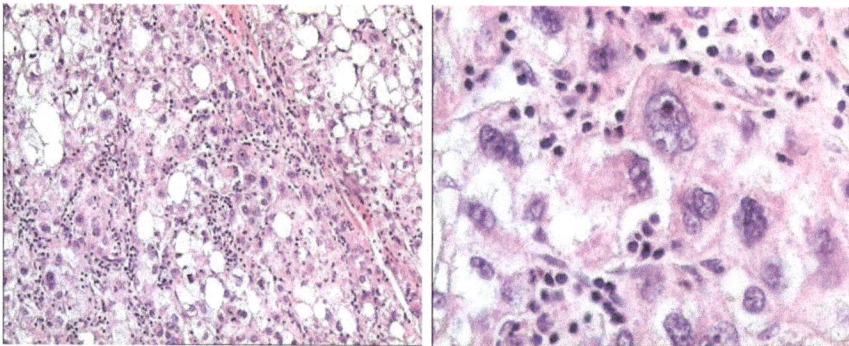

Figure 4. Hepatocellular carcinoma showing nuclear atypia and presence of fat in tumour cells. Haematoxylin-eosin stain, original magnification 100× and 400×.

Hyperinsulinemia causes reduced hepatic synthesis of insulin-like growth factor (IGF)-binding protein-1 and increased bioavailability of IGF1, which further promotes cellular proliferation and inhibits apoptosis [10, 34]. It has been shown recently that elevated fasting insulin, which is inversely related to insulin sensitivity, is an independent risk factor for HCC. Baseline serum levels of C-peptide have also been found to be associated with a higher risk of HCC in the general population independently of obesity and other established liver cancer risk factors [69]. Loss of heterozygosity for IGF2 has been observed in over 60% of HCC cases. This likely coincides with IGF2 overexpression, found in HCC, which has been associated to reduced apoptosis and increased cellular proliferation [68].

The importance of insulin resistance is illustrated by the observations that obesity and type 2 diabetes mellitus comprise increased HCC risk even regardless of the presence or cause of liver cirrhosis [9].

A number of studies have demonstrated a critical role for phosphatase and tensin homolog (PTEN) in the progression of NASH to tumour. *PTEN* deletion results in PKB/Akt activation, promoting proliferation and reducing apoptosis. Insulin-like growth factor 2 mRNA binding protein p62 was reported to be a possible upstream regulator of PTEN. Aberrant microRNAs contribute to carcinogenesis. MiR-21 was found to be another upstream regulator of PTEN participating in NASH-associated cancer induction [10, 14, 70].

The oral iron test has revealed increased absorption of iron compounds in patients affected by NASH [71]. In turn, increased amount of iron in liver tissues is associated with increased risk of HCC in patients affected by NASH-related liver cirrhosis [72]. As the reductive conversion of Fe(III) to Fe(II) necessitates increased oxidation of other compounds, oxidative DNA damage can develop and lead to the malignancy [34, 73]. Iron overload also is known to enhance insulin resistance [74] and to act in concert with other factors damaging liver. The significance of iron overload in hepatic carcinogenesis is shown in several models. The risk of HCC is increased in hereditary haemochromatosis, characterised by excessive iron accumulation in the body and caused by excessive absorption because of homozygous C282Y mutation in *HFE* gene. Almost 8–10% of patients with hereditary haemochromatosis develop HCC. Increased relative risk of HCC (10×) has also been demonstrated in association with long-lasting excess dietary iron intake [37, 74, 75]. Thus, there is significant evidence of the carcinogenic action of iron overload, and evidence of iron accumulation in NAFLD and especially NASH that allows drawing conclusion that iron metabolites are contributing to the development of NASH-related HCC.

The expression profile of *Wnt* signalling genes in NASH strongly suggests inhibition of Wnt pathway. IHC staining of β-catenin shows predominately membrane staining with loss of nuclear staining indicating that β-catenin is not active in NASH. In contrast, 20–90% of HCC cases exhibit active Wnt pathway [76]. Thus, the long-lasting conversion of NASH into HCC hypothetically involves up-regulation of Wnt pathway either by activators or loss of inhibitors [77].

Hepatocyte apoptosis is a prominent feature of NASH (**Figure 5**). The executing mechanism of apoptosis includes activation of characteristic lytic enzymes—the caspases. In an apoptotic hepatocyte, activated caspase-3 is splitting various cell structures, including cytokeratin (CK) 18—the intermediary filament that represents the specific cytoskeleton protein of hepatocytes. Consequently, blood tests can reveal increased concentration of CK18 fragments [70]. In liver tissues, CK8 and CK18-containing Mallory bodies are evident by light microscopy as large, brightly eosinophilic inclusions in liver cell cytoplasm. Although Mallory hyaline is the hallmark of alcohol-induced hepatitis, its development can also be induced by diet rich in saturated fatty acids. The molecular pathways associated with Mallory body development include IL-6, protein p62 that binds ubiquitin in cell cytoplasm, and reduced concentration of HSP72 that prevents protein misfolding. The presence of CK18 in Mallory bodies correlates with plasma CK18 levels [78]. In a longitudinal paired liver biopsy study, the change of CK18 correlated with disease progression. Patients with increased NAFLD activity score 3 years after initial evaluation had greater increase of plasma CK18 compared with those who had stable or decreased activity score [79]. El-Zefzafy et al. proved that CK18 was a sensitive indicator of the severity of liver disease and also could predict the development of HCC. In their study, the sensitivity and specificity of serum CK18 were 95 and 96.7%, respectively, with a cut-off value of 534.5 U/L for HCC diagnosis [80].

In a study by Salomao et al., devoted to HCC in NASH, immunohistochemically there was diffuse loss of cytoplasmic CK8/18 and an increased number of activated hepatic stellate cells within the steatohepatitic HCC, identical to the pattern seen in the surrounding non-neoplastic liver [67, 81].

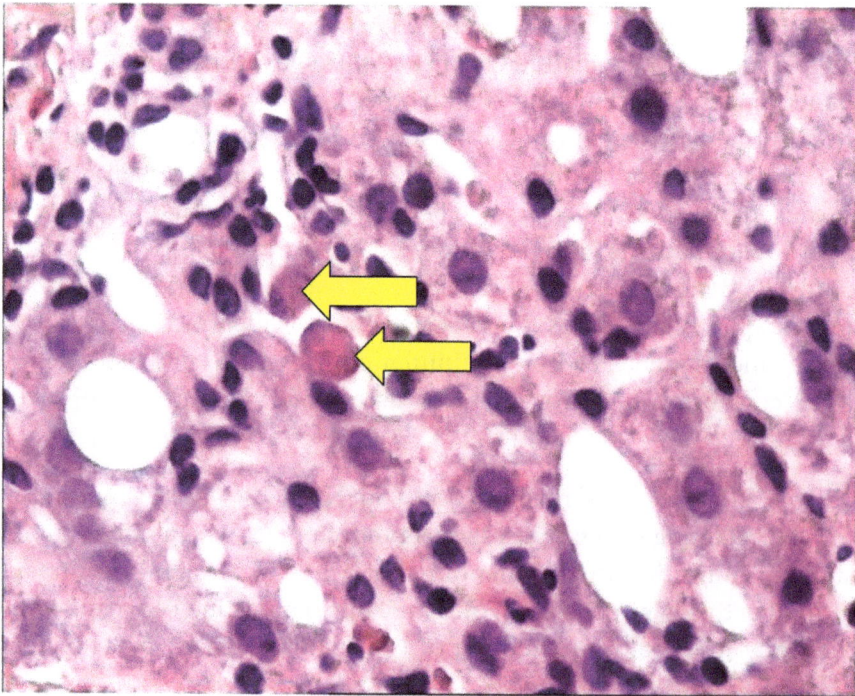

Figure 5. Apoptotic bodies (arrows) in non-alcoholic steatohepatitis. Haematoxylin-eosin stain, original magnification 400×.

The HCC development shows complex associations with telomere shortening. The senescence-associated secretory program of liver stellate cells promotes carcinogenesis. The telomere shortening induces also genomic instability thus facilitating HCC development [41]. Indeed, HCC is characterised by significantly shorter telomeres in comparison to adjacent tissues [82]. However, cancer cells still maintain unlimited proliferation. Evidently, hepatocellular carcinoma cells develop compensatory mechanisms either for telomere extension or for cellular proliferation despite telomere shortening. The elongation of telomeres again can be ensured via diverse mechanisms, including hTERT or alternative lengthening of telomeres via telomerase-independent mechanism seen in 7% of HCC cases [41].

Over the progression of HCC, the telomere length changes in contrary direction. Early liver carcinogenesis is associated with telomere shortening, while disease progression is associated with telomere extension, cell immortalisation and reactivation of telomerase [83]. Longer telomeres in HCC are associated with higher stage (regional or distant spread *versus* localised tumour) and grade (III–IV *versus* lower grade) as well as with worse survival [83, 84]. Telomerase promotes HCC development via several pathways, not limited to maintenance of telomeres and thus cellular proliferation. In addition, hTERT can act as a transcription factor in the Wnt molecular cascade [41]. Experimental data by HCC induction in telomerase-deficient mice have shown increased number of early tumours and reduced incidence of high-grade HCC [85].

Interestingly, shorter telomeres are observed more frequently (telomere length ratio between HCC and surrounding tissues lower than the mean, 70.1% *versus* higher, 29.9%) in HCC that is not related to hepatitis B (50.0% *versus* 50.0%) or C (60.0% *versus* 40.0%), or alcohol abuse (50.0% *versus* 50.0%), although the difference does not reach statistical significance [83]. Telomere shortening can be detected in peripheral blood. Notably, this assay can be used to predict HCC persistence (by telomere shortening) in cases attributable to viral hepatitis B or C but not in HCC attributable to non-infectious causes despite comparable size of patient groups [86].

Genetic predisposition has been studied in NAFLD trying to identify those patients that are at particularly increased risk of HCC. The possible candidate genes could be associated with telomere length and mechanisms involved in preserving telomeres [42]. About 10% of patients affected both by HCC and NASH have germline mutations in *hTERT* in comparison to complete absence of such mutations in NASH patients having cirrhosis and healthy controls [41]. In addition, *PNPLA3* polymorphisms have been studied in NAFLD patients, finding twice increased risk of HCC in association with rs738409 C>G. The proposed mechanism involves retinol metabolism in hepatic stellate cells [34].

The interaction of these pathogenetic mechanisms and genetic predisposition finally results in the increased incidence of HCC in NAFLD that reaches 76–201 per 100,000 contrasting with the incidence of 4.9–16 per 100,000 of the general population [57].

5. Potential treatment strategies

As no specific treatment is approved for NAFLD, lifestyle interventions play the leading role in NAFLD management. Weight loss due to low calorie diet in combination with physical activities is the main therapeutic approach in overweight patients with NAFLD. As hypertriglyceridemia is a frequent and promoting feature of NAFLD [87] reduction of the triglyceride level must be among therapeutic goals. In severe hypertriglyceridemia, total fat consumption should be limited to less than 30 g/day, and carbohydrate amount in daily nutrition should be strictly controlled as well [88].

Physical activity has beneficial effect of reducing triglyceride level, even independently from diet [89]. Thus, at least 30 min of moderate activity most days of the week would be a necessary part of dyslipidemia management [90]. Loss of 5% of body weight decreases hepatic steatosis, but body weight loss of 10% could even improve inflammation and fibrosis in liver [87].

Experimentally investigating hepatocyte-specific PTEN-deficient mouse model, Piguet et al. showed that physical activity could reduce HCC growth in fatty liver. In PTEN-deficient mice, HCC incidence was 71% of exercised mice and 100% of sedentary mice. In addition, liver tumour volume in exercised mice was significantly smaller than that of sedentary mice (444 ± 551 *versus* 945 ± 1007 mm^3) [91]. The physiological substantiation relies on fact that regular physical activity could inhibit mTOR complex, which is engaged in cell growth and proliferation [92].

Increased hepatic free cholesterol accumulation is typical for NASH. Statins are commonly prescribed to reduce cholesterol synthesis in the liver and thus serum levels of free cholesterol [14]. In a recent European multi-centre cohort study, statin use was associated with protection from steatosis (odds ratio, OR 0.09; 95% CI, 0.01–0.32; p = 0.004), steatohepatitis (OR, 0.25; 95% CI, 0.13–0.47; p <0.001), and fibrosis stage F2–F4 (OR, 0.42; 95% CI, 0.20–0.80; p = 0.017). The protective effect of statins on steatohepatitis was stronger in subjects not carrying the I148M PNPLA3 risk variant (p = 0.02), indicating the role of genetic predisposition [93]. Statins also have been associated with reduced risk (range, 0.46–0.79) of HCC [94].

In a meta-analysis, including 4298 patients with HCC, statin use was associated with a 37% reduction in the risk of hepatocellular carcinoma. The effect was stronger in Asian patients but was also present in Western populations. Moreover, the reduction of cancer risk was independent of statin lipid-lowering effects [95]. Several hypotheses have been proposed, including statin ability to inhibit cell proliferation via inhibition of v-myc avian myelocytomatosis viral oncogene homolog protein phosphorylation which seems to play a role in liver carcinogenesis [96], as well as capacity to inhibit the 3-hydroxy-3-methylglutaryl coenzyme A reductase, which activates multiple proliferative pathways [95]. Simvastatin selectively induces apoptosis in cancer, but not in healthy cells. This proapoptotic effect is maintained via RAF/MAPK1/ERK and growth-inhibitory action by suppression of angiogenesis and proteasome pathway [95, 96]. However, data about liver carcinogenesis and statin effects remain controversial. In another large meta-analysis, including 86,936 participants, no beneficial effect of statin in terms of incidence or death from cancer was observed. Even more, in 67,258 patients who received statins, 35 new liver cancers and 24 deaths from liver cancer were reported showing no significant difference from control group, comprising 67,279 patients who received placebo, and developed 33 new liver cancer (p = 0.93) cases leading to 24 deaths (p = 1.00) as analysed by Carrat [97].

Metformin, a widely prescribed drug for treating type 2 diabetes mellitus, is one of the most extensively recognised metabolic modulators which decreases aminotransferase levels and hepatic insulin resistance. It has no beneficial effects on NAFLD histology but still retains an important anti-cancer action [87, 98]. The hypothetic antitumor mechanisms of metformin are believed to be (1) inhibition of mTOR, (2) weight loss and (3) suppressed production of ROS and the associated DNA damage, in combination with (4) reduction of hyperinsulinemia, which is known to lead to cell proliferation [99]. In meta-analysis comprising 105,495 patients with type 2 diabetes, Zhang et al. showed that metformin was associated with an estimated 70% reduction in the risk of developing HCC [98]. The risk reduction in metformin users is significant, regarding both incidence (78%) and mortality (77%) from HCC [100].

The mammalian target of rapamycin (mTOR) promotes growth in a majority of liver cancers, including hepatocellular carcinoma. It participates in the formation of two protein complexes—mTORC1 and mTORC2. mTORC1 is sensitive to rapamycin and has ability to activate downstream targets which regulate cellular growth and metabolism. Prolonged mTORC1 activation is related to liver steatosis and insulin resistance in obese patients [14, 101]. Due to the ability suppress mTORC1, rapamycin and its analogues Everolimus and Temsirolimus have been tested to treat HCC. Unfortunately, results have not been promising. In a phase 3 study of patients with advanced HCC, Everolimus increased the frequency of hepatic injury and showed no improvements regarding survival [14]. After 2 weeks with rapamycin treatment, the lipid droplets in the liver decreased, as well as ROS burden. However, rapamycin treatment promoted liver damage with augmented IL-6 and decreased anti-inflammatory IL-10 production, leading to increased hepatic inflammation and hepatocyte necrosis [101].

Inflammation promotes development of complications in patients with cirrhosis contributing to mortality and to liver insufficiency mediated by pro-inflammatory cytokines. The most recognisable pro-inflammatory cytokine associated with liver damage in case of NAFLD is TNF-α that can be inhibited by pentoxifylline. Lebrec et al. performed randomised, placebo controlled, double-blind trial assessing pentoxifyline effect in 335 patients with cirrhosis. Although pentoxifylline had no effect on short-term mortality, it significantly (p = 0.04) prolonged the complication-free time span [102].

Knowing the important role of NADPH oxidases (NOXs) and production of ROS in liver fibrosis, different strategies to prevent the oxidative damage have been developed [23]. In hepatocytes, NOX4 mediates suppressor effects on TGF-β and can inhibit hepatocyte growth and liver carcinogenesis. In turn, dual NOX4/NOX1 pharmacological inhibitor GKT137831 could decrease both the apparition of fibrogenic markers as well as hepatocyte apoptosis *in vivo* [103].

Currently, multikinase inhibitor sorafenib is the only pharmacological agent that prolongs survival of HCC patients, although the median survival is improved only by 12 weeks [14]. It acts against Raf-1 and B-raf, vascular endothelial growth factor (VEGF) receptors and platelet-derived growth factor receptor kinases [104]. Sorafenib as well as VEGF inhibitors have radiosensitizing effect. However, combined regimens including sorafenib and liver stereotactic radiation or whole liver radiotherapy are characterized by poor tolerability [104]. Various beneficial effects of sorafenib have been reported in liver cirrhosis. As epithelial-mesenchymal transition and TGF-β play crucial roles in liver fibrosis, Ma et al. proved that sorafenib had ability to strikingly suppress TGF-β1 induced epithelial-mesenchymal transition, as well as apoptosis in hepatic stellate cells, in dose-dependent manner [105].

Several treatment strategies might involve the telomere and telomerase complex. In cancer, telomerase inhibitors might arrest tumour growth, prevent further malignisation in surrounding cirrhotic nodules and/or enhance HCC chemosensitivity. In early liver disease, telomerase activation might prevent tissue loss if the etiologic factor cannot be removed. This could be reached via transplantation of liver cells engineered for hTERT expression, direct supply of hTERT to the patient's cells or by small molecules enhancing telomerase activity. However, side effects and enhanced cancer risk must be considered and prevented [41]. The treatment modulating cellular senescence and proliferation control may also target p21 [106–108] and p53 [109] pathways.

The p21 protein, a strong and universal inhibitor of cyclin-dependant kinases, is an important regulator of cell proliferation, apoptosis and senescence [107, 108]. Based on its intracellular location and the molecular background, it can have dual activity. Intranuclear p21 acts as tumour suppressor, as it binds cyclin-dependant kinases and thus suppresses cellular proliferation. Cytoplasmic p21 prevents apoptosis by binding caspases and promotes proliferation and migration of p53-deficient cells. The p21 pathway is also closely associated with senescence. Few small molecular inhibitors of p21 are known, including LLW10, butyrolactone and UC2288. In addition, sorafenib also exhibits anti-p21 activity. LLW10 binds to p21 and induces proteosomal degradation via ubiquitination. Despite the reliable mechanism, the high concentration that is necessary for sufficient activity as well as the instability of LLW10 prevents it from being clinically useful drug. Butyrolactone also induces proteosomal degradation of p21. UC2288 decreases p21 concentration via suppressed transcription and modified posttranscriptional modulation [107]. In turn, upregulation of p21 can be achieved via statins or by anticancer agents including histone deacetylase inhibitors [106]. Induction of senescence would be desirable if the tumour is already present while suppressed senescence might prevent or slow down the development of liver cirrhosis. As was noted, it is possible to modulate p21 level in both directions. However, the net effects must be carefully considered and studied experimentally, knowing the bidirectional activity of p21.

p21 is also an effector of p53-mediated responses in cells maintaining functional p53. In p53-deficient cell, it manifests carcinogenic effects. Thus, restoration of wild-type p53 could be attractive, either in combination with p21-targeted treatment or with other oncological approach. In liver cancer, restoration of p53 activity has resulted in senescence and increased immune response. The therapeutic approaches could include (1) restoration of wild type function to mutant p53 by low molecular weight compounds PRIMA 1 or PRIMA-1MET. The last one has progressed to phase II clinical trials; (2) stabilising p53 due to blocked interaction with MDM2 or MDM4 by nutlins, representing low molecular weight molecules, or by stapled peptides; (3) gene therapy using viral vectors that has already been tested in HCC; (4) induction of synthetic lethality [109].

6. Conclusions

Non-alcoholic steatohepatitis is recognised as the cause of NASH-induced cirrhosis. It has also been associated with a significant fraction of cases previously diagnosed as cryptogenic cirrhosis. Liver cirrhosis can become further complicated by hepatocellular carcinoma, the most frequent primary liver tumour known for serious prognosis and limited treatment options. In addition, the development of HCC in NAFLD patients can precede cirrhosis in a significant fraction of cases. NAFLD is the major hepatic manifestation of obesity and associated metabolic diseases, such as diabetes mellitus. With increasing prevalence of these conditions, NAFLD has become the most common liver disorder worldwide. It affects around 25% of general population and 90% of patients suffering from morbid obesity, i.e., having body mass index equal or greater than 40 kg/m².

The mechanisms of liver steatosis include up-regulation of inflammatory cytokines, as TNF-α, IL-6 and CCL2, released from extrahepatic adipose tissues due to prolonged low-grade inflammation triggered by hypoxia-induced death of fast-growing fat cells. Insulin resistance further contributes to NAFLD and can be aggravated by the pro-inflammatory cytokine background. Free fatty acids and cholesterol cause lipotoxicity due to released reactive oxygen species as well as toxic metabolites generated by non-oxidative biochemical pathways. Decreased level of adiponectin, exaggerated oxidative stress and hepatic iron accumulation also are among the mechanisms of NAFLD.

In the pathogenesis of NAFLD, 20–30% of patients, initially affected by simple liver steatosis, develop hepatic inflammation and thus correspond to the diagnostic criteria of NASH. These cases are at risk to progress to liver cirrhosis and hepatocellular carcinoma. The standardised incidence ratio of HCC in NASH patients reaches 4.4. Regarding the epidemiological profile of hepatocellular carcinoma, the proportion of NASH-related cases is growing and has increased from 8.3 to 13.5% in the time period 2002–2012.

Obesity has been linked to higher frequency of cancers in different organs including the liver. The relative risk of HCC-attributable death in obese patients (body mass index equal or greater than 35 kg/m²) can be as high as 4.5. The underlying mechanisms of carcinogenesis include chronic general low-grade inflammation characterised by elevated levels of TNF-α and IL-6, both of which are tumour-promoting cytokines and major drivers of cell proliferation in NAFLD and NASH. The increased levels of leptin and suppressed production of adiponectin represent another mechanism involved in the progression of NAFLD to HCC in obese individuals. Leptin is a pro-inflammatory, pro-angiogenic and pro-fibrogenic cytokine with a growth-promoting effect. Adiponectin has anti-inflammatory, antiangiogenic and tumour growth-limiting properties. Insulin resistance and hyperinsulinemia lead to excessive cell proliferation. Iron compound deposition has also been related to HCC development in NAFLD-related cirrhosis, possibly due to oxidative DNA damage. Thus, the same molecular pathways that induced NAFLD continue to be active until the development of HCC. These mechanisms are supplemented by critical genetic events including *PTEN* deletion, switch from inactivated to upregulated Wnt pathway and typical mutation pattern in *TP53*. Certain microRNAs, including miR-21, act as molecular switches.

Pathogenetically related molecular markers, e.g., cytokeratin 18, can serve as predictive tests to detect increased risk of HCC.

The molecular pathogenesis of NAFLD is closely related to the selection of treatment targets. NAFLD patients can benefit from low calorie diet, reducing hypertriglyceridemia and potentially reversing steatosis and even fibrosis; physical activity inhibiting mTOR complex;

statins influencing cholesterol synthesis, RAF/MAPK1/ERK and p21 pathway; metformin acting through suppression of mTOR and ROS; pentoxyfillin lowering production of pro-inflammatory cytokines. Multikinase inhibitor sorafenib is indicated in HCC patients. Bidirectional regulation of telomere attrition, senescence, and p21 pathway could be at least theoretically considered in the future. Restoration of wild-type p53 activity becomes possible. The regulation of miRNA machinery also represents a highly attractive future treatment option.

Thus, NAFLD is gaining increasing importance in nowadays medicine as a frequent condition that can lead to such grave complications as liver cirrhosis and hepatocellular carcinoma. Awareness of the molecular profile is helpful to identify the treatment targets and predictive markers.

Acknowledgements

The team of authors gratefully acknowledges artist Ms. Sandra Ozolina for professional preparation of illustrations.

Author details

Dzeina Mezale[1]*, Ilze Strumfa[1], Andrejs Vanags[2], Matiss Mezals[3], Ilze Fridrihsone[1], Boriss Strumfs[4] and Dainis Balodis[1]

*Address all correspondence to: dzeina.mezale@rsu.lv

1 Department of Pathology, Riga Stradins University, Riga, Latvia

2 Department of Surgery, Riga Stradins University, Riga, Latvia

3 Department of Human Physiology and Biochemistry, Riga Stradins University, Riga, Latvia

4 Latvian Institute of Organic Synthesis, Riga, Latvia

References

[1] Tendler DA. Pathogenesis of nonalcoholic fatty liver disease. UpToDate [Internet] Mar 2016 [Updated: Mar 09, 2016]. Available from: http://www.uptodate.com/contents/pathogenesis-of-nonalcoholic-fatty-liver-disease [Accessed: Mar 03 ,2017]

[2] White DL, Kanwal F, El-Serag HB. Association between nonalcoholic fatty liver disease and risk for hepatocellular cancer, based on systematic review. Clinical Gastroenterology and Hepatology. 2012;10(12):1342-1359.e2. DOI: 10.1016/j.cgh.2012.10.001

[3] El-Serag HB, Kanwal F. Epidemiology of hepatocellular carcinoma in the United States: Where are we? Where do we go? Hepatology. 2014;60(5):1767-1775. DOI: 10.1002/hep.27222

[4] Michelotti GA, Machado MV, Diehl AM. NAFLD, NASH and liver cancer. Nature Reviews Gastroenterology and Hepatology. 2013;**10**(11):656-665. DOI: 10.1038/nrgastro. 2013.183

[5] Younossi ZM, Koenig AB, Abdelatif D, Fazel Y, Henry L, Wymer M. Global epidemiology of nonalcoholic fatty liver disease. Meta-analytic assessment of prevalence, incidence, and outcomes. Hepatology. 2016;**64**(1):73-84. DOI: 10.1002/hep.28431

[6] Marengo A, Jouness RI, Bugianesi E. Progression and natural history of nonalcoholic fatty liver disease in adults. Clinical Liver Disease. 2016;**20**(2):313-324. DOI: 10.1016/j. cld.2015.10.010

[7] Fingas CD, Best J, Sowa JP, Canbay A. Epidemiology of nonalcoholic steatohepatitis and hepatocellular carcinoma. Clinical Liver Disease. 2016;**8**(5):119-122. DOI: 10.1002/cld.585

[8] Younossi ZM, Otgonsuren M, Henry L, Venkatesan C, Mishra A, Erario M, Hunt S. Association of nonalcoholic fatty liver disease (NAFLD) with hepatocellular carcinoma (HCC) in the United States from 2004 to 2009. Hepatology. 2015;**62**(6):1723-1730. DOI: 10.1002/hep.28123

[9] Pais R, Barritt AS 4th, Calmus Y, Scatton O, Runge T, Lebray P, et al. NAFLD and liver transplantation: Current burden and expected challenges. Journal of Hepatology. 2016;**65**(6):1245-1257. DOI: 10.1016/j.jhep.2016.07.033

[10] Baffy G, Brunt EM, Caldwell SH. Hepatocellular carcinoma in non-alcoholic fatty liver disease: An emerging menace. Journal of Hepatology. 2012;**56**(6):1384-1391. DOI: 10.1016/j.jhep.2011.10.027

[11] Sheth SG, Sanjiv C. Natural history and management of nonalcoholic fatty liver disease in adults. UpToDate [Internet]. Nov 2016 [Updated: Nov 08, 2016]. Available from: http://www.uptodate.com/contents/natural-history-and-management-of-nonalcoholic-fatty-liver-disease-in-adults [Accessed: Mar 03, 2017]

[12] Agrawal S, Duseja AK. Non-alcoholic fatty liver disease: East versus West. Journal of Clinical and Experimental Hepatology. 2012;**2**(2):122-134. DOI: 10.1016/S0973-6883(12)60101-7

[13] Day CP, James OF. Steatohepatitis: A tale of two "hits"? Gastroenterology. 1998;**114**(4): 842 845

[14] Charrez B, Qiao L, Hebbard L. Hepatocellular carcinoma and non-alcoholic steatohepatitis: The state of play. World Journal of Gastroenterology. 2016;**22**(8):2494-2502. DOI: 10.3748/wjg.v22.i8.2494

[15] Tilg H, Moschen AR. Evolution of inflammation in nonalcoholic fatty liver disease: The multiple parallel hits hypothesis. Hepatology. 2010;**52**(5):1836-1846. DOI: 10.1002/ hep.24001

[16] Wong RJ, Cheung R, Ahmed A. Nonalcoholic steatohepatitis is the most rapidly growing indication for liver transplantation in patients with hepatocellular carcinoma in the U.S. Hepatology. 2014;**59**(6):2188-2195. DOI: 10.1002/hep.26986

[17] Hao C, Zhu PX, Yang X, Han ZP, Jiang JH, Zong C, et al. Overexpression of SIRT1 pro-
      motes metastasis through epithelial-mesenchymal transition in hepatocellular carci-
      noma. BMC Cancer. 2014;**14**:978. DOI: 10.1186/1471-2407-14-978

[18] Schwartz JM, Carithers RL. Clinical features and diagnosis of primary hepatocellular
      carcinoma. UpToDate [Internet]. Dec 2016 [Updated: Dec 20, 2016]. Available from:
      https://www.uptodate.com/contents/clinical-features-and-diagnosis-of-primary-hepa-
      tocellular-carcinoma [Accessed: Mar 03, 2017]

[19] Polyzos SA, Toulis KA, Goulis DG, Zavos C, Kountouras J. Serum total adiponectin in
      nonalcoholic fatty liver disease: A systematic review and meta-analysis. Metabolism.
      2011;**60**(3):313-326. DOI: 10.1016/j.metabol.2010.09.003

[20] Wang Y, Liu Z, Zou W, Hong H, Fang H, Tong W. Molecular regulation of miRNAs and
      potential biomarkers in the progression of hepatic steatosis to NASH. Biomarkers in
      Medicine. 2015;**9**(11):1189-1200. DOI: 10.2217/bmm.15.70

[21] Kolb R, Sutterwala FS, Zhang W. Obesity and cancer: Inflammation bridges the two.
      Current Opinion in Pharmacology. 2016;**29**:77-89. DOI: 10.1016/j.coph.2016.07.005

[22] Cusi K. Role of insulin resistance and lipotoxicity in non-alcoholic steatohepatitis.
      Clinical Liver Disease. 2009;**13**(4):545-563. DOI: 10.1016/j.cld.2009.07.009

[23] Friedman SL. Pathogenesis of hepatic fibrosis. UpToDate [Internet]. Nov 24, 2015
      [Updated: Nov 24, 2015]. Available from: http://www.uptodate.com/contents/pathogen-
      esis-of-hepatic-fibrosis [Accessed: Mar 03, 2017]

[24] Sharifnia T, Antoun J, Verriere TG, Suarez G, Wattacheril J, Wilson KT et al. Hepatic
      TLR4 signaling in obese NAFLD. American Journal of Physiology. Gastrointestinal and
      Liver Physiology. 2015;**309**(4):G270-278. DOI: 10.1152/ajpgi.00304.2014

[25] Novo E, Busletta C, Bonzo LV, Povero D, Paternostro C, Mareschi K, et al. Intracellular
      reactive oxygen species are required for directional migration of resident and bone
      marrow-derived hepatic pro-fibrogenic cells. Journal of Hepatology. 2011;**54**(5):964-974.
      DOI: 10.1016/j.jhep.2010.09.022

[26] Pietrangelo A. Iron in NASH, chronic liver diseases and HCC: How much iron is too
      much? Journal of Hepatology. 2009;**50**(2):249-251. DOI: 10.1016/j.jhep.2008.11.011

[27] Zimmermann A, Zimmermann T, Schattenberg J, Pöttgen S, Lotz J, Rossmann H, et
      al. Alterations in lipid, carbohydrate and iron metabolism in patients with non-alco-
      holic steatohepatitis (NASH) and metabolic syndrome. European Journal of Internal
      Medicine. 2011;**22**(3):305-310. DOI: 10.1016/j.ejim.2011.01.011

[28] Seki E, Brenner DA. Recent advancement of molecular mechanisms of liver fibrosis.
      Journal of Hepato-Biliary-Pancreatic Sciences. 2015;**22**(7):512-518. DOI: 10.1002/jhbp.
      245

[29] Trautwein C, Friedman SL, Schuppan D, Pinzani M. Hepatic fibrosis: Concept to treat-
      ment. Journal of Hepatology. 2015;**62**(1 Suppl):S15-24. DOI: 10.1016/j.jhep.2015.02.039

[30] Mercado-Irizarry A, Torres EA. Cryptogenic cirrhosis: Current knowledge and future directions. Clinical Liver Disease. 2016;7(4):69-72. DOI: 10.1002/cld.539

[31] Rinaldi L, Nascimbeni F, Giordano M, Masetti C, Guerrera B, Amelia A, et al. Clinical features and natural history of cryptogenic cirrhosis compared to hepatitis C virus-related cirrhosis. World Journal of Gastroenterology. 2017;23(8):1458-1468. DOI: 10.3748/wjg.v23.i8.1458

[32] Alamo JM, Bernal C, Barrera L, Marin LM, Suarez G, Serrano J, et al. Liver transplantation in patients with cryptogenic cirrhosis: Long term follow-up. Transplantation Proceedings. 2011;43(6):2230-2232. DOI: 10.1016/j.transproceed.2011.05.017

[33] Hashemi SJ, Hajiani E, Masjedizadeh A, Makvandi M, Shayesteh AA, Alavinejad SP, et al. Occult hepatitis B infection in patients with cryptogenic liver cirrhosis in southwest of Iran. Jundishapur Journal of Microbiology. 2015;8(3):e16873. DOI: 10.5812/jjm.16873

[34] Margini C, Dufour JF. The story of HCC in NAFLD: From epidemiology, across pathogenesis, to prevention and treatment. Liver International. 2016;36(3):317-324. DOI: 10.1111/liv.13031

[35] Michitaka K, Nishiguchi S, Aoyagi Y, Hiasa Y, Tokumoto Y, Onji M; Japan Etiology of Liver Cirrhosis Study Group. Etiology of liver cirrhosis in Japan: A nationwide survey. Journal of Gastroenterology. 2010;45(1):86-94. DOI: 10.1007/s00535-009-0128-5

[36] Nayak NC, Jain D, Vasdev N, Gulwani H, Saigal S, Soin A. Etiologic types of end-stage chronic liver disease in adults: Analysis of prevalence and their temporal changes from a study on native liver explants. European Journal of Gastroenterology & Hepatology. 2012;24(10):1199-1208. DOI: 10.1097/MEG.0b013e32835643f1

[37] West J, Card TR, Aithal GP, Fleming KM. Risk of hepatocellular carcinoma among individuals with different aetiologies of cirrhosis: A population-based cohort study. Alimentary Pharmacology & Therapeutics. 2017;45(7):983-990. DOI: 10.1111/apt.13961

[38] Sorensen HT, Friis S, Olsen JH, Thulstrup AM, Mellemkjaer L, Linet M, et al. Risk of liver and other types of cancer in patients with cirrhosis: A nationwide cohort study in Denmark. Hepatology. 1998;28(4):921-925

[39] Singal AK, Hasanin M, Kaif M, Wiesner R, Kuo YF. Nonalcoholic steatohepatitis is the most rapidly growing indication for simultaneous liver kidney transplantation in the United States. Transplantation. 2016;100(3):607-612. DOI: 10.1097/TP.0000000000000945

[40] Kong D, Zhang F, Zhang Z, Lu Y, Zheng S. Clearance of activated stellate cells for hepatic fibrosis regression: Molecular basis and translational potential. Biomedicine & Pharmacotherapy. 2013;67(3):246-250. DOI: 10.1016/j.biopha.2012.10.002

[41] Donati B, Valenti L. Telomeres, NAFLD and chronic liver disease. International Journal of Molecular Sciences. 2016;17(3):383. DOI: 10.3390/ijms17030383

[42] Carulli L, Anzivino C. Telomere and telomerase in chronic liver disease and hepatocarcinoma. World Journal of Gastroenterology. 2014;**20**(20):6287-6292. DOI: 10.3748/wjg.v20. i20.6287

[43] Calado RT, Brudno J, Mehta P, Kovacs JJ, Wu C, Zago MA, et al. Constitutional telomerase mutations are genetic risk factors for cirrhosis. Hepatology. 2011;**53**(5):1600-1607. DOI: 10.1002/hep.24173

[44] Hartmann D, Srivastava U, Thaler M, Kleinhans KN, N'kontchou G, Scheffold A, et al. Telomerase gene mutations are associated with cirrhosis formation. Hepatology. 2011;**53**(5):1608-1617. DOI: 10.1002/hep.24217

[45] Laish I, Mannasse-Green B, Hadary R, Biron-Shental T, Konikoff FM, Amiel A, Kitay-Cohen Y. Telomere dysfunction in nonalcoholic fatty liver disease and cryptogenic cirrhosis. Cytogenetic and Genome Research. 2016;**150**(2):93-99. DOI: 10.1159/ 000454654

[46] Siriwardana RC, Niriella MA, Dassanayake AS, Liyanage C, Gunathilaka B, Jayathunge S, de Silva HJ. Clinical characteristics and outcome of hepatocellular carcinoma in alcohol related and cryptogenic cirrhosis: A prospective study. Hepatobiliary & Pancreatic Diseases International. 2015;**14**(4):401-405

[47] Hlady RA, Tiedemann RL, Puszyk W, Zendejas I, Roberts LR, Choi JH, et al. Epigenetic signatures of alcohol abuse and hepatitis infection during human hepatocarcinogenesis. Oncotarget. 2014;**5**(19):9425-9443. DOI: 10.18632/oncotarget.2444

[48] Alsohaibani F, Porter G, Al-Ashgar H, Walsh M, Berry R, Molinari M, Peltekian KM. Comparison of cancer care for hepatocellular carcinoma at two tertiary-care referral centers from high and low endemic regions for viral hepatitis. Journal of Gastrointestinal Cancer. 2011;**42**(4):228-235. DOI: 10.1007/s12029-010-9200-x

[49] Paradis V, Zalinski S, Chelbi E, Guedj N, Degos F, Vilgrain V, et al. Hepatocellular carcinomas in patients with metabolic syndrome often develop without significant liver fibrosis: A pathological analysis. Hepatology. 2009;**49**(3):851-859. DOI: 10.1002/hep. 22734

[50] Chang CY, Hernandez-Prera JC, Roayaie S, Schwartz M, Thung SN. Changing epidemiology of hepatocellular adenoma in the United States: Review of the literature. International Journal of Hepatology 2013;**2013**:604860. DOI: 10.1155/2013/604860

[51] Feng J, Wu J, Zhu R, Feng D, Yu L, Zhang Y, et al. Simple risk score for prediction of early recurrence of hepatocellular carcinoma within the Milan criteria after orthotopic liver transplantation. Scientific Reports. 2017;**7**:44036. DOI: 10.1038/srep44036

[52] Takuma Y, Nouso K, Makino Y, Gotoh T, Toshikuni N, Morimoto Y, et al. Outcomes after curative treatment for cryptogenic cirrhosis-associated hepatocellular carcinoma satisfying the Milan criteria. Journal of Gastroenterology and Hepatology. 2011;**26**(9):1417-1424. DOI: 10.1111/j.1440-1746.2011.06775.x

[53] Kimura T, Kobayashi A, Tanaka N, Sano K, Komatsu M, Fujimori N, et al. Clinicopathological characteristics of non-B non-C hepatocellular carcinoma without past hepatitis B virus infection. Hepatology Research. 2017; **47**(5):405-418. DOI: 10.1111/hepr.12762

[54] Tokushige K, Hashimoto E, Horie Y, Taniai M, Higuchi S. Hepatocellular carcinoma in Japanese patients with nonalcoholic fatty liver disease, alcoholic liver disease, and chronic liver disease of unknown etiology: Report of the nationwide survey. Journal of Gastroenterology. 2011;**46**(10):1230-1237. DOI: 10.1007/s00535-011-0431-9

[55] Yasui K, Hashimoto E, Komorizono Y, Koike K, Arii S, Imai Y, et al. Characteristics of patients with nonalcoholic steatohepatitis who develop hepatocellular carcinoma. Clinical Gastroenterology and Hepatology. 2011;**9**(5):428-433. DOI: 10.1016/j.cgh.2011.01.023

[56] Duan XY, Qiao L, Fan JG. Clinical features of nonalcoholic fatty liver disease-associated hepatocellular carcinoma. Hepatobiliary & Pancreatic Diseases International. 2012;**11**(1): 18-27. DOI: 10.1016/S1499-3872(11)60120-3

[57] Leung C, Yeoh SW, Patrick D, Ket S, Marion K, Gow P, Angus PW. Characteristics of hepatocellular carcinoma in cirrhotic and non-cirrhotic non-alcoholic fatty liver disease. World Journal of Gastroenterology. 2015;**21**(4):1189-1196. DOI: 10.3748/wjg.v21.i4.1189

[58] Farges O, Ferreira N, Dokmak S, Belghiti J, Bedossa P, Paradis V. Changing trends in malignant transformation of hepatocellular adenoma. Gut. 2011;**60**(1):85-89. DOI: 10.1136/gut.2010.222109

[59] Hirabayashi S. The interplay between obesity and cancer: A fly view. Disease Models & Mechanisms. 2016;**9**(9):917-926. DOI: 10.1242/dmm.025320

[60] Kyrgiou M, Kalliala I, Markozannes G, Gunter MJ, Paraskevaidis E, Gabra H, et al. Adiposity and cancer at major anatomical sites: Umbrella review of the literature. BMJ. 2017;**356**:j477. DOI: 10.1136/bmj.j477

[61] Karagozian R, Derdák Z, Baffy G. Obesity-associated mechanisms of hepatocarcinogenesis. Metabolism. 2014;**63**(5):607-617. DOI: 10.1016/j.metabol.2014.01.011

[62] Park EJ, Lee JH, Yu GY, He G, Ali SR, Holzer RG, et al. Dietary and genetic obesity promote liver inflammation and tumorigenesis by enhancing IL-6 and TNF expression. Cell. 2010;**140**(2):197-208. DOI: 10.1016/j.cell.2009.12.052

[63] Nakagawa H, Umemura A, Taniguchi K, Font-Burgada J, Dhar D, Ogata H, et al. ER stress cooperates with hypernutrition to trigger TNF-dependent spontaneous HCC development. Cancer Cell. 2014;**26**(3):331-343. DOI: 10.1016/j.ccr.2014.07.001

[64] Catrysse L, van Loo G. Inflammation and the metabolic syndrome: The tissue-specific functions of NF-κB. Trends in Cell Biology. 2017;**27**(6):417-429. DOI: http://dx.doi.org/10.1016/j.tcb.2017.01.006

[65] Saxena NK, Sharma D, Ding X, Lin S, Marra F, Merlin D, Anania FA. Concomitant activation of the JAK/STAT, PI3K/AKT, and ERK signaling is involved in leptin-mediated promotion of invasion and migration of hepatocellular carcinoma cells. Cancer Research. 2007;**67**(6):2497-2507. DOI: 10.1158/0008-5472.CAN-06-3075

[66] Dalamaga M, Diakopoulos KN, Mantzoros CS. The role of adiponectin in cancer: A review of current evidence. Endocrine Reviews. 2012;33(4):547-594. DOI: 10.1210/er.2011-1015

[67] Salomao M, Remotti H, Vaughan R, Siegel AB, Lefkowitch JH, Moreira RK. The steatohepatitic variant of hepatocellular carcinoma and its association with underlying steatohepatitis. Human Pathology. 2012;43(5):737-746. DOI: 10.1016/j.humpath.2011.07.005

[68] Page JM, Harrison SA. NASH and HCC. Clinical Liver Disease. 2009;13(4):631-647. DOI: 10.1016/j.cld.2009.07.007

[69] Chettouh H, Lequoy M, Fartoux L, Vigouroux C, Desbois-Mouthon C. Hyperinsulinaemia and insulin signalling in the pathogenesis and the clinical course of hepatocellular carcinoma. Liver International. 2015;35(10):2203-2217. DOI: 10.1111/liv.12903

[70] Yu J, Shen J, Sun TT, Zhang X, Wong N. Obesity, insulin resistance, NASH and hepatocellular carcinoma. Seminars in Cancer Biology. 2013;23(6 Pt B):483-491. DOI: 10.1016/j.semcancer.2013.07.003

[71] Hoki T, Miyanishi K, Tanaka S, Takada K, Kawano Y, Sakurada A, et al. Increased duodenal iron absorption through up-regulation of divalent metal transporter 1 from enhancement of iron regulatory protein 1 activity in patients with nonalcoholic steatohepatitis. Hepatology. 2015;62(3):751-761. DOI: 10.1002/hep.27774

[72] Sorrentino P, D'Angelo S, Ferbo U, Micheli P, Bracigliano A, Vecchione R. Liver iron excess in patients with hepatocellular carcinoma developed on non-alcoholic steato-hepatitis. Journal of Hepatology. 2009;50(2):351-357. DOI: 10.1016/j.jhep.2008.09.011

[73] Fargion S, Valenti L, Fracanzani AL. Role of iron in hepatocellular carcinoma. Clinical Liver Disease. 2014;3(5):108-110. DOI: 10.1002/cld.350

[74] Kew MC. Hepatic iron overload and hepatocellular carcinoma. Liver Cancer. 2014;3(1):31-40. DOI: 10.1159/000343856

[75] Sikorska K, Bernat A, Wroblewska A. Molecular pathogenesis and clinical consequences of iron overload in liver cirrhosis. Hepatobiliary & Pancreatic Diseases International. 2016;15(5):461-479. DOI: 10.1016/S1499-3872(16)60135-2

[76] Thompson MD, Monga SP. WNT/beta-catenin signaling in liver health and disease. Hepatology. 2007;45(5):1298-1305. DOI: 10.1002/hep.21651

[77] Clarke JD, Novak P, Lake AD, Shipkova P, Aranibar N, Robertson D, et al. Characterization of hepatocellular carcinoma related genes and metabolites in human nonalcoholic fatty liver disease. Digestive Diseases and Sciences. 2014;59(2):365-374. DOI: 10.1007/s10620-013-2873-2879

[78] Takaki A, Kawai D, Yamamoto K. Molecular mechanisms and new treatment strategies for non-alcoholic steatohepatitis (NASH). International Journal of Molecular Sciences. 2014;15(5):7352-7379. DOI: 10.3390/ijms15057352

[79] Wong VW, Wong GL, Choi PC, Chan AW, Li MK, Chan HY, et al. Disease progression of non-alcoholic fatty liver disease: A prospective study with paired liver biopsies at 3 years. Gut. 2010;59(7):969-974. DOI: 10.1136/gut.2009.205088

[80] El-Zefzafy W, Eltokhy H, Mohamed NA, Abu-Zahab Z. Significance of serum cytokeratin-18 in prediction of hepatocellular carcinoma in chronic hepatitis C infected Egyptian patients. Open Access Macedonian Journal of Medical Sciences. 2015;3(1):117-123. DOI: 10.3889/oamjms.2015.021

[81] Knudsen ES, Gopal P, Singal AG. The changing landscape of hepatocellular carcinoma: etiology, genetics, and therapy. American Journal of Pathology. 2014;184(3):574-583. DOI: 10.1016/j.ajpath.2013.10.028

[82] Zhang Y, Shen J, Ming-Whei, Lee YP, Santella RM. Telomere length in hepatocellular carcinoma and paired adjacent non-tumor tissues by quantitative PCR. Cancer Investigation. 2007;25(8):668-677

[83] Lee HW, Park TI, Jang SY, Park SY, Park WJ Jung SJ, Lee JH. Clinicopathological characteristics of TERT promoter mutation and telomere length in hepatocellular carcinoma. Medicine (Baltimore). 2017;96(5):e5766. DOI: 10.1097/MD.0000000000005766

[84] Yang B, Shebl FM, Sternberg LR, Warner AC, Kleiner DE, Edelman DC, et al. Telomere length and survival of patients with hepatocellular carcinoma in the United States. PLoS One. 2016;11(11):e0166828. DOI: 10.1371/journal.pone.0166828

[85] Farazi PA, Glickman J, Jiang S, Yu A, Rudolph KL, DePinho RA. Differential impact of telomere dysfunction on initiation and progression of hepatocellular carcinoma. Cancer Research. 2003;63(16):5021-5027

[86] Feng W, Yu D, Li B, Luo OY, Xu T, Cao Y, Ding Y. Paired assessment of liver telomere lengths in hepatocellular cancer is a reliable predictor of disease persistence. Bioscience Reports. 2017;37(2):pii: BSR20160621. DOI: 10.1042/BSR20160621

[87] Lonardo A, Bellentani S, Argo CK, Ballestri S, Byrne CD, et al. Non-alcoholic Fatty Liver Disease Study Group, Epidemiological modifiers of non-alcoholic fatty liver disease: Focus on high-risk groups. Digestive and Liver Disease. 2015;47(12):997-1006. DOI: 10.1016/j.dld.2015.08.004

[88] European Association for Cardiovascular Prevention & Rehabilitation, Reiner Z, Catapano AL, De Backer G, Graham I, Taskinen MR, et al. ESC/EAS Guidelines for the management of dyslipidaemias: The Task Force for the management of dyslipidaemias of the European Society of Cardiology (ESC) and the European Atherosclerosis Society (EAS). European Heart Journal. 2011;32(14):1769-1818. DOI: 10.1093/eurheartj/ehr158

[89] Vanhees L, Geladas N, Hansen D, Kouidi E, Niebauer J, Reiner Z, et al. Importance of characteristics and modalities of physical activity and exercise in the management of cardiovascular health in individuals with cardiovascular risk factors: Recommendations

from the EACPR. Part II. European Journal of Preventive Cardiology. 2012;**19**(5):1005-1033. DOI: 10.1177/1741826711430926

[90] Corey KE, Chalasani N. Management of dyslipidemia as a cardiovascular risk factor in individuals with nonalcoholic fatty liver disease. Clinical Gastroenterology and Hepatology. 2014;**12**(7):1077-1084. DOI: 10.1016/j.cgh.2013.08.014

[91] Piguet AC, Saran U, Simillion C, Keller I, Terracciano L, Reeves HL, Dufour JF. Regular exercise decreases liver tumors development in hepatocyte-specific PTEN-deficient mice independently of steatosis. Journal of Hepatology. 2015;**62**(6):1296-1303. DOI: 10.1016/j.jhep.2015.01.017

[92] Degasperi E, Colombo M. Distinctive features of hepatocellular carcinoma in non-alcoholic fatty liver disease. The Lancet Gastroenterology & Hepatology. 2016;**1**(2):156-164. DOI: 10.1016/S2468-1253(16)30018-8

[93] Dongiovanni P, Petta S, Mannisto V, Mancina RM, Pipitone R, Karja V, et al. Statin use and non-alcoholic steatohepatitis in at risk individuals. Journal of Hepatology. 2015;**63**(3):705-712. DOI: 10.1016/j.jhep.2015.05.006

[94] El-Serag HB, Johnson ML, Hachem C, Morgana RO. Statins are associated with a reduced risk of hepatocellular carcinoma in a large cohort of patients with diabetes. Gastroenterology. 2009;**136**(5):1601-1608. DOI: 10.1053/j.gastro.2009.01.053

[95] Singh S, Singh PP, Singh AG, Murad MH, Sanchez W. Statins are associated with a reduced risk of hepatocellular cancer: A systematic review and meta-analysis. Gastroenterology. 2013;**144**(2):323-332. DOI: 10.1053/j.gastro.2012.10.005

[96] Noureddin M, Rinella ME. Nonalcoholic fatty liver disease, diabetes, obesity, and hepatocellular carcinoma. Clinical Liver Disease. 2015;**19**(2):361-379. DOI: 10.1016/j.cld.2015.01.012

[97] Carrat F. Statin and aspirin for prevention of hepatocellular carcinoma: What are the levels of evidence? Clinics and Research in Hepatology and Gastroenterology. 2014;**38**(1):9-11. DOI: 10.1016/j.clinre.2013.09.007

[98] Zhang ZJ, Zheng ZJ, Shi R, Su Q, Jiang Q, Kip KE. Metformin for liver cancer prevention in patients with type 2 diabetes: A systematic review and meta-analysis. The Journal of Clinical Endocrinology & Metabolism. 2012;**97**(7):2347-2353. DOI: 10.1210/jc.2012-1267

[99] Jara JA, López-Muñoz R. Metformin and cancer: Between the bioenergetic disturbances and the antifolate activity. Pharmacological Research. 2015;**101**:102-108. DOI: 10.1016/j.phrs.2015.06.014

[100] Zhang P, Li H, Tan X, Chen L, Wang S. Association of metformin use with cancer incidence and mortality: A meta-analysis. Cancer Epidemiology. 2013;**37**(3):207-218. DOI: 10.1016/j.canep.2012.12.009

[101] Umemura A, Park EJ, Taniguchi K, Lee JH, Shalapour S, Valasek MA, et al. Liver damage, inflammation, and enhanced tumorigenesis after persistent mTORC1 inhibition. Cell Metabolism. 2014;**20**(1):133-144. DOI: 10.1016/j.cmet.2014.05.001

[102] Lebrec D, Thabut D, Oberti F, Perarnau JM, Condat B, Barraud H, et al. Pentoxifylline does not decrease short-term mortality but does reduce complications in patients with advanced cirrhosis. Gastroenterology. 2010;**138**(5):1755-1762. DOI: 10.1053/j.gastro.2010.01.040

[103] Crosas-Molist E, Fabregat I. Role of NADPH oxidases in the redox biology of liver fibrosis. Redox Biology. 2015;**6**:106-111. DOI: 10.1016/j.redox.2015.07.005

[104] Goody RB, Brade AM, Wang L, Craig T, Brierley J, Dinniwell R, et al. Phase I trial of radiation therapy and sorafenib in unresectable liver metastases. Radiotherapy & Oncology. 2017;**123**(2):234-239. DOI: 10.1016/j.radonc.2017.01.018

[105] Ma R, Chen J, Liang Y, Lin S, Zhu L, Liang X, Cai X. Sorafenib: A potential therapeutic drug for hepatic fibrosis and its outcomes. Biomedicine & Pharmacotherapy. 2017;**88**:459-468. DOI: 10.1016/j.biopha.2017.01.107

[106] Abbas T, Dutta A. p21 in cancer: Intricate networks and multiple activities. Nature Reviews Cancer. 2009;**9**(6):400-414. DOI: 10.1038/nrc2657

[107] Liu R, Wettersten HI, Park SH, Weiss RH. Small-molecule inhibitors of p21 as novel therapeutics for chemotherapy-resistant kidney cancer. Future Medicinal Chemistry. 2013;**5**(9):991-994. DOI: 10.4155/fmc.13.56

[108] Georgakilas AG, Martin OA, Bonner WM. p21: A two-faced genome guardian. Trends in Molecular Medicine. 2017;**23**(4):310-319. DOI: 10.1016/j.molmed.2017.02.001

[109] Duffy MJ, Synnott NC, McGowan PM, Crown J, O'Connor D, Gallagher WM. p53 as a target for the treatment of cancer. Cancer Treatment Reviews. 2014;**40**(10):1153-1160. DOI: 10.1016/j.ctrv.2014.10.004

Permissions

All chapters in this book were first published in ASCITES&LC, by InTech Open; hereby published with permission under the Creative Commons Attribution License or equivalent. Every chapter published in this book has been scrutinized by our experts. Their significance has been extensively debated. The topics covered herein carry significant findings which will fuel the growth of the discipline. They may even be implemented as practical applications or may be referred to as a beginning point for another development.

The contributors of this book come from diverse backgrounds, making this book a truly international effort. This book will bring forth new frontiers with its revolutionizing research information and detailed analysis of the nascent developments around the world.

We would like to thank all the contributing authors for lending their expertise to make the book truly unique. They have played a crucial role in the development of this book. Without their invaluable contributions this book wouldn't have been possible. They have made vital efforts to compile up to date information on the varied aspects of this subject to make this book a valuable addition to the collection of many professionals and students.

This book was conceptualized with the vision of imparting up-to-date information and advanced data in this field. To ensure the same, a matchless editorial board was set up. Every individual on the board went through rigorous rounds of assessment to prove their worth. After which they invested a large part of their time researching and compiling the most relevant data for our readers.

The editorial board has been involved in producing this book since its inception. They have spent rigorous hours researching and exploring the diverse topics which have resulted in the successful publishing of this book. They have passed on their knowledge of decades through this book. To expedite this challenging task, the publisher supported the team at every step. A small team of assistant editors was also appointed to further simplify the editing procedure and attain best results for the readers.

Apart from the editorial board, the designing team has also invested a significant amount of their time in understanding the subject and creating the most relevant covers. They scrutinized every image to scout for the most suitable representation of the subject and create an appropriate cover for the book.

The publishing team has been an ardent support to the editorial, designing and production team. Their endless efforts to recruit the best for this project, has resulted in the accomplishment of this book. They are a veteran in the field of academics and their pool of knowledge is as vast as their experience in printing. Their expertise and guidance has proved useful at every step. Their uncompromising quality standards have made this book an exceptional effort. Their encouragement from time to time has been an inspiration for everyone.

The publisher and the editorial board hope that this book will prove to be a valuable piece of knowledge for researchers, students, practitioners and scholars across the globe.

List of Contributors

Marcus Hollenbach
Department of Medicine, Neurology, and Dermatology, Division of Gastroenterology and Rheumatology, University of Leipzig, Leipzig, Germany

Tomomi Kogiso, Kuniko Yamamoto, Mutsuki Kobayashi, Yuichi Ikarashi, Kazuhisa Kodama, Makiko Taniai, Nobuyuki Torii, Etsuko Hashimoto and Katsutoshi Tokushige
Department of Internal Medicine, Institute of Gastroenterology, Tokyo Women's, Medical University, Shinjuku-ku, Tokyo, Japan

Andra-Iulia Suceveanu and Adrian-Paul Suceveanu
Faculty of Medicine, Department of Gastroenterology, Emergency Hospital of Constanta, Ovidius University, Constanta, Romania

Laura Mazilu
Faculty of Medicine, Department of Internal Medicine, Emergency Hospital of Constanta, Ovidius University, Constanta, Romania

Irinel-Raluca Parepa
Faculty of Medicine, Department of Cardiology, Emergency Hospital of Constanta, Ovidius University, Constanta, Romania

Felix Voinea
Faculty of Medicine, Department of Surgery, Emergency Hospital of Constanta, Ovidius University, Constanta, Romania

Patricia Huelin, Jose Ignacio Fortea, Javier Crespo and Emilio Fábrega
Gastroenterology and Hepatology Department, Marqués de Valdecilla University Hospital, Infection, Immunity and Digestive Pathology Group, Research Institute Marqués de Valdecilla

(IDIVAL), Grupo Clínico Vinculado al Centro de Investigación Biomédica en Enfermedades Hepáticas y Digestivas (CIBEREHD), Santander, Spain

Alexander Giakoustidis
Department of HPB Surgery, Royal London Hospital, London, UK

Dimitrios E. Giakoustidis
Division of Transplant Surgery, Department of Surgery, School of Health Sciences, Aristotle University of Thessaloniki, Thessaloniki, Greece

Abdulrahman Bendahmash
Department of Pediatrics, King Faisal Specialist Hospital & Research Center, Riyadh, Saudi Arabia

Hussien Elsiesy
Department of Liver Transplantation, King Faisal Specialist Hospital & Research Center, Riyadh, Saudi Arabia
Department of Medicine, Alfaisal University, Riyadh, Saudi Arabia

Waleed K. Al-hamoudi
Department of Liver Transplantation, King Faisal Specialist Hospital & Research Center, Riyadh, Saudi Arabia
Department of Medicine, College of Medicine, King Saud University, Riyadh, Saudi Arabia

Alexander A. Vitin
Department of Anesthesiology, University of Washington, Seattle, WA, USA

Dana Tomescu
Department of Anesthesia and Intensive Care "Carol Davila", University of Medicine and Pharmacy, Fundeni Clinical Institute, Bucharest, Romania

Leonard Azam irei
University of Medicine and Pharmacy Tîrgu Mureş, Tîrgu Mureş, Romania

Aziza Ajlan
Department of Pharmacy, King Faisal Specialist Hospital & Research Center, Riyadh, Saudi Arabia

Kazuyuki Suzuki
Department of Nutritional Science, Morioka University, Takizawa, Japan

Ryujin Endo
Division of Hepatology, Department of Internal Medicine, Iwate Medical University, Morioka, Japan

Akinobu Kato
Department of Gastroenterology, Morioka Municipal Hospital, Morioka, Japan

Berna Karakoyun
Department of Basic Health Sciences, Faculty of Health Sciences, Marmara University, Istanbul, Turkey

Dzeina Mezale, Ilze Strumfa, Ilze Fridrihsone and Dainis Balodis
Department of Pathology, Riga Stradins University, Riga, Latvia

Andrejs Vanags
Department of Surgery, Riga Stradins University, Riga, Latvia

Matiss Mezals
Department of Human Physiology and Biochemistry, Riga Stradins University, Riga, Latvia

Boriss Strumfs
Latvian Institute of Organic Synthesis, Riga, Latvia

Index

www.ingramcontent.com/pod-product-compliance
Lightning Source LLC
Chambersburg PA
CBHW061946190326
41458CB00009B/2804

* 9 7 8 1 6 3 2 4 2 6 7 9 6 *